STUDENT WORKBOOK FOR

CLINICAL PRACTICE

OF THE

DENTAL

HYGIENIST

10th EDITION

STUDENT WORKBOOK FOR

CLINICAL PRACTICE
OF THE
DENTAL
HYGIENIST

10th EDITION

Charlotte J. Wyche, RDH, MS

Department of Periodontology and Dental Hygiene
University of Detroit Mercy School of Dentistry
Detroit, Michigan

Esther M. Wilkins, BS, RDH, DMD

Department of Periodontology
Tufts University School of Dental Medicine
Boston, Massachusetts

Wolters Kluwer | Lippincott Williams & Wilkins
Health

Philadelphia · Baltimore · New York · London
Buenos Aires · Hong Kong · Sydney · Tokyo

Acquisitions Editor: Barrett Koger
Managing Editor: Kevin C. Dietz
Marketing Manager: Nancy Bradshaw
Production Editor: Kevin Johnson
Design Coordinator: Stephen Druding
Compositor: Aptara

DISCLAIMER

Care has been taken to confirm the accuracy of the information present and to describe generally accepted practices. However, the authors, editors, and publisher are not responsible for errors or omissions or for any consequences from application of the information in this book and make no warranty, expressed or implied, with respect to the currency, completeness, or accuracy of the contents of the publication. Application of this information in a particular situation remains the professional responsibility of the practitioner; the clinical treatments described and recommended may not be considered absolute and universal recommendations.

The authors, editors, and publisher have exerted every effort to ensure that drug selection and dosage set forth in this text are in accordance with the current recommendations and practice at the time of publication. However, in view of ongoing research, changes in government regulations, and the constant flow of information relating to drug therapy and drug reactions, the reader is urged to check the package insert for each drug for any change in indications and dosage and for added warnings and precautions. This is particularly important when the recommended agent is a new or infrequently employed drug.

Some drugs and medical devices presented in this publication have Food and Drug Administration (FDA) clearance for limited use in restricted research settings. It is the responsibility of the healthcare provider to ascertain the FDA status of each drug or device planned for use in their clinical practice.

DEDICATION

To every student who has ever asked a question.
By challenging us, you teach your teachers more
than you can know.

AND

To every teacher who has ever helped a student
find the answer to a question. You have taught that
student well.

CONTENTS

SECTION IV   DENTAL HYGIENE DIAGNOSIS AND CARE PLANNING   139

SECTION V   IMPLEMENTATION: PREVENTION   151

SECTION VI   IMPLEMENTATION: CLINICAL TREATMENT   223

There is no doubt that each student learns differently. Therefore, the aim of this workbook is to provide a variety of types of exercises so that you will be able to find something here to help you learn important concepts that are the foundation of the dental hygiene practice. You are always encouraged, of course, to create additional learning experiences and activities that fit with your own learning style.

HOW TO USE THIS WORKBOOK

Some general guidelines for the exercises in the workbook are described below. Most of the exercises provide lines for you to write your answers. In some cases, additional pages or a copy of the *Patient-Specific Dental Hygiene Care Plan* template from Appendix D will be required to provide a complete answer. You should also know that your instructor will be able to find "answers" to the questions or ideas for discussion points on a faculty Web site that accompanies the workbook.

■ **KNOWLEDGE** exercises in each chapter will help you target important information and help you master the introductory material provided in the textbook. You will define terms, concepts, and principles in your own words; list the components of larger ideas; and reorganize information from the textbook in a variety of ways. Knowledge exercises comprise the largest, but by no means the most important, portion of this workbook.

■ **COMPETENCY** questions are found in each chapter and also in Section Summary areas of this workbook. These exercises will ask you to use critical thinking skills to apply basic knowledge to clinical situations, analyze patient assessment data, or document patient care activities. You will also create dental hygiene care plans based on a variety of patient case scenarios.

■ **DISCOVERY** activities are found in some of the chapters and also in each Section Summary. These exercises will take you beyond the basic knowledge of

dental hygiene practice. The Discovery activities will direct you to find and analyze current information about a topic introduced in the textbook by, for example, doing a scientific literature search, a Web-based internet search, or a dental product analysis.

■ **QUESTIONS PATIENTS ASK** are also intended to encourage you to practice evidence-based decision making skills by thinking about ways you can look beyond the textbook and information provided by your instructors to address specific patient concerns.

■ **EVERYDAY ETHICS** scenarios will challenge you to apply ethical principles. Many of these scenarios were created using real-life ethical situations faced by practicing dental hygienists. Questions and discussion points are included to lead you as you think about, write about, discuss, or role play each situation.

■ **FACTORS TO TEACH THE PATIENT** cases ask you to outline a conversation to teach your patient using patient-appropriate language and knowledge gained from the textbook. Those brief conversations can then be compared with conversations written by your student colleagues, used for "role play" exercises, or placed in your portfolio to illustrate your expertise in patient education.

■ **FOR YOUR PORTFOLIO** suggestions are located in each Section Summary. A learning portfolio is a collection of student work and reflection that is organized in such a way that it demonstrates an increase in student knowledge and professional competence over time. A student portfolio can be compiled simply and creatively using a three-ring binder with tabbed separators to organize the material into appropriate sections.

Development of a portfolio provides an opportunity for you to reflect on your growth as a dental hygiene professional. A portfolio that highlights your unique talents and provides evidence of special skills, competencies, or learning that goes beyond the requirements of your educational program can be useful after graduation during employment interviews.

EVIDENCE-BASED DENTAL HYGIENE PRACTICE

The workbook contains a ***Primer for Evidence-Based Decision Making*** (EBDM) that will help you begin to understand the skills necessary for providing patient care based on sound scientific principles. There is a global movement in all the health science disciplines to provide therapies and preventive measures for patients based on scientific evidence of efficacy and safety. In dental hygiene practice, that means that you will be challenged to know about the latest research findings, and also to use that information to make clinical decisions regarding each individual patient's care.

To that end, it becomes imperative that you are able to search for information using scientific journal databases and internet search techniques. Not only that, you must be competent in the process of analyzing the information you find in order to make decisions regarding "best practices" for maintaining each patient's oral health. EBDM is based on current research findings, each individual patient's situation, and your own good clinical judgment. You can use EBDM to recommend, or decide not to recommend, a variety of therapies, techniques, and oral health products.

The best way to develop these skills is, of course, to practice them. The Primer and the Discovery exercises in each chapter of this workbook will help you.

COMPETENCIES FOR THE DENTAL HYGIENIST

The American Dental Education Association (ADEA) Competencies outline the areas in which a new graduate dental hygienist is expected to be able to apply knowledge to ensure that safe and effective patient care is provided. The title page for each section of this workbook lists specific ADEA competencies supported by learning the information from chapters included in that section of the textbook. The complete list of competency statements found in Appendix A will provide a reference point to help you understand why learning specific concepts from each chapter is important for becoming a professional dental hygienist.

As you read the ADEA competency statements, you should note that your school may have adapted them somewhat for use in your dental hygiene program. Your school's competencies may be organized in a slightly different manner but will probably be very similar. You should make a point of receiving a copy of your school's competency statements for reference.

I encourage you to enjoy the process of learning and I hope that this workbook offers activities that will help you.

Sincerely,
Charlotte J. Wyche, RDH, MS
Dental Hygiene Educator

A Primer for Evidence-Based Decision Making (EBDM)

Judi S. Luxmore, RDH, MS and Charlotte J. Wyche, RDH, MS

The main goal of clinical dental hygiene practice is to improve the oral health of the patient. Many questions and/or problems that arise on a daily basis need current and reliable information in order to provide the best treatment for patients. To that end, a systematic method is recommended to wade through the myriad of research. Evidence-Based Decision Making will assist healthcare professionals in formulating objective recommendations to improve patient outcomes.

I. What is EBDM?

1. Many definitions exist for evidence-based decision making.
   - A simple definition states, "Evidence-based clinical practice is an approach to decision making in which the clinician uses the best evidence available, in consultation with the patient, to decide upon the option which suits that patient best."[1]
   - The ability to access and understand current research findings is important when using EBDM to plan dental-hygiene care. However, other factors are also taken into consideration. Figure 1 illustrates how four crucial elements combine to form the EBDM process.[2]
2. Skills needed to implement EBDM include:
   - **Understanding of EBDM**
     - A variety of tutorials that inform about EBDM are available on the Internet.
   - **Self-directed learning**
     - Continuing education
     - Scientific literature
   - **Reading and understanding research**
     - The ability to recognize reliable versus unreliable material in relation to publications, articles, and/or research
   - **Computer/Internet literacy**
     - The ability to evaluate Web-based information
     - The ability to search the literature via databases of biomedical references efficiently

II. A Systematic Approach

A systematic method is crucial to the development of good EBDM skills. The following is a step-by-step procedure for using an evidence-based approach to patient care.[2,3]

1. **Start with the patient: What is the clinical problem or question related to a specific patient case?**
   - Asking the right question to research is fundamental—and critical—to the evidence-based decision-making process.
   - Include important characteristics of the patient (i.e., age, gender, etc.)
2. **Develop a well-built clinical question concerning that case.**
   - A well-built question, sometimes referred to as a **PICO**[2,4] question, includes four parts:

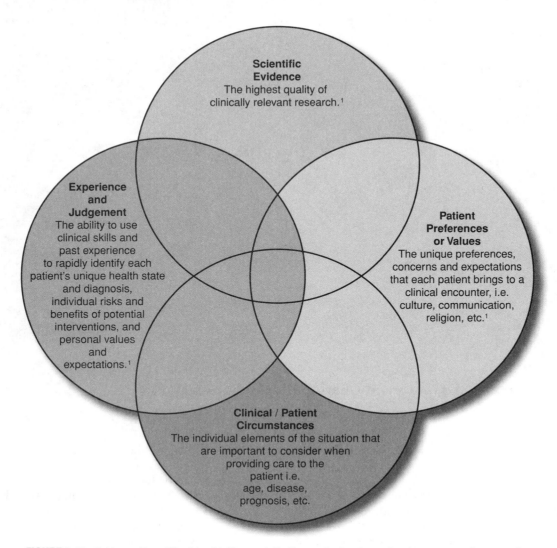

FIGURE 1 The Evidence-Based Decision Making model indicates the four interrelated components important for applying scientific evidence to patient-care decisions. (Forrest J, Miller S, Newman MG, Overman P. *Evidence-based decision making: a translational guide for dental professionals.* Baltimore: Lippincott Williams & Wilkins;2008: in press).

- Patient problem or population (**P**)
  - What are the most important characteristics of the patient?
- Intervention (**I**)
  - Which main intervention, prognostic factor, or exposure are you considering?
- Comparison (**C**)
  - What is the main alternative to compare with the intervention?
  - Your clinical question does not always need a specific comparison.
- Outcome (**O**)
  - What can you hope to accomplish, measure, improve, or affect?
3. **Select an appropriate resource, and conduct a search of scientific literature.**[2,5]
   - **MEDLINE** (Pub Med)
     - A biomedical database offered free from the U.S. National Library of Medicine.

- **CINAHL** (Cumulative Index to Nursing and Allied Health Literature)
  - A bibliographic database that includes abstracts of nursing and allied health articles.
- **Cochrane Library** (The Cochrane Collaboration)
  - An international nonprofit and independent organization; produces and disseminates systematic reviews of healthcare interventions and promotes the search for evidence in the form of clinical trials and other studies of interventions.
- Other resources, including individual journals, newsletters, guidelines, the COT research register, software, Internet resources, e-mail discussion lists, and library resources.
4. **Analyze the evidence for validity (closeness to the truth) and value (usefulness in clinical practice).**[6,7]

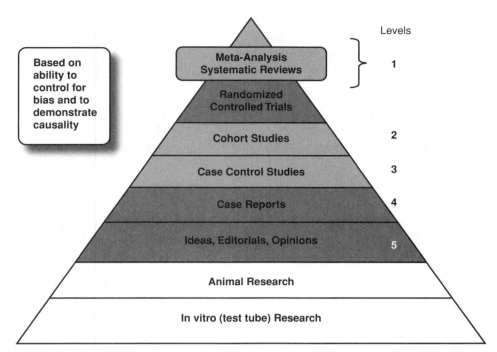

FIGURE 2 The Levels of Evidence triangle illustrates the relative strength and availability of types of evidence available for making clinical decisions. (Forrest J, Miller S, Newman MG, Overman P. *Evidence-based decision making: a translational guide for dental professionals.* Baltimore: Lippincott Williams & Wilkins;2008: in press).

5. **Return to the patient: Apply the evidence along with your clinical expertise/experience and the patient's preferences.**
6. **Evaluate the results**
   - If patient outcome is unsuccessful, begin process again.

III. Evaluating Research[7–9]

The number of scientific research studies is growing. Some studies might not be appropriate for answering your clinical question. Using a hierarchy to judge the suitability of each type of research is helpful. The concept of **levels of evidence** can be used to evaluate the strength (**scientific rigor and quality**) of the evidence. Figure 2 represents the relative strength and availability of the types of evidence.

Systematic reviews, which combine and analyze findings from several research studies, are considered the strongest evidence. The most clinically relevant research types appear at the top of the triangle; the less relevant types of research follow in descending order. The top three levels represent actual clinical research; the bottom levels are most useful as background resources.

IV. Evaluating Web Sites[10–13]

Internet-based information is overwhelming in its composition. Finding the appropriate information from the appropriate site takes an understanding of both content and location.

1. **Choose a search engine that is right for the job.**
   - Many databases lead to newspaper and magazine articles. Scientific literature databases/articles will not be found by using search engines or directories such as *Google* or *Yahoo*.
   - Biomedical information comes from:
     - Search engines such as EviDents (http://medinformatics.uthscsa.edu/)
     - Databases such as:
       - MEDLINE (http://www.ncbi.nlm.nih.gov/entrez/query.fcgi?DB=pubmed)
       - Cochrane Collaboration (http://www.cochrane.co.uk/en/index.htm)
2. **Determine the purpose of the site (e.g., to educate, entertain, or market products)**
   Be familiar with *domain names* and what they mean.
   - .edu and .gov are considered reliable sites for educational and governmental information.
   - .org indicates nonprofit organizations. An understanding of the mission and purpose of the organization is important.
   - .com and .net tend to be from special interest groups and advertising (possibly for profit).
3. **Analyze the information to make sure it is relevant to your topic.**
   - Topic covered in-depth?
   - Bibliography present?

- References to other Web sites included?
- All points of view covered?

4. **Determine who is responsible for the information (i.e., author and publisher)**
   - Author: Credentials and contact information given?
   - Publisher of the site: To locate the publisher, look at the site address (URL) and under links such as "About Us" or "Our Mission," or at the bottom of the page.

5. **Determine accuracy and objectivity of the site:**
   - Accuracy
     - Information similar to other sources (text books/journal articles)?
     - References given?
   - Objectivity
     - Conflicts of interest and/or bias apparent?
     - All points of view discussed?
     - Credentials of the author and publisher (to determine the underlying connection) given?

6. **Note how well the site is maintained.**
   - Currency
     - Last update indicated? Is this important for your topic?
   - Quality control
     - Links current and working?
     - Grammar and spelling errors?

7. **Putting it all together** (strengths and weaknesses of site)
   - Weigh the appropriateness of all the above areas to determine if the site is worthwhile in relation to your topic.

V. Conclusion

Perfecting basic research strategies will allow the dental hygiene practitioner to locate reliable and appropriate healthcare information in an efficient manner. Ultimately, a systematic approach to evaluating and analyzing the content and location of research materials will lead to better and improved patient care. Some resources for further study about EBDM are listed at the end of this section.

VI. References

1. Muir Gray JA. *Evidence-based healthcare: how to make health policy and management decisions.* London: Churchill Livingstone; 1997.
2. Forrest JL, Miller SA. Evidence-based decision making in action: Part 1. Finding the best clinical evidence. *J Contemp Dent Pract* 2002;3(3): 10–26.
3. Pwee KH. What is this thing called EBM? *Singapore Med J* 2004;45(9):413–417.
4. Sackett DL, Richardson WS, Rosenberg W, et al. *Evidence-based medicine: how to practice and teach EBM.* London: Churchill Livingstone; 1997.
5. Bidwell SR. Finding the evidence: resources and skills for locating information on clinical effectiveness. *Singapore Med J* 2004;45(12):548–550.
6. Sutherland SE. Evidence-based dentistry: Part V. Critical appraisal of the dental literature: papers about therapy. *J Can Dent Assoc* 2001;67(8): 442–445.
7. Forrest JL, Miller SA. Evidence-based decision making in action: Part 2. Evaluating and applying the clinical evidence. *J Contemp Dent Pract* 2003;4(1):42–52.
8. Sutherland SE. Evidence-based dentistry: Part IV. Research design and levels of evidence. *J Can Dent Assoc* 2001;67(7):375–378.
9. SUNY Health Sciences. Guide to research methods: the evidence pyramid [Internet]. SUNY (State University of New York) Evidence Based Medicine Course; 2004 January 6 [cited 12 December 2006]. Available at: http://library. downstate.edu/EBM2/2100.htm.
10. North Virginia Community College Library Research Tools: Website evaluation: a brief guide to evaluating websites [Internet]. 2006 October 20 [cited 11 December 2006]. Available at: http://www.nvcc.edu/library/.
11. Health on the Net Foundation: HON code of conduct (HONcode) for medical and health web sites [Internet]. 2006 December 6 [cited 11 December 2006]. Available at: http://www.hon. ch/HONcode/Conduct.html.
12. Barker J, Saifon O. Evaluating Web pages: questions to ask and strategies for getting the answers [Internet]. University of California Berkeley Library; 2005 March 22 [cited 11 December 2006]. Available at: http://www.lib.berkeley.edu/ TeachingLib/Guides/Internet/Evaluate.html.
13. Kapoun J. Teaching undergrads WEB evaluation: a guide for library instruction [Internet]. *C&RL News* 1998;522–523. [cited 12 December 2006]. Available at: http://www.library.cornell.edu/olinuris/ ref/research/webcrit.html.

VII. Resources For Further Study
Evidence-Based Tutorials:

1. University of North Carolina
   - http://www.hsl.unc.edu/services/tutorials/ ebm/welcome.htm
2. University of Rochester Medical Center
   - http://www.urmc.rochester.edu/hslt/miner/ resources/evidence_based/index.cfm
3. State University of New York
   - http://library.downstate.edu/EBM2/contents. htm

Online Databases

1. PubMed (free) MEDLINE
   - http://www.ncbi.nlm.nih.gov/entrez/query.fcgi? DB=pubmed
     (Tutorials: **MEDLINE in OVID,** use the OVID tutorial at http://www.mclibrary.duke.edu/training/ovid
     MEDLINE in PubMed, go to http://www.nlm.nih.gov/bsd/pubmed_tutorial/m1001.html)
2. MedlinePlus
   - http://medlineplus.gov/
3. The Cochrane Library
   - http://www3.interscience.wiley.com/cgi-bin/mrwhome/106568753/HOME? CRETRY=1&SRETRY=0
4. National Guideline Clearing House
   - http://www.guideline.gov
5. CINAHL® Database (nursing, allied health, biomedicine, and health care)
   - http://www.cinahl.com/

Evidence-Based Centers

1. Evidence-Based News, National Center for Dental Hygiene, University of Southern California
   - http://www.usc.edu/hsc/ebnet/
2. Centre for Evidence-Based Dentistry, Oxford
   - http://www.cebd.org/
3. Centre for Evidence-Based Medicine, Oxford
   - http://www.cebm.net/

Web Site Evaluation

1. Health on the Net Foundation, HONcode Principles
   - www.hon.ch/HONcode/Conduct.html
2. UC Berkeley Library, Evaluating Web Pages
   - http://www.lib.berkeley.edu/TeachingLib/Guides/Internet/Evaluate.html
3. Cornell Library, Five Criteria for Evaluating Web Pages
   - http://www.library.cornell.edu/olinuris/ref/research/webcrit.html

ACKNOWLEDGMENTS

Joan McClintok, RDH, MEd
(original author for workbook chapters 6, 7, and 10 to 19 in the first edition)

Tina Daniels, RDH, BS
(Guidelines for Conversation during Patient Education)

Judi Luxmore, RDH, MS
(Evidence-based Primer)

Textbook contributing authors who also provided new ideas, feedback, suggestions for learning exercises, or cases for "their chapters" in this addition of the workbook:

Nancy Sisty-Lepeau, RDH, MS, MA *(Chapters 45–46)*
Karen A. Raposa, RDH, MBA *(Chapter 25)*
Stacy A. Matsuda, RDH, BS *(Chapters 36-37)*
Terri Tillis, RDH, MS, MA *(Chapter 41)*
Debbie Manne, RDH, RN, MSN, OCN *(Chapter 52)*
Deborah Mancinelli Lyle, RDH, BS, MA *(Chapter 27)*
Marilyn Cortell, RDH MS *(Chapter 40)*
Janet Towle, RN, RDH, BS, Med *(Chapters 49, 60)*

Thank you all for your help in making this workbook possible.

Orientation to Clinical Dental Hygiene Practice

Chapter 1

■ SECTION I LEARNING OBJECTIVES

Completing the exercises in this section of the workbook will prepare you to:

1. Identify the characteristics of a dental hygiene professional.
2. Apply ethical, legal, cultural, and personal professional standards to the practice of dental hygiene.

■ COMPETENCIES FOR THE DENTAL HYGIENIST (APPENDIX A)

The following ADEA competencies are supported by the learning in Section I.

Core Competencies: C1, C2, C5, C6, C9, C11

Health Promotion and Disease Prevention Competencies: HP2, HP4, HP5

Professional Growth and Development Competencies: PGD1, PGD3

The Professional Dental Hygienist

Chapter Outline

Learning Objectives

Upon successful completion of these exercises, you will be able to:

1. Identify and define key terms and concepts related to the professional dental hygienist.
2. Define the scope of dental hygiene practice.
3. Identify and define the components of the Dental Hygiene Process of Care.
4. Identify cultural considerations that can affect delivery of dental hygiene care.
5. Identify and apply components of the Dental Hygiene Code of Ethics.
6. Explain legal, ethical, and personal factors affecting dental hygiene practice.
7. Apply concepts in ethical decision making.

KNOWLEDGE EXERCISES

1. Identify and (in your own words) briefly define the healthcare–related roles that your dental hygiene education will prepare you to fulfill.

   _____

   _____

   _____

   _____

   _____

2. How is the role of public health related to the other roles?

   _____

   _____

   _____

   _____

3. Describe a dental hygienist using the terminology associated with integrated practice roles, healthcare focus, and services provided by dental hygienists.

_____

_____

_____

_____

_____

4. Identify three personal factors that affect the way in which an individual dental hygienist is perceived as a representative of the entire profession of dental hygiene.

_____

_____

_____

5. Define _dental hygiene care_.

_____

_____

_____

6. Identify three types of services provided by the dental hygienist.

_____

_____

_____

7. Define _health promotion_.

_____

_____

_____

8. What dental hygienist role was emphasized by Dr. A. C. Fones, who is considered the father of dental hygiene?

_____

_____

_____

9. What is the primary goal of each dental hygienist with respect to patient care?

_____

_____

_____

10. List at least three objectives for professional dental hygiene practice.

_____

_____

_____

11. In what way is the dental hygienist a co-therapist?

_____

_____

_____

12. In your own words, explain the three types of prevention.

_____

_____

_____

13. List three ways, other than formal advanced education, in which a dental hygienist can specialize.

_____

_____

_____

14. The Dental Hygiene Process of Care provides the framework for offering individualized dental hygiene services based on identified patient needs. In your own words, briefly define each of the five phases of the Dental Hygiene Process of Care.

■ _Assessment_

_____

_____

_____

■ _Diagnosis_

_____

_____

■ _Planning_

_____

_____

_____

■ _Implementation_

_____

_____

_____

■ *Evaluation*

_____

_____

_____

15. Both _____ (observed) and _____ (perceived) data are collected in the assessment phase of the Dental Hygiene Process of Care.

16. Identify three factors involved in analyzing assessment data before formulating the dental hygiene diagnosis.

_____

_____

_____

17. In your own words, describe the purpose of dental hygiene diagnosis statements.

_____

_____

_____

18. What is a dental hygiene care plan?

_____

_____

_____

19. Identify the steps that are important to include when you are planning dental hygiene care.

_____

_____

_____

_____

_____

20. Define *oral hygiene.*

_____

_____

_____

21. Define *dental hygiene intervention.*

_____

_____

22. Define *dental hygiene prognosis.*

_____

_____

_____

23. Dental hygienists usually provide dental hygiene care under the supervision of a dentist. Identify and briefly define four levels of supervision.

_____

_____

_____

_____

_____

24. When is a patient's continuing care interval determined?

_____

_____

25. In what ways are the assessment and the evaluation phases of the dental hygiene process of care similar?

_____

_____

_____

26. Identify at least one way that ethnic or cultural background can affect your patient's health status or the way they respond to your dental hygiene interventions.

_____

_____

_____

27. _____ is a skill that can be developed by exploring and learning to appreciate the wide variety of differences among the individuals who are your patients.

28. Cultural competence, which includes respect and responsiveness to the unique culturally related characteristics, values, and needs of each patient, will help you provide _____ oral health care.

29. Providing handouts written in a plain and easily understandable way for your patients whose primary

language is different from the dominant local language is one component of _____.

30. What six special factors apply to members of a group defined as having professional status?

_____

_____

_____

_____

_____

_____

31. What is a code of ethics?

_____

_____

_____

32. Name at least two professional organizations that have developed codes of ethics for the practice of dental hygiene.

_____

_____

33. In your own words, briefly define each of the seven core values in dental hygiene.

_____

_____

_____

_____

34. As a dental hygienist, you are responsible for approaching ethical decisions in a thorough and logical manner. The textbook defines two components, the steps in Table 1-2 and a sequence for a logical approach, that can be used together to form a framework for making ethical decisions.

   ▓ *Identify the four steps (components) in the framework for making decisions.*

   _____

   _____

   _____

   ▓ *Identify the six steps that formulate a logical approach to the four steps (components) in the Table 1-2 framework.*

   _____

   _____

   _____

_____

_____

_____

35. As a professional dental hygienist, what is your primary responsibility?

_____

_____

_____

COMPETENCY EXERCISES

1. Provide examples from dental hygiene practice, education, and licensure to explain why a dental hygienist can be considered a primary healthcare professional. In your discussion, refer to the definition of *primary healthcare* and to the definition of a *profession* (Box 1-1 in the textbook).

   _____

   _____

   _____

2. Explain why the notion of lifelong learning is considered to be an ethical component of dental hygiene practice.

   _____

   _____

   _____

3. Core values in dental hygiene practice include **autonomy and respect.** An example of this value is that you, as the dental hygienist, must respect your patient's right to refuse dental hygiene treatment, even when your professional opinion is that doing so may cause deterioration of their oral health status.

   Select another one of the core values in dental hygiene practice and give an example to illustrate it. Discuss your example with student colleagues.

   _____

   _____

   _____

4. Dental hygiene interventions play a major role in all levels of prevention of oral disease. Give examples (different from those included in the textbook) of a dental hygienist's role in each level of prevention.

   _____

   _____

_____

_____

_____

_____

5. Identify an expression, gesture, or movement that you commonly make (see Box 1-4 for some ideas). Explain how your action can have unintended meaning or be the cause of a misunderstanding that will have a negative effect on the relationship you are developing with a patient of cultural background that is different than your own.

_____

_____

_____

_____

_____

_____

6. David Martin is a 13-year-old who chews bubble gum and sips a sugar-sweetened carbonated beverage all day long, especially when he is studying. An oral examination indicates that he has extensive dental decay. Write a dental hygiene diagnosis statement for David.

Problem _____

Related to _____

7. Mrs. Jenkins is a new patient. It is policy in this clinic that every new patient receives a complete radiographic survey as part of an initial examination because Dr. Graves, the dentist, believes that she cannot make a complete diagnosis without radiographs.

Mrs. Jenkins refuses to have the radiographs made even after you have carefully explained the need for radiographs for complete diagnosis and discussed research findings regarding the safety of current x-ray techniques (see Chapter 9, Factors to Teach the Patient, page 179)

Dr. Graves decides that if Mrs. Jenkins continues to refuse, she will be asked to go elsewhere for her treatment. Do you consider this an ethical issue or an ethical dilemma? Justify your answer. Determine your response to this situation and discuss it with a student colleague.

_____

_____

_____

DISCOVERY EXERCISES

1. Box 1-4 in the textbook lists questions for self-assessing personal values. Write out brief answers for each of the five questions. Identify how your personal values relate to your future as a dental hygiene professional.

2. Obtain a copy of the rules or laws that govern the practice of dental hygiene in your state or country. Answer the following questions.
   - _What type of supervision must dental hygienists have when they provide care for the public?_
   - _What specific services are the dental hygienists in your state or area licensed to provide?_
   - _What are continuing education requirements for dental hygienists who practice in your state or country?_

Everyday Ethics

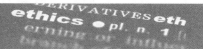

Refer to the Codes of Ethics (Appendices I, II, and III in the textbook) and the Framework for Making Decisions (Table 1-2 in the textbook) as you discuss the following scenario with your classmates.

The first term of the dental hygiene curriculum has just finished. The instructor asks for student volunteers to help at the college's health fair to provide basic routine brushing and flossing directions to people who stop at the dental hygiene information table. Three students—Alice, Annette, and Josephine—sign up to volunteer for this community service. The day before the health fair, which takes place on a Saturday, Annette is asked to work in the dental office where she is employed part-time. Because she really needs the money, she decides not to attend the health fair and instead goes to work without telling anyone.

Questions for Consideration
1. In general, would this situation be described as a professional issue or an ethical dilemma? Why?
2. Discuss Annette's actions in terms of the core ethical values.
3. What aspects of the Dental Hygiene Code of Ethics can you use to support your choice of action?

3. Find a contact person for the dental hygiene professional association nearest to you and ask questions about membership, continuing education, and leadership opportunities.

4. Explore *The Provider's Guide to Quality and Culture: Health Disparities* Web site (available from the Managers Electronic Resource Center at: www.erc.msh.org). Click on the link to the Provider's Guide on the left hand side of the page. Take the quiz to identify misconceptions you have about characteristics common to individuals of other cultures. Return to this Web site to review more specific information when you are planning care for a patient whose cultural background is different from your own.

QUESTIONS PATIENTS ASK

What sources of information can you identify that will help you answer your patient's questions in this scenario?

Your patient, Jessica Miles, who is a junior in high school, comments, "My mom and I were talking about where I will be going to college after next year. She said to ask you where you went. She thinks what you do would be real cool. Did you have to take a lot of sciences? Do they have dental chairs and all the equipment right in the school and do people come in for you to learn from? I know you clean our teeth—why do you like working in people's mouths?"

FOR YOUR PORTFOLIO

Use the basic information in this chapter to write a personal philosophy of dental hygiene practice. Describe

Factors To Teach The Patient

Sarah, your really good friend, has agreed to be a patient for your first clinical experience as a dental hygiene student. When you call her to remind her of her appointment tomorrow, she asks you a bit about what you will do during the appointment. You excitedly begin to explain the procedures.

Sarah interrupts saying that it all sounds pretty boring to her. She asks you to tell her why you are studying so hard to become a dental hygienist. Using the example of a patient conversation in Appendix B as a guide, write a statement explaining your knowledge and interest in dental hygiene practice to Sarah.

This scenario is related to the following factors:

■ The role of the dental hygienist as co-therapist with each patient and with members of the dental profession
■ The moral and ethical nature of becoming a dental hygiene professional person
■ The patient's potential state of oral health and how it can be improved and maintained

how you believe yourself to be as a dental hygiene professional. Identify characteristics that describe the way you will provide dental hygiene care. Do this at the beginning of your training just after you complete these chapter exercises, and then do it again just before you graduate (don't peek at what you wrote the first time, please). Finally write a summary of how these two documents reveal your personal growth during your training as a professional.

Preparation for Dental Hygiene Appointments

■ SECTION II LEARNING OBJECTIVES

Completing the exercises in this section of the workbook will prepare you to:

1. Apply concepts of infection/exposure control to protect the safety of self and patient during the dental hygiene appointment.

2. Position self, patient, and equipment to promote comfort, safety, and efficiency during the dental hygiene appointment.

■ COMPETENCIES FOR THE DENTAL HYGIENIST (APPENDIX A)

The following ADEA competencies are supported by the learning in Section II.

Core Competencies: C2, C3, C4, C5, C6, C8, C10, C11

Health Promotion and Disease Prevention: HP2, HP3, HP4, HP6

Patient/Client Care: PC1, PC2, PC3, PC4, PC5

CHAPTER 2

Infection Control: Transmissible Diseases

Chapter Outline

Learning Objectives

Upon successful completion of these exercises, you will be able to:

1. Identify and define key terms and concepts related to control of infectious diseases.
2. Explain the infectious process and discuss methods of preventing transmission of infection.
3. Identify and distinguish pathogens transmissible by the oral cavity.
4. Identify oral lesions related to various infectious agents.

KNOWLEDGE EXERCISES

Please also be sure to refer to textbook Appendix IV, "The CDC 2003 Guidelines for Infection Control in Dental Health-Care Settings," as you complete the exercises in this chapter.

Standard Precautions Crossword Puzzle

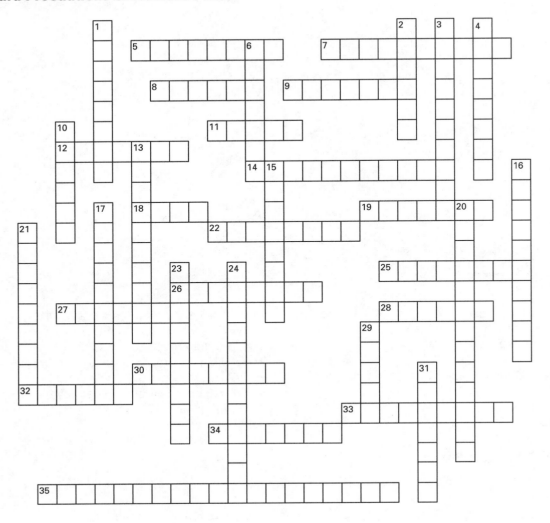

Across

5 Refers to a widespread, extensive, or worldwide epidemic.

7 A subcutaneous, intramuscular, or intravenous injection.

8 Refers to an infection in which the causative agent remains inactive for a period of time within certain body cells.

9 Someone who harbors a specific infectious agent but shows no clinical signs of disease.

11 A genetic entity that contains either DNA or RNA or both; replicates inside living cells.

12 Constant presence of a disease within a geographic area.

14 The factor that identifies a specific disease in a laboratory blood test (two words).

18 Refers to increased likelihood of infection.

19 Suspended microbial particles; less than 50 mm in diameter.

22 Most infective stage of the HSV virus; characterized by burning, stinging sensation before the appearance of vesicles.

25 Refers to a vector that is a living organism, such as an insect; infecting organisms multiply in the body of this vector before becoming infective to other recipients.

26 A natural or acquired resistance against disease.

27 Particles that are airborne a short time and drop onto other objects; usually greater than 50 mm in diameter.

28 An inanimate object on which disease-producing agents can be conveyed.

30 Refers to the presence of a virus in certain body secretions, excretions, or surface lesions.

32 Refers to a viral infection that resides in the ganglia of nerves and reactivates at a later date.

33 Inflammation of the parotid gland.

34 The type of immunity that is transferred from the mother or acquired by inoculation of protective antibodies.

35 An infection control approach in which the dental health care provider treats all human blood and body fluids as if known to be infectious (two words).

Down

1 A soluble protein molecule secreted in response to, and able to bind to, a specific antigen.

2 Inability to react to skin-test antigen because of immunosuppression.

3 A virus with RNA as its core genetic material.

4 A virus, microorganism, or other substance that causes disease.

6 Another term used for jaundice.

10 A carrier that transfers an infectious microorganism from one host to another.

13 The microscopic living organisms.

15 Widespread occurrence of more than the usual number of cases of a particular disease.

16 By way of, or through, a mucous membrane.

17 Refers to the period of time between initial contact with an infectious agent and the appearance of clinical symptoms of the disease.

20 Refers to a pathogen that causes disease only when the host's resistance is lowered.

21 Early or premonitory symptom (adjective).

23 The disease-evoking power of an infectious agent.

24 Continuous observation of the patterns of a disease in order to try to control it.

29 A laboratory test to detect antibody in the blood serum.

31 A substance that induces an immune response.

Several tables in Chapter 2 of the textbook provide excellent summaries of infectious agents and diseases. You should study these tables carefully. Ask your instructor to tell you how thoroughly (or to what level of detail) you will need to study the information in these tables at this point in your dental hygiene program.

The following exercises will help you identify information that is of special concern to you as a dental healthcare provider.

1. The first step in providing safe patient care is for the dental team to attend to sterilization/disinfection of instruments and equipment. What additional step is required to prevent cross-infections?

   _____

   _____

   _____

2. List six factors that are necessary for transmission of disease.

   _____

   _____

   _____

   _____

   _____

   _____

3. Preventing disease transmission requires breaking the chain of transmission. The use of standard precautions breaks the chain at every point. Identify additional ways that the dental team can break the chain and prevent transmission of infection.

   _____

   _____

   _____

4. Identify items in the dental setting that can serve as reservoirs for infectious agents.

   _____

   _____

   _____

5. Identify factors that influence whether an infection develops after exposure to an infectious agent.

   _____

   _____

   _____

6. Identify conditions that can affect your patient's normal defenses against infection and may require you to take extra precautions during dental hygiene treatment.

   _____

   _____

   _____

   _____

7. Identify ways that infectious particles can become airborne in the dental setting.

   _____

   _____

8. Identify ways of controlling airborne transmission of infection in the dental setting.

   _____

   _____

   _____

   _____

9. Chapter 2 and Section IX-K of the CDC recommendations (see textbook Appendix _____) both mention tuberculosis as an infectious disease that is of concern for dental healthcare providers. Identify the microorganism that causes tuberculosis.

   _____

10. In what way is tuberculosis infection most commonly transmitted?

    _____

11. What is XDR?

    _____

12. In the textbook, Tables 2-1 and 2-3, the text of Chapter 2, and Section IIA of the CDC recommendations (see textbook Appendix IV) each contains information about hepatitis viruses. Use Infomap 2-1 on the next page to compare disease process and modes of prevention for each type of hepatitis virus.

13. Which virus occurs in periodontal pockets with relatively high prevalence?

    _____

14. Which of the herpes viruses can establish a latent infection in the trigeminal nerve ganglion that can reactivate and erupt in a surface lesion later?

    _____

INFOMAP 2-1	HEPATITIS	
HEPATITIS VIRUS TYPE	**DISEASE INCUBATION AND PROCESS**	**METHODS FOR REVENTION**
Hepatitis A		
Hepatitis B		
Hepatitis C		
Hepatitis D		
Hepatitis E		

15. Many viral infections are associated with intraoral findings. Complete Infomap 2-2, writing a brief description of oral conditions you might identify while providing an intraoral examination for a patient who is infected with each of these types of viruses. For each virus, spell out the full name in the space next to the acronym.

16. Which virus type is associated with lesions on hands and eyes?

_____

17. AIDS is associated with infection by the _____ virus.

18. A patient's HIV status can be classified by using a combination of a laboratory count of _____ cells and identification of related symptoms.

19. As the count of indicator cells decreases, the symptoms of disease and the incidence of oral infections or oral lesions related to the HIV infection _____.

INFOMAP 2-2	
VIRUS TYPE	**ASSOCIATED ORAL CONDITIONS**
HHV1	
HSV2	
HHV3	
HHV4	
HHV5	
HHV6	
HHV7	
HHV8	

20. A thorough oral examination can reveal oral lesions that indicate a change in the health status of your patient with HIV infection. Give an example of each of the three following types of infection that you will look for each time you provide an oral examination.

▓ *Fungal*

_____

▓ *Viral*

_____

▓ *Bacterial*

_____

21. In your own words, briefly describe three types of acute gingival/periodontal infections that may be observed in your patient with HIV infection.

_____

_____

_____

22. Identify situations in which children are at risk for HIV infections.

_____

_____

_____

23. Why do medications prepared for children with an HIV-positive status increase the risk for dental disease?

_____

_____

_____

COMPETENCY EXERCISES

1. The CDC 2003 Guidelines for Infection Control in Dental Health Care Settings (Appendix IV in the textbook) provides evidence-based recommendations for dental healthcare providers. Each recommendation is categorized according to a specific system that is outlined in the first section. Use the information provided in CDC Guidelines to discuss, in your own words, what each of the recommendation categories means.

_____

_____

_____

_____

_____

_____

_____

_____

2. In your own words, write a paragraph or two summarizing the recommendations (in Section II of CDC Guidelines) for preventing transmission of blood-borne pathogens. What category of evidence supports these recommendations?

_____

_____

_____

_____

_____

_____

Everyday Ethics

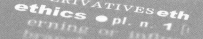

Refer to the Codes of Ethics (Appendices I, II, and III in the textbook) and Framework for Making Decisions (Table 1-2 in the textbook) as you discuss the following scenario with your classmates.

Mr. Sands, a patient returning for his regular maintenance appointment, is scheduled with Jenny, one of the two dental hygienists available that day. Mr. Sands has a history of hepatitis C. When Jenny reviewed the history before seating the patient, she immediately makes up an excuse and asks Marilyn, the other hygienist, to treat this patient while she attends to the two pedodontic patients in a different treatment room.

Questions for Consideration
1. What does Jenny need to understand about refusing to treat the patient with a hepatitis C history?
2. Using the decision framework in Table 1-2 (page 14), list alternative solutions or outcomes that apply to this situation.
3. How is the principle of justice related to Jenny's actions?

Factors To Teach The Patient

Your patient, Ms. Janette Whitlow, arrives just on time for her dental hygiene appointment, and you greet her cheerfully. As you update her health history, she mentions that she is grumpy because she is getting another cold sore and her lip itches and burns. You look closely and observe a reddened, slightly swollen area on her lower lip that is just beginning to get small bumps. As she talks, Janette slowly rubs her hand up across her face and eyes and up into her hair.

Using the information about HSV infections in Chapter 2 and the example of a patient conversation in Appendix B as guides, write a conversation explaining to Janette why you recommend postponing her appointment until another day. Also explain why she should not touch or scratch the sore area on her lip.

Ask a student colleague or dental hygiene instructor to give feedback on the conversation you create, and then modify the conversation based on what you learned from the feedback.

This scenario is related to the following factors:

■ Reasons for postponing an appointment when a herpes lesion (fever blister or cold sore) is present on the lip or in the oral cavity

■ Importance of not touching or scratching the lesion because of self-infection to the fingers or eyes, for example

■ How the viruses can survive on objects and transfer infection to other people

3. In your own words, identify clinical management procedures to follow if your patient's medical history raises concerns about tuberculosis infection.

CHAPTER 3

Exposure Control: Barriers for Patient and Clinician

Chapter Outline

Learning Objectives

Upon successful completion of these exercises, you will be able to:

1. Identify and define key terms and concepts related to exposure control, clinical barriers, and latex allergies.
2. Apply and remove clinical barrier materials without cross-contamination.
3. Identify and explain the rationale for hand washing and other exposure-control techniques used during patient care.
4. Identify criteria for selecting appropriate protective barrier materials.

KNOWLEDGE EXERCISES

Be sure also to refer to textbook Appendix IV, CDC 2003 Guidelines for Infection Control in Dental Health-Care Settings, as you complete the exercises for this chapter.

1. An organized system for exposure control that treats body fluids of all patients as though they were infectious is a description of _____.

2. What is considered the single most important procedure for the prevention of cross-contamination?

   _____

3. Identify the term or concept related to each of the following statements.

   ▪ Physically blocks exposure to bodily fluids to prevent disease transmission.

   _____

   ▪ A specific, potentially health-threatening bodily contact with infectious material while you are providing dental hygiene care.

   _____

■ Contact with infectious material that is reasonable to expect as a component of providing dental hygiene care.

_____

4. Identify three purposes for having a written exposure control plan.

_____

_____

_____

5. Define the following terms in your own words.

■ *Immunization*

_____

_____

■ *Inoculation*

_____

_____

_____

■ *Toxoid*

_____

_____

_____

■ *Vaccine*

_____

_____

_____

■ *Vaccination*

_____

_____

_____

■ *HCP*

_____

_____

_____

6. Unscramble the following words; definitions are included to help you.

■ *hiiinrts (inflammation of the mucous membrane of the nose)*

_____

■ *toxmanu (a test for the presence of active or inactive tuberculosis)*

_____

■ *bcmytaercoiumr cykitbreysos (droplet nuclei, ranging from 0.5 to 1 μm, that are a risk in healthcare settings)*

_____

7. Updating immunizations against a number of diseases is an important protective factor for DHCP. What is a booster immunization?

_____

_____

_____

8. List the vaccines recommended for DHCP.

_____

_____

_____

9. What regular tests are recommended to monitor DHCP exposure to infectious diseases?

_____

_____

_____

10. List the factors that describe an appropriate clinic gown or uniform.

_____

_____

_____

11. If your protective covering (clinic gown) becomes visibly soiled during patient care, what should you do?

_____

_____

_____

12. During patient care, long hair should be fastened back and facial hair should be covered by _____.

13. Write a one- or two-word phrase that will help you remember each of the seven criteria of an ideal face mask. (Box 3-2 in texbook.)

_____

_____

_____

_____

_____

_____

_____

14. Particles in aerosols smaller than _____ can remain suspended up to 24 hours.

15. What size particle can penetrate to the alveoli of lungs when inhaled?

_____

16. What size are the tuberculosis-causing bacterium particles?

_____

17. The CDC guidelines recommend changing a mask between patients or during patient care if the mask becomes _____.

18. When should you wear a shield over your regular mask during patient care?

_____

_____

_____

19. Who wears protective eyewear during dental hygiene care?

_____

_____

_____

20. List types of eyewear appropriate for wear during patient care.

_____

_____

_____

21. List three steps you can use to disinfect and provide care for eyewear worn during patient care.

_____

_____

_____

22. Identify the glove safety factors that are important for both the patient and the dental hygienist during dental hygiene care.

_____

_____

_____

23. When you are selecting the type of gloves to use during patient care, which glove comfort factors are primarily important to the dental hygienist?

_____

_____

_____

24. The cuffs of your gloves should be positioned _____ the cuffs of your long-sleeved clinic wear to provide a complete barrier to contamination.

25. After positioning your gloves before patient care, you should touch only _____.

26. List the factors that affect the ability of gloves to provide a complete aseptic barrier.

_____

_____

_____

_____

_____

27. Long fingernails can harbor microorganisms. What is the best way to clean under your fingernails before patient care?

_____

_____

_____

28. Identify additional potential effects of having long fingernails when providing dental hygiene care.

_____

_____

_____

29. What recommendation is included in the CDC 2003 guidelines regarding hand jewelry?

_____

_____

_____

30. If your gloves become torn, cut, or punctured during patient care, what should you do?

_____

_____

_____

31. In your own words, describe the characteristics of an ideal sink for handwashing before patient care.

_____

_____

_____

32. During clinical practice, you will wash your hands many, many times each day. List the indications for washing your hands.

_____

_____

_____

33. List the sequence of steps used for the antiseptic handwashing procedure you will perform before patient care.

_____

_____

_____

_____

_____

34. In the CDC 2003 guidelines, Section III, an alternative hand hygiene method for hands that are not visibly soiled is given the highest category (IA) recommendation. What is the method recommended for hands that are not visibly soiled?

_____

_____

_____

35. Match each term with the correct description. Write the letter of the appropriate description in the space next to the term it refers to.

TERM	DESCRIPTION
_____ Standard mask filtration _____ Surgical soap _____ Antiseptic hand-wash _____ Handwashing _____ Wide-coverage eyewear _____ Resident bacteria _____ Transient bacteria _____ Skin integrity _____ Gloves _____ Glove integrity _____ Eyewash station	A. Relatively stable on skin; reduced by washing B. Blocks particles with greater than 95% efficiency C. Used before patient care D. Most important in preventing cross-contamination E. Never at the sink used for patient-care handwashing F. Used by both clinician and patient G. Contains antimicrobial agent H. Contaminates skin if contacted; reduced by washing I. Available in nonsterile and presterilized forms J. Affected by many things, including length of time worn K. Can be protected by covering abrasions with a liquid bandage

36. In your own words, define the following terms related to a latex allergic response.

▪ *Allergen*

_____

_____

▪ *Hypoallergenic*

_____

_____

▪ *Atopy*

_____

_____

▪ *Type I reaction*

_____

_____

▪ *Type IV hypersensitivity*

_____

_____

_____

METHOD	PREPARATION	LATHERING METHOD	SITUATION IN WHICH THE TECHNIQUE IS RECOMMENDED
Routine handwash			
Antiseptic handwash			
Surgical antisepsis			
Antiseptic hand rub			

37. List five pieces of equipment that you use when providing dental hygiene care (other than gloves) that may contain latex.

_____

_____

_____

_____

_____

COMPETENCY EXERCISES

1. Fill out the Infomap (located above) to compare the methods of handwashing. Then use the information in the Infomap to verbally describe the differences between the methods to a fellow student or a patient.

2. Use the information in Chapter 3 to develop a step-by-step checklist, in proper sequence, for getting ready to provide patient care. Consider the sequence for handwashing as well as applying all of the personal protective barriers that you use in your clinic. Pay careful attention to creating a detailed system that minimizes the possibility of cross-contamination.

   Compare your checklist with the lists that other students have created or with one provided by your instructor. Refine your list and use it as part of your own personal written exposure-control plan.

_____

_____

_____

_____

_____

_____

_____

_____

_____

_____

_____

Everyday Ethics

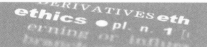

Refer to the Codes of Ethics (Appendices I, II, and III in the textbook) and Framework for Making Decisions (Table 1-2 in the textbook) as you discuss the following scenario with your classmates.

After Mr. Green's dental hygiene treatment is completed, the dentist, Dr. Root, is notified so that the final examination can be made. Dr. Root comes in shortly and sits down next to the patient. He browses through the notations made in the patient's chart and then picks up the mirror and explorer to proceed with a clinical examination. It is apparent that he has not washed his hands or donned a new pair of gloves. This situation has happened occasionally before.

Questions for Consideration
1. Mabel, the dental hygienist, notes that the dentist did not change his gloves or wash his hands. What choices of action are there to take in such a situation?
2. As the situation is analyzed, would this be considered an ethical issue or an ethical dilemma? Why?
3. How is beneficence for this patient threatened?

Factors To Teach The Patient

Mrs. Johnson is bringing her 3-year-old son, Jimmy, in for his first dental hygiene appointment. She states that he is frightened by the mask and asks you not to wear it during the appointment. She is also concerned because she has never been asked to wear glasses during previous dental hygiene appointments at another dental office. She states that Jimmy will probably protest at having to wear the child-size glasses you have ready.

Using the example conversation provided in Appendix B as a guide, write a paragraph you will use to explain to Mrs. Johnson the importance of, and the rationale for, using these barriers. Include some comments that will help explain their use to Jimmy.

This scenario is related to the following factors:

■ Necessity for use of barriers (face mask, protective eyewear, and gloves) by the clinician for the benefit of the patient
■ Importance of eye protection

3. Give examples of at least three ways you can prevent cross-contamination during handwashing before patient care in a clinic setting.

_____

_____

_____

4. Practice removing gloves using the system illustrated in Figure 3-4 in the textbook. Explain how this procedure will prevent cross-contamination.

CHAPTER 4

Infection Control: Clinical Procedures

Chapter Outline

Learning Objectives

Upon successful completion of these exercises, you will be able to:

1. Identify and define key terms and concepts related to clinical procedures for infection control.
2. Identify basic considerations, guidelines, procedures, and methods for prevention of disease transmission.
3. Describe characteristics of an optimal treatment room and instrument-processing center.
4. Select appropriate disinfection, sterilization, and storage methods for clinical instruments and materials.
5. Identify procedures for management of an exposure incident.

KNOWLEDGE EXERCISES

Be sure also to refer to Appendix IV in the textbook (CDC 2003 Guidelines for Infection Control in Dental Health-Care Settings) as you complete the following exercises.

1. Define *asepsis* in your own words.

_____

_____

_____

2. How are biofilm and bioburden similar?

_____

_____

_____

3. What does *infection control* mean?

_____

_____

_____

4. Define *nosocomial infection*. (Textbook, Box 4-1, pg 69)

_____

_____

_____

5. State the reason for maintaining proper infection-control procedures when you are providing dental hygiene care.

_____

_____

_____

6. List three infection-control components that are all necessary for preventing transmission of infection and eliminating cross-infection.

_____

_____

_____

7. In your own words, describe the processing steps you follow before you sterilize instruments used for patient care.

Step   **Description**

_____

_____

_____

_____

_____

8. The CDC guidelines recommend (section VI-A) that you use only FDA-cleared medical devices and that you follow manufacturer's instructions for sterilization. The category for this recommendation is 1B. What does a category 1B recommendation mean?

_____

_____

_____

9. Identify three approved sterilization methods and list the time requirement that ensures adequate sterilization for each method.

Sterilization method   **Time requirement**

_____

_____

_____

_____

10. Which method of sterilization processes instruments at the highest temperature?

_____

_____

_____

11. How does the method of sterilization you identified in question 10 affect or act on microorganisms?

_____

_____

_____

12. What organism is in the biologic indicator strips that are used weekly to test the efficiency of the sterilization method identified in question 10?

_____

_____

_____

13. List two disadvantages of the dry-heat method of sterilization.

_____

_____

_____

14. Chemical vapor sterilization cannot be used for materials and objects that _____; it also cannot be used for heavy, tightly wrapped packages that _____.

15. Chemical vapor sterilization systems should not be used in a small room because _____ is required for safe use.

16. A chemical vapor sterilization system is tested weekly with biologic indicator strips containing _____.

17. What is the purpose of pressure during moist heat autoclave sterilization?

_____

_____

_____

18. Moist heat sterilizes dental instruments in approximately 15 minutes. Under what conditions do you increase the sterilization time?

_____

_____

_____

19. Identify two contraindications or special considerations to think about before using steam autoclaving as a method for sterilization.

_____

_____

_____

20. Describe the action of moist heat on microorganisms.

_____

_____

_____

21. *Geobacillus stearothermophilus* in _____ or _____ or on _____ is used as a biologic indicator to test the efficiency of steam autoclave sterilizing systems.

22. When is spore testing done?

_____

_____

_____

23. Briefly describe a system for remembering to regularly monitor sterilization effectiveness.

_____

_____

_____

24. List three factors that could result in a failed monitoring test during sterilization of instruments.

_____

_____

_____

25. To keep your instruments contamination free, you should store them in the _____.

26. Describe a type of chemical indicator that is used each time on packaging to identify instruments that have been processed.

_____

_____

_____

27. What is a disinfectant?

_____

_____

_____

28. List three uses for chemical disinfectants.

_____

_____

_____

29. Describe the three levels of chemical disinfectants.

_____

_____

_____

30. List the factors you will consider when selecting a chemical disinfectant for use in your dental hygiene treatment room.

_____

_____

_____

31. What information on a product label tells you about the effectiveness of the chemical agent you use for disinfection?

_____

_____

_____

32. What is a sporicide?

_____

_____

_____

33. List the product label items to look for when you prepare and use a chemical disinfectant.

_____

_____

_____

34. Identify the way in which each of the four main types of chemical disinfectants destroys microorganisms.

Type of disinfectant   **Method of action**

_____

_____

_____

_____

35. Care is required when you are using chemical disinfectants. Which of the main types of disinfectants have potentially harmful or damaging effects?

Type   **Potential effects**

_____

_____

_____

_____

36. Identify two reasons why it is difficult to maintain asepsis of instruments that have been processed by immersion in a chemical disinfectant.

_____

_____

_____

37. When you are cleaning your dental hygiene treatment room after a dental hygiene visit, infectious waste, such as contaminated disposable gowns, masks, gloves, and soiled gauze, are placed in a trash can inside of a _____. Some other types of waste products are disposed of in a more rigorous manner.

38. Define each of the following types of waste.

   ■ *Infectious waste*

   _____

   _____

   _____

■ *Contaminated waste*

_____

_____

■ *Hazardous waste*

_____

_____

■ *Toxic waste*

_____

_____

■ *Regulated waste*

_____

_____

_____

39. Items such as needles are disposed of in a _____.

40. The CDC 2003 guidelines recommend use of _____-level chemical disinfectants on clinical surfaces that are visibly contaminated with blood.

41. When you are disinfecting surfaces such as the dental chair and countertops, you will spray the surface with the appropriate chemical agent, wipe or scrub the entire surface, and then _____ to leave the surface wet.

42. Water lines are flushed for _____ at the beginning of the day and, according to the CDC 2003 guidelines, for _____ between patients to reduce microbial counts.

43. Identify two oral procedures that can reduce microbial counts before dental hygiene treatment.

_____

_____

_____

44. What three components regarding infection control are included in an office policy manual?

_____

_____

Everyday Ethics

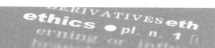

Refer to the Codes of Ethics (Appendices I, II, and III in the textbook) and Framework for Making Decisions (Table 1-2 in the textbook) as you discuss the following scenario with your classmates.

Kimberly, the dental hygienist, begins to scale and then notices that the indicator tape on the sterilizing package had not changed color. She excuses herself and finds out from the receptionist that a call to the repair service has been made because the autoclave has been shutting down before completion of the cycle. It is after 1:00 PM and patients are scheduled all afternoon.

Questions for Consideration

1. When proper sterile technique is not followed, what ethical principles and core values are involved? Explain Kimberly's duty to her patients.
2. Offer possible solutions for this situation. Describe how it could be defended to the patient, the dentist, and other dental team members.
3. What roles can the dental hygienist play to ensure that it does not happen again?

45. Identify two situations that would cause you to initiate the exposure management process.

_____

_____

_____

COMPETENCY EXERCISES

1. **Putting it all together:** Write brief statements or lists to summarize all of the procedures you can follow every day to maintain the chain of asepsis and prevent disease transmission in each of the following categories.

   ▨ *You and your colleagues*

   _____

   _____

   _____

   ▨ *Your patient*

   _____

   _____

   _____

   ▨ *The clinic*

   _____

   _____

   _____

   ▨ *During treatment*

   _____

   _____

   _____

▨ *Posttreatment*

_____

_____

_____

2. Explain the difference between decontamination, disinfection, and sterilization.

_____

_____

_____

Factors To Teach The Patient

Mrs. Norton is on the telephone again. She has just made a first dental appointment for Daniella, her 3-year-old daughter, and she is clearly nervous about it. This is the second time she has called in with questions. This time, she wants to be assured that her daughter will not be exposed to any infectious diseases during dental hygiene treatment.

Using the information you learned in Chapters 3 and 4 of the textbook and the example of a patient conversation in Appendix B as a guide, write a statement explaining standard precautions to Mrs. Norton.

This scenario is related to the following factors:

■ The meaning of *standard precautions* and what is included under the term; how these precautions protect the patient and the dental team members
■ Methods for sterilization of instruments, including handpieces, and how the autoclave or other sterilizer is tested daily or weekly

3. Identify specific ways that planning ahead can ensure that you will maintain asepsis and eliminate cross-contamination during patient treatment in your school clinic.

_____

_____

_____

4. The textbook describes features of dental treatment room equipment that facilitate optimum infection control. Describe the features in your school clinic that meet these criteria.

_____

_____

_____

5. Describe the procedure you will follow immediately if you experience a puncture wound exposure in the clinic at your school.

_____

_____

_____

Patient Reception and Ergonomic Practice

Learning Objectives

Upon successful completion of these exercises, you will be able to:

1. Identify and define key terms and concepts related to patient reception and ergonomic practice.

2. Prepare the treatment room for patient reception.
3. Identify and discuss components of safe and efficient patient positioning.
4. Identify and practice factors that contribute to ergonomic dental hygiene practice.

KNOWLEDGE EXERCISES

1. Identify three treatment room factors that you will prepare before your patient arrives for the dental hygiene appointment.

   _____

   _____

   _____

2. List two factors you will include when you are welcoming your patient to the dental hygiene treatment room.

   _____

   _____

3. The more attention you pay to ergonomics and good body mechanics, the more likely you are to avoid cumulative trauma injuries during your dental hygiene career. In your own words, define the following terms.

   ■ *Ergonomics*

   _____

   _____

   _____

   ■ *Body mechanics*

   _____

   _____

   _____

■ *Cumulative trauma*

_____

_____

_____

4. The main objectives in the preferred patient positioning discussed in this chapter are that both you and your patient are as _____ as possible during dental hygiene treatment and that visibility and access during care are enhanced.

5. In your own words, describe the characteristics of an ideal dental chair.

_____

_____

_____

_____

_____

6. Explain how the dental chair is arranged before each patient is seated when he or she arrives for treatment.

_____

_____

_____

7. List the proper sequence of steps that you would use to adjust the dental chair and patient to the final working position after the patient is seated.

_____

_____

_____

_____

_____

_____

8. Describe the supine position.

_____

_____

_____

9. Your patient is positioned in the dental chair with her brain 40° lower than her heart, and her legs and feet are raised. What is this position called?

_____

_____

10. List three reasons for placing your patient in a semi-upright position (contraindications for the supine position).

_____

_____

_____

11. After completing dental hygiene treatment and raising the dental chair to an upright position, what important step should you include to ensure patient safety?

_____

_____

_____

12. What is postural hypotension?

_____

_____

_____

13. Identify the characteristics of an acceptable clinician's stool.

_____

_____

14. Identify the components of neutral seated posture for the dental hygiene clinician.

_____

_____

_____

_____

_____

_____

15. When both you and your patient are in the correct position during dental hygiene treatment, your relaxed elbows are at the same level as _____ and the distance between your eyes and your patient's mouth is about _____.

16. Clock-hour positioning for the dental hygiene clinician is associated with enhanced access to:

_____

_____

17. Flexibility of both the clinician's and patient's positioning during dental hygiene care can increase both _____ and _____ to oral structures for the dental hygienist.

18. Identify two ways to enhance the clinician's visual access to the oral cavity while providing dental hygiene care.

     _____

     _____

     _____

19. List the characteristics of a good dental light.

     _____

     _____

     _____

20. Identify the major components of ergonomic dental hygiene practice and self-care principles for health and well-being.

     _____

     _____

     _____

21. Identify the three components of the triad of musculoskeletal health.

     _____

     _____

     _____

COMPETENCY EXERCISES

1. Practice each of the functional movement exercises shown in Figure 5-7 in the textbook. (Doesn't that feel good? Let's do it again!)

2. Explain how ergonomically designed power-driven equipment can help prevent physical occupational disorders.

3. Describe ways in which the layout of your personal clinical work area can contribute to negative health outcomes for you.

4. A treatment room that is completely prepared when each patient arrives demonstrates professionalism and inspires patient confidence. The dental hygiene instruments are arranged for each patient with the sterile packaging sealed until the patient is seated and the appointment has started. Explain how your body language and the way the treatment room is arranged can affect a patient's impression of your professionalism as you welcome him or her to your clinic.

     _____

     _____

     _____

     _____

     _____

     _____

5. Mrs. Virginia Weatherbee, a 50-year-old with a charming smile, is a new patient in your clinic. Write a statement in which you properly introduce yourself to her as you greet her in the reception room for the first time.

     _____

     _____

     _____

     _____

     _____

     _____

Everyday Ethics

Refer to the Codes of Ethics (Appendices I, II, and III in the textbook) and Framework for Making Decisions (Table 1-2 in the textbook) as you discuss the following scenario with your classmates.

Hygienist Celia has developed chronic pain in her neck, back, and hands. As a result, she knows that her instrumentation is affected and patients are not receiving definitive scaling at their appointments.

Questions for Consideration

1. How does this health hazard affect the clinician; the patient?
2. Why is this an ethical situation?
3. What are the ergonomic risk factors that may have been the primary contributors to Celia's condition?
4. What safe work practices should she have practiced to avoid the problems she is having?
5. What preventive strategies can she integrate into her practice to improve her condition?

6. Mrs. Weatherbee grins and asks you to please call her Ginny. Right after you get your patient settled in the dental chair, Dr. Grey's 19-year-old daughter, Gina, who is home from college for the summer working in the clinic as the dental hygiene assistant, peeks in to ask you a question. Introduce Gina to your patient.

_____

_____

_____

_____

_____

_____

7. Just after you finish going over the health history with your patient, Dr. Grey, who happens to be in his 70s, walks into your treatment room to meet the new patient. Introduce your patient to the dentist.

_____

_____

_____

_____

_____

_____

Factors To Teach The Patient

The patient in your chair today is a curious and very fidgety 10-year-old boy named Nathan. Even before you get him seated in the dental chair, he starts asking you questions about how things work and the function of each button and switch. He just can't seem to sit still.

Using the example of a patient conversation in Appendix B as a guide, write a statement explaining the dental chair and how it helps keep both Nathan and you safe and comfortable. Use the conversation you create to role play this situation with a fellow student. If you are the patient in the role play, be sure to ask questions. If you are the dental hygienist in the role play, try to anticipate questions and answer them in your explanation—and remember as you talk that Nathan is only 10 years old.
This scenario is related to the following factors:

■ How patient cooperation makes it possible for the dental hygienist to practice with less stress and strain to prevent musculoskeletal discomfort and pain, and deliver better patient care

DISCOVERY EXERCISES

1. Ask a student colleague to observe you periodically as you provide care to a patient or practice instrumentation in your preclinic labs. What risk factors for physical occupational disorders does your colleague identify in the way you are practicing? What steps will you need to take to help maintain personal wellness throughout your career?

Preparation for Dental Hygiene Appointments

▉ Chapters 2–5

COMPETENCY EXERCISES

1. Compile a personal immunization log. Identify any missing immunizations and make arrangements to receive them.

2. Examine the personal protective barrier equipment (protective eyewear, masks, gloves, etc.) that you have selected for your own use in clinic and describe how they meet the characteristics of acceptable exposure-control barriers.

3. Locate the eyewash station in your clinic that is nearest to your treatment area. Practice using it.

4. This is a first-ever dental appointment for Jean Luc Aristide, age 11, who has emigrated recently from Haiti. He speaks very little English, but his bright smile and curious gaze capture your attention and make you smile back at him. He is accompanied to his dental appointment by Marge Black, a social worker who speaks English and has been helping the family receive health care for Jean Luc at a nearby teaching hospital. Jean Luc is HIV positive. What questions will you ask to determine Jean Luc's health status before planning dental hygiene care?

5. What steps will you take to protect both Jean Luc and yourself while you are providing dental hygiene care and oral health instructions?

DISCOVERY EXERCISES

1. Search online or in the library to discover the purpose and function of each of the following federal, state, and local government organizations and discuss how they relate to the practice of dental hygiene.
   - ▉ CDC
   - ▉ EPA
   - ▉ FDA
   - ▉ OSAP
   - ▉ OSHA
   - ▉ *Department of Community Health*

2. The CDC 2003 Guidelines for Infection Control in Dental Health-Care Settings in Appendix IV in the textbook contains only the outlined recommendations, not the full text of the report. You can access the complete report in your library by looking for the Centers for Disease Control and Prevention's *Guidelines for Infection Control in Dental Health Settings—2003* (MMWR 2003;52, no. RR-17) or online at www.cdc.gov/mmwr/indrr_2003.html. Explore the full report to find and read the section titled "Contact Dermatitis and Latex Hypersensitivity." Write a brief summary of what you learned. When you have time, explore the information in other sections of the report.

3. Investigate the sterilization methods and procedures that are used at your school clinic.

4. Imagine that you have been asked to select a new handwashing soap that will be used in your clinic. Search for scientific evidence of effectiveness of antibacterial agents commonly used in handwashing soaps that are available for use by dental hygienists. Select the best alternative, and explain why you made your selection. (*Hint:* Check the soap that is currently in use in your clinic as well as some dental supplier catalogs to find the most commonly used antibacterial agents, and then develop a PICO question that will help you review the scientific literature for research evidence of effectiveness.)

5. Investigate dental supply catalogs to determine the types of gloves available for use in dental clinics and the cost of each type. What scientific evidence is available to help you determine which type of glove provides the most effective barrier to microorganisms you are likely to encounter during patient care?

FOR YOUR PORTFOLIO

1. Develop a personal, written exposure-control plan. Don't forget to include an appropriate reference list to indicate that you have based your personal plan on scientific evidence. Consider making the plan in a format that could be easily updated and adapted to any setting later on when you are a practicing dental hygienist.

2. List your personal selections/recommendations for handwashing soap, gloves, and any other infection-control supplies used in dental hygiene care. Support each recommendation with a brief written summary of product characteristics and how the product meets criteria for acceptability.

3. Develop a personal, written long-term plan to avoid cumulative trauma injuries related to dental hygiene practice. Update this plan yearly as you learn more about working conditions that compromise your comfort and effectiveness when you are providing dental hygiene care.

Assessment

■ SECTION III LEARNING OBJECTIVES

Completing the exercises in this section of the workbook will prepare you to:

1. Identify components of a complete patient assessment.
2. Apply a variety of assessment methods to gather data and document the patient's health status.
3. Determine community oral health status using a variety of dental indices.

■ COMPETENCIES FOR THE DENTAL HYGIENIST (APPENDIX A)

The following ADEA competencies are supported by the learning in Section III.

Core Competencies: C5, C8, C9, C10

Health Promotion and Disease Prevention Competencies: HP3, HP4, HP5, HP6

Community Involvement Competencies: CM1, CM2, CM6

Patient/Client Care Competencies: PC1, PC5

Documentation

Learning Objectives

Upon successful completion of these exercises, you will be able to:

1. Identify and define key terms and concepts that relate to written and computerized dental records and charting.
2. Describe concepts related to ensuring maintenance of confidentiality and privacy of patient information.
3. Discuss the various uses of the patient health record.
4. Discuss multiple patient examination methods.
5. Compare three tooth numbering systems.
6. Explain multiple strategies for record documentation and data collection.

KNOWLEDGE EXERCISES

1. Identify the important components of the patient record.

   _____

   _____

   _____

2. List the uses of the patient record.

   _____

   _____

   _____

3. What actions regarding a patient record are essential to ensure accurate documentation of patient care in case the record is needed during a legal action?

   _____

   _____

   _____

4. Define the term *sign*. Is a sign an objective or a subjective symptom?

   _____

   _____

   _____

5. Give one example of a subjective symptom.

   _____

6. A sign or symptom that is unique to a particular disease is a _____ sign or symptom.

7. *Match the following types and methods of examination with the correct definition or description.*

TYPES AND METHODS OF EXAMINATION	DEFINITION/ DESCRIPTION
_____ Complete _____ Screening _____ Limited _____ Follow-up _____ Maintenance _____ Visual _____ Palpation _____ Instrumentation _____ Percussion _____ Electrical test _____ Auscultation	A. Tapping with fingers or an instrument B. A complete reassessment after completion of treatment C. Limited examination to observe the effects of treatment D. Detects the presence or absence of vital pulp tissue E. Uses observation, radiographs, and light F. A thorough, comprehensive study G. Uses the sense of touch through tissue manipulation or pressure H. An examination usually made for an emergency I. An explorer and probe are used for specific examination of the teeth and periodontal tissues J. Uses sound K. A brief examination used for initial assessment and classification

8. In your own words, define the following types of visual observation:

   ■ *Direct observation*

   _____

   _____

   _____

   ■ *Radiographic examination*

   _____

   _____

   _____

   ■ *Transillumination*

   _____

   _____

   _____

9. Identify the purposes for complete and accurate charting in patient records.

   _____

   _____

   _____

10. What materials and instruments will you use when you are charting your patient's dentition?

    _____

    _____

    _____

11. Identify the types of chart forms that can be used to record your patient's dental charting.

    _____

    _____

    _____

12. When you record your patient's dental chart, you first enter basic information (name, birthdate, today's date), and then you use a systematic procedure to accomplish an accurate charting.

    ■ *Define* systematic procedure.

    _____

    _____

    _____

    ■ *List* the sequence of recommended items to be noted during a charting appointment.

    _____

    _____

    _____

    _____

    _____

    _____

13. In your own words, briefly describe the clinical observations that are included in your patient's periodontal charting.

    ■ *Gingival changes*

    _____

    _____

    _____

    ■ *Items charted*

    _____

    _____

    _____

INFOMAP 6-1

TOOTH NUMBERING SYSTEM	ORGANIZATION (ARCHES OR QUADRANTS)	PERMANENT DENTITION	PRIMARY DENTITION	ADDITIONAL FEATURES	EXAMPLE: PERMANENT MAXILLARY RIGHT CENTRAL INCISOR
Palmer System Tooth Numbering					
International Tooth Numbering (Fédération Dentaire Internationale)					
Universal Tooth Numbering (American Dental Association)					

▓ *Deposits*

_____

_____

_____

▓ *Occlusal factors*

_____

_____

_____

▓ *Radiographic findings*

_____

_____

_____

14. Because different tooth numbering systems are used in dental offices and clinics, it is necessary for you to be familiar with all of them. Refer to Figures 6-1, 6-2, and 6-3 in the textbook to complete Infomap 6-1 on the next page of this workbook. Completing this infomap will help you compare the three types of tooth numbering systems.

Everyday Ethics

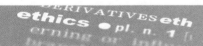

Refer to the Codes of Ethics (Appendices I, II, and III in the textbook) and Framework for Making Decisions (Table 1-2 in the textbook) as you discuss the following scenario with your classmates.

Mrs. Belvedere, the office manager in Dr. Grain's office, has online access to all electronic patient records from her computer at home. With Dr. Grain's permission, she often uses her home e-mail to contact patients and insurance companies regarding treatment plans, insurance coverage, or financial records. Patients receive HIPAA information about confidentiality and security of their information, but are not told that Mrs. Belvedere has access to their records at her home. Hanna, who is a new dental hygienist in the office, inadvertently finds out that sensitive patient information is being sent out from the same home e-mail account that is used by both Mrs. Belvedere's husband and her adult son. When Hanna approaches Dr. Grain about the potential breach in security of patient information, he seems unconcerned.

Questions for Consideration
1. What dental hygiene core values are being compromised if Hanna decides not follow through to try to change the situation?
2. What standards of professional responsibility, identified in the ADHA code of ethics, apply in this situation?
3. Describe how ethical theory (Table III-1, page 100) can support Hanna as she decides how to approach Mrs. Belvedere and Dr. Grain to make changes in the way patient records and information are handled.
4. Role play ways that Hanna can approach Dr. Grain to resolve the issues related to security of patient information.

COMPETENCY EXERCISES

1. You are volunteering at a collegewide wellness expo. You are working with your student colleagues and a dentist faculty member to provide oral cancer examinations and tobacco cessation information. Explain to the patient who is sitting in your chair the type of examination you will be conducting and what he or she should expect.

   _____

   _____

   _____

   _____

   _____

2. Mrs. Alverez has just called the dental clinic you are practicing in to say that she has a severe toothache. You have an opening in your schedule and are asked to examine her and to report your findings to Dr. Greenwood. What type of examination will you conduct, and what examination methods will you use to collect the necessary information?

   _____

   _____

   _____

   _____

   _____

3. Caroline Lacy is your patient at 10 o'clock. She is 3 years old and has never had her teeth charted. Just for practice, identify the correct tooth number for the two teeth listed below using each of the tooth numbering systems.

	MANDIBULAR LEFT PRIMARY FIRST MOLAR	MAXILLARY LEFT PRIMARY FIRST MOLAR
Palmer		
FDI	_____	_____
Universal	_____	_____

Factors To Teach The Patient

Review the individualized care plan for Mrs. Lorna Patel in Appendix D. You have just seated Mrs. Patel, who is new to the practice and is very surprised that you collected so much information. She wants to know why you needed so many details about her medical history and what those numbers mean on her periodontal charting.

Use the example of a patient conversation in Appendix B of this workbook as a guide to create a conversation to explain to Mrs. Patel the implications of the data collected on her medical history as well as on the periodontal findings. Compare your conversation with a student colleague to identify any missing information

This scenario is related to the following factors:

- Interpretation of all recordings; meaning of all numbers used, such as for probing depths
- The importance of making a complete study of the patient's oral problems before beginning treatment
- Advantages of cooperation and patience in furnishing information that will help dental personnel to interpret observations accurately so that the correct diagnosis and appropriate treatment plan can be made

4. The dentist you practice with has decided to change from a chart that uses anatomic drawings of the complete teeth to a chart that contains only geometric diagrams. The plan is to record both restorative and periodontal findings on the new form. You are asked for your opinion at the staff meeting. What will you say?

   _____

   _____

   _____

Personal, Dental, and Medical Histories

Learning Objectives

Upon successful completion of these exercises, you will be able to:

1. Identify and define key terms and concepts related to preparing patient histories.
2. Discuss the purposes of the personal, medical, and dental histories.
3. List and discuss the types, systems, forms used, question types, and styles used to collect patient history data.
4. Recognize considerations for patient care that are identified by various items recorded on the patient history.

KNOWLEDGE EXERCISES

1. List the purposes of the personal, medical, and dental histories.

   _____

   _____

   _____

2. In your own words, describe the systems for obtaining the patient's history.

■ *Preappointment information*

   _____

   _____

   _____

■ *Brief history*

   _____

   _____

   _____

■ *Self-history*

_____

_____

■ *Complete history*

_____

_____

_____

3. List the characteristics of an adequate patient history form.

_____

_____

_____

4. Why is it important to record contact information for the patient's physician in the personal history?

_____

_____

_____

5. Why is it important to record a patient's family dental history or culturally related health practices in the dental history?

_____

_____

_____

6. What limitations may affect the accuracy of a patient history?

_____

_____

_____

7. Describe each type of patient-history questionnaires in your own words.

■ *System oriented*

_____

_____

_____

■ *Disease oriented*

_____

_____

_____

■ *Symptom oriented*

_____

_____

_____

■ *Culture oriented*

_____

_____

_____

8. Identify the advantages or disadvantages associated with each method of collecting patient data.

METHODS OF DATA COLLECTION	ADVANTAGE OR DISADVANTAGE
Each answer may be used more than one time. A. Questionnaire B. Interview	_____ Patient may be embarrassed to talk about personal conditions and may hold back significant information _____ Legal aspect of a written record with patient's signature _____ Consistent _____ Personal contact contributes to development of rapport for future appointments _____ Time-saving _____ Flexibility for individual needs; details obtained can be adapted for supplementary questioning

COMPETENCY EXERCISES

1. You have just seated your patient, Mrs. Lorna Patel. Refer to Appendix D to review her care plan. Take some time to review the significant findings listed in the medical and dental history sections. Link each item in the significant findings column of her care plan to a specific patient history item recorded in her medical or dental history. Refer to Tables 7-2 and 7-3 in the textbook when answering this question.

_____

_____

_____

_____

_____

_____

2. Would you request a medical consultation for Mrs. Patel? Explain why or why not.

_____

_____

_____

_____

_____

_____

3. You review Mrs. Patel's dental history with her. Suggest one follow-up question for each answer she has given.

   ▣ *1.5 years since last recall*

   _____

   _____

   _____

   ▣ *Flosses daily*

   _____

   _____

   _____

   ▣ *Rinses with alcohol-based mouthrinse*

   _____

   _____

   _____

▣ *Uses mints and candy for dry mouth*

_____

_____

_____

▣ *Uses bottled water with no fluoride content*

_____

_____

_____

▣ *Mouth is dry all the time*

_____

_____

_____

4. Mrs. Patel presents with a history of previous infective endocarditis. You are scheduled to take impressions and radiographs today. Mrs. Patel is not premedicated. Should you continue to treat her? Why or why not?

_____

_____

_____

_____

_____

Everyday Ethics

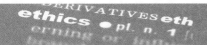

Refer to the Codes of Ethics (Appendices I, II, and III in the textbook) and Framework for Making Decisions (Table 1-2 in the textbook) as you discuss the following scenario with your classmates.

Chris, the dental hygienist, was waiting for her new patient at 1:00. All she knew was that Irina was 70 years old, from Russia, and could speak and understand English fairly well. Chris heard the front door to the office open and went out to greet her patient. The little lady was on the arm of a teenage boy who quickly helped Irina to a chair and turned to leave after saying to Chris (pointing to the patient) "Just back from hospital. Car not parked." Then to his grandmother "Back in an hour," before he rushed out.

   Chris ushered her into the treatment room and helped her into the chair, then started the history questions with "What were you in the hospital for?" Irina grabs Chris's arm and firmly requests, "Want teeth cleaned." Chris attempts to explain why she is asking the questions about her health.

Then she asks for her physician's name and permission to call the physician to obtain the information. Irina points to her heart, but just becomes more agitated and keeps repeating "Want teeth cleaned" and refuses to give approval to call her doctor. Chris is alarmed at the possibility that she may have had a type of heart surgery that needs premedication.

Questions for Consideration

1. Professionally and ethically, what are a dental hygienist's responsibilities to ensure that a patient understands the seriousness of an illness?
2. In the light of the possible language barrier between Chris and Irina, what actions can Chris take to find out the necessary information and prepare this patient for the dental hygiene appointment? Are there procedures that do not require premedication that could be accomplished?
3. Which of the dental hygiene core values apply to Chris's actions for the patient's benefit?

_____

_____

_____

5. Review the patient history questionnaire form used in your practice setting (your dental hygiene program or the dental practice where you receive care). Identify the type of patient-history questionnaire that is used, and critique the effectiveness of this method of data collection.

_____

_____

_____

_____

_____

DISCOVERY EXERCISES

1. Search on line to find patient health history questionnaires in languages other than English.

2. Explore the American Dental Association Web site (_http://www.ada.org_) to find their version of the most current guidelines for antibiotic premedication of dental patients.

Factors To Teach The Patient

You are just starting to treat Jon Wojeckick, who is 37 years old. You begin to ask questions about his medical history. You notice he has stopped making eye contact and is hesitating over some of the answers. You have a feeling that he is not giving you accurate information, and you want to be sure you are obtaining all the data you need to provide optimum safe care. You know from studying Tables 7-1, 7-2, and 7-3 in the textbook that items from the patient history have a connection to how you provide dental hygiene care for your patient.

Use the example of a patient conversation in Appendix B of this workbook as a guide to write a statement explaining the relationship between oral health and physical health and the need for accurate information to facilitate treatment planning. Include at least three examples of appointment considerations that are linked to items in the patient history. Be sure to assure Mr. Wojeckick that recorded histories are kept in strict professional confidence.

This scenario is related to the following factors:

■ The need for obtaining the personal, medical, and dental history before performing dental and dental hygiene procedures and the need for keeping the histories up to date

■ The assurance that recorded histories are kept in strict professional confidence

■ The relationship between oral health and general physical health

■ The interrelationship of medical and dental care

Vital Signs

Chapter Outline

Learning Objectives

Upon successful completion of these exercises, you will be able to:

1. Identify and define key terms and concepts related to recording vital signs.
2. Identify four vital signs and describe the range of expected values.
3. Describe procedures for determining and recording a patient's temperature, pulse, respiration, and blood pressure.
4. Discuss the importance of regular determination of vital signs for a patient receiving dental hygiene care.

KNOWLEDGE EXERCISES

Signs of Life Word Search Puzzle

To solve the puzzle, first use the clues to determine the words; then find the words in the grid. Words in the grid can run across, down, or diagonally and can start at the right or left, or top or bottom.

```
N N F B L P M D K K K K B C M X M S B J T V M
P J N H T Q Y T V D B H W M B R T C C W J V M
C C C B L G G L L T T K N R P E I L H U T L Y
M T V I T A L S I G N S N X T L L Y B B F N C
K B Y Y B H T B Q X Y V L H O K P B F P N F G
M Z K M M T N H R J R C O T P O L F M E R C F
E T R C P G N Z X A Y S S Z T R O L L A Q X X
R C R N M A F B K J C A R H R K N O D R H R J
C V T H L M N R A O I H E H T R T I N C Y R M
U D B Y L J C I P D A R I O R S A P G Q P F R
R B R X F O X E C N M U R A A L D J E F E X P
Y Z A Q R O H Q P I H O S I L I X L G L R G Y
L N D E N K C N A U K Y D C T T O N G R T T R
D C Y A V H W J F B L D P O U T G X K S H T E
Y Y C L K F M J N L H S R E S L Q D Y C E R X
Y R A L N D P Y F R Q A E Y R M T S Q T R H I
B D R M W V N F C J C W S R X T T A L Q M Y A
U T D N O R M O T E N S I V E O E B T K I T F
L Y I L X R B D C G R M J L L L N N N I A H R
B N A V H D I U R N A L X I Y Z K M S C O M T
N V M K D J J L N T Z R C Q C M N N N I M N L
B T A C H Y C A R D I A P N E A R H L X O L J
L Q S P H Y G M O M A N O M E T E R P P P N G
```

Word Search Clues

Identify each term described below.
- All four; body temperature, pulse, respiratory rate, and blood pressure.
- Artery in the neck that is the site for taking a pulse during cardiopulmonary resuscitation.
- Blood pressure machine consisting of inflatable cuff, two tubes, a bulb, and a pressure gauge.
- A contraction of the heart ventricles during which blood is forced into the aorta and the pulmonary artery.
- A count of heartbeats; can also refer to the pressure that is the difference between systolic and diastolic blood pressure (40 mmHg).
- Element used in a device that records body temperature and also in a device that records blood pressure.
- Fever; temperature values greater than 37.5°C or 99.5°F.
- Heartbeat at a rate greater than 100 beats per minute.
- Higher-than-normal body temperature; values greater than 41.0°C.
- Inflatable component of a sphygmomanometer that wraps around the patient's arm during recording of a blood pressure.
- Listening for sounds produced within the body.
- The lower number in a recorded blood pressure fraction; marks the pressure at the last distinct tap heard on the sphygmomanometer.
- Lower-than-normal body temperature; values below 96.0°F.
- Normal tension or tone; pertaining to having normal blood pressure.
- Noted along with irregularities of strength and quality when counting the pulse rate.
- Oxygen deficiency, potentially leading to increased pulse rate and impairment of coordination.
- The peak or highest pressure recorded when determining a blood pressure.
- Pertaining to or occurring during the daytime or period of light.
- The phase of the cardiac cycle in which the heart relaxes between contractions and the two ventricles are dilated by the blood flowing into them.
- The pressure hand control component of the sphygmomanometer.
- Pulse taken using fingertips placed at the wrist.
- The relatively constant temperature of deep tissues of the body.
- The site used to find the pulse for an infant.
- Sounds originating within the blood passing through the vessel or produced by vibratory motion of the arterial wall.
- A systolic blood pressure of 140 mmHg or greater and diastolic blood pressure of 90 mmHg or greater.
- Temporary cessation of spontaneous respirations.
- A type of thermometer that is gently inserted into the ear canal.
- Unusually slow heartbeat and pulse; below 50 beats per minute.
- Used to carry the sound when recording blood pressure.

Procedures and Techniques

1. The vital signs patient record stamp that is illustrated in Figure 8-1 in the textbook suggests recording a fifth vital sign. What is it?

   _____

   _____

   _____

2. Describe how you will position your patient to explain and record vital signs.

   _____

   _____

   _____

3. If your patient's vital signs are not within normal range, what should you do?

   _____

   _____

   _____

4. What are the normal adult ranges for all vital signs?

   _____

   _____

   _____

5. What factors should you consider when you are deciding whether to take your patient's temperature?

   _____

   _____

   _____

6. Normal average temperature varies among individuals, but in general, the average temperature of an adult older than 70 years is slightly _____ than the adult average, and the temperature of a child younger than 5 years may be slightly _____.

7. List three factors that can increase body temperature.

   _____

   _____

   _____

8. The most common location for taking a temperature is the mouth. What contraindications would lead you to select another method?

   _____

   _____

   _____

9. What emergency situations may cause your patient to exhibit an increased pulse rate? (*Hint:* See Tables 66-4 and 66-5 in the textbook.)

   _____

   _____

   _____

   _____

   _____

   _____

10. In your own words, describe how to obtain and record your patient's pulse.

    _____

    _____

    _____

11. Define a respiration.

    _____

    _____

    _____

12. Describe five factors to observe while you are counting your patient's respiration rate.

    _____

    _____

    _____

13. Describe the procedure for counting respirations.

    _____

    _____

    _____

14. What emergency situations can cause a change in your patient's respiration?

    _____

    _____

    _____

15. Blood pressure depends on what factors?

    _____

    _____

    _____

16. Emergencies such as fainting, blood loss, and shock will cause blood pressure to _____.

17. The blood pressure cuff comes in four sizes. You should select a cuff width that is _____ than the diameter of your patient's arm. If the cuff you select does not cover at least two thirds of your patient's upper arm, the blood pressure reading will be too _____.

18. Why is it a good idea to present a very brief introduction to the procedure before recording a patient's blood pressure?

    _____

    _____

    _____

19. When taking a patient's blood pressure, position either the right or left arm, slightly flexed, with the whole lower arm supported at the level of the patient's heart (the arm of the dental chair works great for this). How do you determine where to place the lower edge of the cuff?

    _____

    _____

    _____

20. How do you determine where to place the stethoscope end piece?

    _____

    _____

    _____

21. Before you position the stethoscope end piece, you will close the needle valve attached to the hand-control bulb and inflate the cuff. Where is the maximum inflation level (MIL)?

    _____

    _____

    _____

22. In your own words, describe what happens after you position the stethoscope end piece on the patient's arm.

    _____

    _____

    _____

23. The mercury _____ is the gauge on which the blood pressure interval is read.

24. What information is recorded in the patient's record about the results of the blood pressure reading?

    _____

    _____

    _____

25. What action should you take if your patient's blood pressure is at a prehypertension level or above?

    _____

    _____

    _____

26. How frequently should your patient's blood pressure be taken and recorded during dental hygiene treatment?

    _____

    _____

    _____

COMPETENCY EXERCISES

1. You have just seated Maura Kennedy in the dental chair for her dental hygiene maintenance appointment. You read in her patient record that she is 33 years old, has no remarkable health problems, and is taking no medications. She reports that the only change in her health history today is that she has had a sinus infection for the last 2 weeks. She reports that she started taking antibiotics the day before yesterday and is feeling a bit better, but her nasal passages are still all stuffed up. Write a brief statement that you will use to inform Maura that

Everyday Ethics

Refer to the Codes of Ethics (Appendices I, II, and III in the textbook) and Framework for Making Decisions (Table 1-2 in the textbook) as you discuss the following scenario with your classmates.

Gracie was having a very busy day and at 10:15 was already late for the 10:00 patient, Mr. McElroy, who had arrived early and was waiting in the reception area. While completing his history, to save time, she copied over the blood pressure recording from his previous appointment just 2 weeks ago. It had been 130/83, only slightly into the prehypertension level.

The appointment was planned for the maxillary left quadrant with anesthesia. After the scaling was complete and Mr. McElroy was climbing out of the dental chair, looking a bit unsteady as he stood up, he casually remarked: "I just remembered while you were working that

my Doc gave me a new prescription—I suppose I should have told you before. But it is only one pill a day—for keeping the blood pressure down. I don't have any trouble anyway, he just wanted to be sure."

Questions for Consideration

1. Explain how the principles of beneficence and maleficence apply to Gracie's actions with Mr. McElroy's examination and charting procedures.
2. Has Gracie placed the office at risk for a possible medical emergency given Mr. McElroy's physical status? Answer by describing the rights and duties of both the hygienist and the patient.
3. Who is responsible for ensuring that accurate documentation has been completed on all patients from an ethical and a quality assurance perspective?

you are going to determine and record her vital signs.

_____

_____

_____

_____

_____

_____

2. When you take Maura's temperature, you find that it is normal. Her pulse rate is 70 bpm; while you still have your fingers on her wrist, you count her respirations. Her respiration is slightly fast, 25 per minute, and you note that she takes several shallow breaths followed by one or two gulps of air and that she wheezes a bit when she exhales. However, you note that her color is good, so she must not be having any real problem with air exchange, and her breathing problems may just be the result of her stuffy nose. You wrap the blood pressure cuff around her right arm, pump it up, and place the stethoscope. You hear the sounds begin at the 122 mark on the manometer and the last sound you hear is at 83.

Factors To Teach The Patient

Mr. Borman Gorbachov, the CEO of a large manufacturing firm, is always in a hurry. He simply can't seem to sit still for his whole appointment and is always chiding you that you should work faster so that he can be done and get back to work. Today he sighs heavily and then protests loudly when you tell him that you are going to take and record his vital signs. He states that he just had his blood pressure taken a month or so ago at his doctor's office and there is nothing wrong with him. You look in his patient record to discover that the previous blood pressure, taken almost 2 years ago, was normal.

Use the example of a patient conversation in Appendix B as a guide to prepare a conversation you can use to educate Mr. Gorbachov about the reasons you determine a patient's vital signs at each appointment. Use the conversation you create to educate a patient or friend, and then modify it based on what you learned from the interaction.

This scenario is related to the following factors:

■ How vital signs can influence dental and dental hygiene appointments
■ The importance of having a blood pressure determination at regular intervals

After a discussion with Maura and with Dr. Ichero, you all decide to reschedule Maura for her maintenance visit in a couple of weeks when her sinus infection is gone.

Using your institution's guidelines for writing in patient records, document in the space that you assessed Maura's vital signs at this appointment.

Date	Comments	Signature

3. Create a brief step-by-step guide for determining and recording all of the vital signs on a 3-by-5-inch card (this is sometimes called a "job aid"). If you can laminate your job aid, you will be able to disinfect it to use during patient care. Practice using your step-by-step guide to determine and record vital signs for family members, friends, or student colleagues. If you practice with a dental hygiene instructor as your patient, you can receive valuable feedback on your techniques!

Dental Radiographic Imaging

Chapter Outline

Learning Objectives

Upon successful completion of these exercises, you will be able to:

1. Identify and define key terms, abbreviations, and concepts related to exposing and processing dental radiographs.
2. Describe procedures for producing and processing x-rays and digital x-ray images.
3. Identify measures to protect yourself and your patient from ionizing radiation.
4. Select film size and type, film-holding devices, and clinical radiographic techniques for patient surveys.
5. Describe the positioning of individual intraoral film packets based on area of the mouth and clinical technique.
6. Use guidelines to determine the indication for exposure of dental radiographs.
7. Identify probable causes of common radiographic inadequacies.

KNOWLEDGE EXERCISES

Key Words, Concepts, and Abbreviation Crossword Puzzle

Across

2 Tungsten filament, which is a coiled wire heated to generate a cloud of electrons; has a negative charge.

4 The emission and propagation of energy through space or a material medium in the form of waves or particles.

5 Increases or decreases the incoming voltage.

7 Radiation that escapes through the protective shielding of the x-ray unit tube head.

9 Milliampere second.

10 The dose of radiation that is lethal for 50% of the population in a specified period of time.

11 1/1000 of an ampere.

13 Millisievert

19 The art and science of making radiographs.

20 A type of scatter radiation that attacks a loosely bound electron and proceeds in a different direction as scatter radiation.

21 Refers to the entire body with the exclusion of germ cells.

23 Extension cone paralleling.

25 The dose of radiation that produces the appearance of redness on human skin.

31 The appearance of dark images on a radiograph as a result of the greater amount of radiation that penetrates low-density objects.

33 Radiation particles or photons produced by the interaction of primary radiation with matter.

35 Roentgen equivalent man.

37 A term for radiation forms of energy, propagated by wave motion as photons that differ widely in wavelength, frequency, and photo energy.

39 As low as reasonably achievable.

41 A form of secondary radiation that during passage through a substance has been deviated in direction and may have been modified by an increase in wavelength.

42 The absorbed dose delivered by a beam of radiation to the surface through which the beam emerges from an object.

43 Radiation that comes directly from the target of the anode of an x-ray machine.

44 The secondary shadow that surrounds the periphery of the primary shadow; a blurred margin.

45 Radiation that serves no useful purpose; includes leakage, secondary and scatter radiation.

46 A light-tight container, usually backed with lead, in which x-ray films are placed for exposure.

47 The dose delivered by a radiation beam and backscatter at the point where the central ray passes through the superficial layer of the object; the surface-absorbed dose.

48 An error of technique that results when the beam of radiation does not completely cover the film being exposed.

Down

1 A finite bundle of energy of visible light or electromagnetic radiation.

2 The technique used for controlling the size and shape of the radiation beam.

3 A card or plastic sheet coated with fluorescent material that produces visible light, adding to the latent image produced directly by radiation.

6 Milligray.

8 Kilovolt peak.

10 The invisible change produced in an x-ray film emulsion by the action of x-radiation or light from which the visible image is subsequently developed and fixed chemically.

12 The amount of energy imparted by ionizing radiation to a unit mass of irradiated material at a specific exposure point.

14 The appearance of light (white) images on a radiograph as a result of the amount of radiation that is absorbed by dense objects.

15 The minimum dose of radiation that produces a detectable degree of any effect.

16 A measure of film exposure time; the burst of radiation generated during a half cycle of alternating current.

17 The dose of radiation that is, or could be, sufficient to cause death.

18 The scattering of relatively low-energy x-rays by elastic collisions without loss of photon energy.

19 A visible image on a radiation-sensitive film emulsion produced by chemical processing after exposure to ionizing radiation.

22 Rate of exposure.

24 Short-wavelength electromagnetic radiation of nuclear origin similar to x-rays, but usually of higher energy.

26 The maximum dose equivalent that a person (or specified parts of that person) is allowed to receive in a stated period of time.

27 That branch of science that deals with the use of radiant energy in the diagnosis and treatment of disease.

28 Radiation produced by electron transitions from higher orbitals to replace ejected electrons of inner electron orbitals.

29 A tungsten target embedded in a copper stem, positioned at an angle to the electron beam; has a positive charge

30 The unit of absorbed dose.

31 An intensifying screen system that is considered to be a "fast" exposure system for x-ray imaging.

32 The art and science of protecting human beings from injury by radiation.

34 The window where the useful beam emerges from the tube; covered with a permanent seal of glass.

36 Radiation absorbed dose.

38 Milliampere impulse.

40 The process by which a beam of radiation is reduced in intensity when passing through some materials.

Exposing and Processing Radiographs

1. In your own words, state two important objectives of dental radiology.

   _____

   _____

   _____

   _____

2. Using the diagrams and descriptions in the textbook as a reference, describe in your own words how x-rays are produced after the power switch on the x-ray machine is activated.

   _____

   _____

   _____

   _____

   _____

   _____

3. Collimation refers to:

   _____

   _____

   _____

4. How does a change in mA affect the final radiographic image?

   _____

   _____

   _____

5. Identify how increasing the kilovoltage affects the image density.

   _____

   _____

   _____

6. How is image contrast affected by increasing the kilovoltage?

   _____

   _____

   _____

7. List two advantages of high kVp.

   _____

   _____

   _____

8. List three advantages of lengthening the target-to-film distance during exposure of patient radiographs.

   _____

   _____

   _____

9. How is the target-to-film distance lengthened on an individual x-ray unit?

   _____

   _____

   _____

10. Identify three components to consider when selecting dental radiograph film.

    _____

    _____

    _____

11. What are the advantages of using digital radiography?

    _____

    _____

    _____

12. Correctly sequence the following steps in producing an INDIRECT digital radiograph, numbering them from 1 to 5 (1 = first step; 5 = final step).

    _____ Electronic charge activates the sensor.

    _____ Image is scanned using a laser scanner.

    _____ Image is stored on the PSP plate.

    _____ Sensor is placed in the patient's mouth.

    _____ Image is displayed on the computer.

13. What type of digital imaging uses a sensor with a cord attached?

    _____

    _____

14. The digital radiograph captures an image using _____ shades of gray.

Radiation Safety

1. Identify three factors that influence the biologic effects of radiation on cells.

   _____

   _____

   _____

2. List human tissues and organs that are highly radiosensitive.

   _____

   _____

   _____

3. List three ways to protect yourself from primary and leakage radiation while making patient radiographs.

   _____

   _____

   _____

4. Relative to your patient's head, where can you best stand to protect yourself from secondary radiation?

   _____

   _____

   _____

5. List the ways you can protect your patient during exposure of dental radiographs.

   _____

   _____

   _____

Clinical Techniques

1. Describe a complete dental radiographic survey.

   _____

   _____

   _____

2. When a rectangular position-indicating device (PID) is used for beam collimation when you expose dental radiographs, how do you adjust the x-ray machine to accommodate both horizontal and vertical film positioning?

   _____

   _____

   _____

3. Match the area of the mouth or teeth listed below with the radiographic film size most frequently used.

_____ Overlapping anterior teeth	A. Film size no. 0
_____ Permanent dentition bitewings	B. Film size no. 1
_____ Primary teeth	C. Film size no. 2
_____ Adult posterior (periapical view)	
_____ Child maxillary (occlusal view)	

4. Select one correct answer to complete the following statement. When exposing a periapical film of tooth 12, directing the central ray with too much vertical angle will produce an image of the tooth that has:

   A. Overlapping of the root of the tooth with the roots of adjacent teeth

   B. Roots that appear much longer then they really are

   C. Roots that appear very short

5. Identify three reasons why the paralleling technique usually produces better images with increased patient safety than the bisecting-angle technique.

   _____

   _____

   _____

6. When positioning the film inside the patient's mouth, the stippled or colored side of the film packet is placed:

   _____

   _____

   _____

7. To maintain a visually open contact on a bitewing x-ray, the horizontal angle of the central beam is directed:

   _____

   _____

   _____

8. How do you position the patient's head when you are making an occlusal survey image of the mandibular teeth?

   _____

   _____

   _____

9. When you are using the paralleling technique to expose periapical radiographs, the patient's head may be in any position convenient for you and comfortable for the patient as long as:

_____

and

_____

10. List the reasons why images of oral structures on a panoramic x-ray may have poor detail or be distorted even if you are very careful to use proper techniques when exposing the radiograph.

_____

_____

_____

11. Identify one reason that a panoramic image may be ordered instead of or in addition to periapical films for an individual patient.

_____

_____

In and Out of the Darkroom

1. Exposure to radiation changes the silver halide crystals coating x-ray film to _____ and _____ ions.

2. After developing the film, only the amount of _____ corresponding to radiolucency and radiopacity remains.

3. The fixer solution removes the _____ crystals that were not exposed to radiation.

4. Correct processing temperature and time for optimal manual processing are _____ °F for _____ minutes.

5. If the temperature of the solutions is higher than the optimal, the amount of time that the film remains in the developer should be _____.

6. What kind of safelight filter is used in a darkroom when processing both intraoral and extraoral films?

_____

_____

_____

7. Match the image inadequacy commonly found on dental x-rays (first column) with the most probable cause of the problem (second column).

_____ Dark lines across film	A. Extreme increase in vertical angle
_____ Double image	
_____ Foreshortening	B. Film exposed twice
_____ Large dark stain on one end of the film	C. Bent film
_____ Light image with a pattern overlaying the image	D. Unsafe safelight
	E. Sudden temperature change in processing solutions
_____ Puckered surface	F. Static electricity
_____ Stretched appearance of images	G. Film placed backward in mouth
_____ Whole film too dark	H. Overlap of film in developer

8. List anatomic landmarks (besides the teeth) that you might locate on an x-ray of your patient's mandibular incisor area.

_____

_____

_____

9. Name a mandibular structure that could appear on a maxillary third molar x-ray.

_____

_____

_____

10. Identify the factors that will enhance interpretation of images on patient radiographs.

_____

_____

_____

_____

COMPETENCY EXERCISES

1. In your own words, describe the difference between direct and indirect imaging of oral structures.

_____

_____

_____

_____

_____

_____

2. In your own words, explain the relationship between the tooth, the film, and the central beam of radiation when using the paralleling technique. (_Hint:_ Use your hands as a three-dimensional way to "draw" the images so you can visualize them.)

_____

_____

_____

_____

_____

3. Mrs. Honey Davis, age 42, presents in your clinic for her initial appointment. She states that she has come because she needs her teeth cleaned and because a tooth on the upper left side of her mouth has been bothering her. She has not been to visit a dentist for 2 years. She states that she had a lot of x-rays taken when she was last examined by her previous dentist just before she moved to your town, but that she did not bring them with her today.

   When collecting your initial assessment data, you identify no positive clinical signs/symptoms of periodontal disease and no clinical evidence of active dental caries. She has six small amalgam restorations in her posterior teeth; only tooth 19 has a restoration on a proximal surface. However, Mrs. Davis reports intermittent use of mint candy to combat a feeling of dry mouth caused by a medication she takes. You also note an accumulation of biofilm on proximal tooth surfaces.

You are planning to ask Dr. Gray, your employer, to examine Mrs. Davis. You know that he will probably order some radiographs. Using Table 9-5, Guidelines for Prescribing Dental Radiographs, in the textbook, determine which films would be recommended for Mrs. Davis and why.

_____

_____

_____

_____

_____

_____

4. When you are ready to expose the films prescribed by Dr. Gray, you position Mrs. Davis's head so that her occlusal plane is parallel to the floor. You know that the appropriate vertical angle of the central ray when exposing bitewing films is set at +8° to +10°. Describe what you notice about the slant of the position-indicating device (PID) when the x-ray unit is appropriately positioned near the patient's face.

_____

_____

_____

5. While exposing a periapical radiograph of Mrs. Davis's tooth 15 using the paralleling technique:

   A. The front edge of the film should rest approximately at the mesial edge of tooth _____.

   B. The film should be placed _____ to the long axis of tooth 15 and parallel to the mesial/distal line of the tooth.

Everyday Ethics

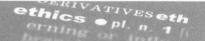

Refer to the Codes of Ethics (Appendices I, II, and III in the textbook) and Framework for Making Decisions (Table 1-2 in the textbook) as you discuss the following scenario with your classmates.

A new patient to the practice, Mr. Glazier, brings a full series of radiographs (16 PAs and 4 BWs) from the previous dentist, prepared just 3 months ago. Following the oral examination, the dentist instructs the dental hygienist to make a panoramic radiograph and 4 BWs.

Mr. Glazier inquires why additional exposures are needed at this time.

Questions for Consideration
1. How will the dental hygienist question the prescriptive request by the dentist for additional radiographs? What would an appropriate response be? How can it be phrased?
2. What ethical standards of care and/or risks should be considered on behalf of the patient? Identify the moral duty of a dental hygienist in this situation.

C. The central beam of radiation is directed _____ to the long axis of tooth 15.

D. The _____ cusp of tooth 15 should rest in slot B (the break-off point) of a disposable Styrofoam film holder.

6. After you take all of the films prescribed for Mrs. Davis and place them in a paper cup, you will go into the darkroom to process the films. Sequence the steps below to follow the process of x-ray development, correctly numbering them from 1 to 9 (1 = first step; 9 = last step).

_____ Darkroom safe-lighting activated

_____ Disinfection of all darkroom areas and equipment used

_____ Infection protocol followed to disinfect film covering

_____ Film placed in fixer solution

_____ Plastic or paper coating removed from film

_____ Film placed in developer solution

_____ Film placed in water bath

_____ Film thoroughly dried

7. In spite of your attempts to reassure him of the appropriateness and safety of the bitewing x-rays prescribed by the dentist, your patient, Jeff Darlington, has refused to have any x-rays taken at his recall appointment. Using your institution's guidelines for writing in patient records, document that he refused the recommended exposures.

Date	Comments	Signature

Factors To Teach The Patient

As you talk with Mr. Glazier, you realize that not only is he concerned about why additional x-rays are necessary, but he is extremely concerned about the safety and negative effects of the additional dose of radiation he will receive. Using the example of a patient conversation from Appendix B as a guide, write a statement explaining all of the safety factors in place in your clinic to protect him from excessive exposure to radiation.

Use the conversation you create to role play this situation with a fellow student. If you are the patient in the role play, be sure to ask questions. If you are the dental hygienist, try to anticipate questions and answer them in your explanation.

This scenario is related to the following factor:

■ When the patient asks about the safety of radiation

8. Gather a variety of dental radiographs taken in your clinic that are currently not being used for patient care. Place them in x-ray mounts for easy viewing. Evaluate the radiographs using Table 9-2, Characteristics of an Acceptable Radiograph, in the textbook.

Identify any errors in technique or processing and describe possible causes and corrections you can make to eliminate the problem. Compare your evaluation of the films with those made by one or two of your student colleagues. Discuss any differences in the way you each evaluated the same x-ray or the corrective measure you described for an error.

Extraoral and Intraoral Examination

Learning Objectives

Upon successful completion of these exercises, you will be able to:

1. Identify and define key terms and concepts related to providing an intraoral and extraoral patient examination.
2. List and describe the objectives of the examination of the oral cavity and adjacent structures by the dental hygienist.
3. List and describe the steps for a thorough examination.
4. Accurately describe conditions and lesions found during an oral examination.
5. List the warning signs of oral cancer and discuss the follow-up procedure for a suspicious lesion.

KNOWLEDGE EXERCISES

1. List a dental hygienist's objectives for the extraoral and intraoral examinations.

   _____

   _____

   _____

   _____

   _____

   _____

   _____

   _____

2. As you get ready to perform an examination for your patient, you should:

   ■ *Review* _____ *and* _____.

   ■ *Examine* _____.

   ■ *Explain* _____.

3. In your own words, explain the advantages of using a systematic sequence for the examination.

   _____

   _____

   _____

4. Match the types of palpation with the appropriate definition and description. There are two answers for each type of palpation.

TYPES OF PALPATION	DEFINITION/DESCRIPTION
Digital _____ _____	A. Use of finger or fingers and thumb from each hand applied simultaneously in coordination
Bimanual _____ _____	B. Use of a finger C. Two hands used at the same time to examine corresponding structures on opposite sides of the body
Bilateral _____ _____	D. Use of finger and thumb of the same hand E. Palpation of the lips F. Index finger applied to the inner border of the mandible beneath the canine-premolar area to determine the presence of a torus mandibularis
Bidigital _____ _____	G. Index finger of one hand palpates the floor of the mouth inside, while a finger or fingers from the other hand press on the same area from under the chin externally H. Fingers placed beneath the chin to palpate the submandibular lymph nodes

5. In your own words, define the following types of information recorded for an oral lesion.

■ *History*

_____

_____

_____

■ *Location and extent*

_____

_____

_____

_____

■ *Size and shape*

_____

_____

_____

■ *Color*

_____

_____

_____

■ *Surface texture*

_____

_____

_____

■ *Consistency*

_____

_____

_____

6. The term *induration* _____ means.

7. Early oral cancer takes many forms. Write a brief description of the characteristics you might observe for each of the five basic forms listed below.

■ White areas:

_____

_____

_____

■ Red areas:

_____

_____

_____

■ Ulcers:

_____

_____

■ Masses:

_____

_____

■ Pigmentation:

_____

_____

_____

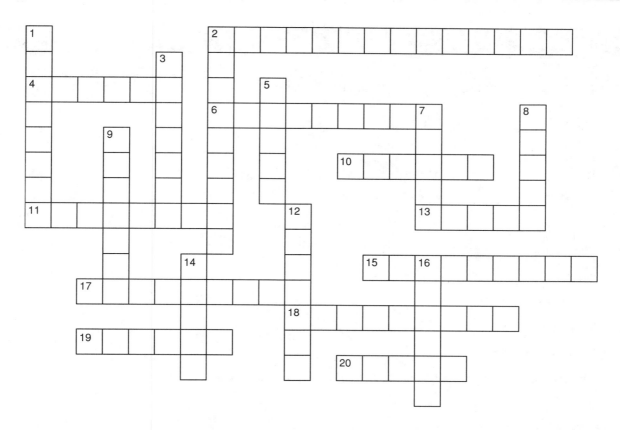

Use Tables 10-2, 10-3, and 10-4

Across

2 Loose membranous layer of exudates.
4 Larger than a papule (greater than 5 mm but less than 1 cm).
6 Growing outward.
10 Circumscribed area not elevated above the surrounding skin or mucosa.
11 Red area of variable size and shape.
13 General swelling or enlargement, 2 cm or greater in width.
15 Resembling a small, nipple-shaped projection or elevation.
17 Rough, wartlike.
18 Hardened.
19 Small solid lesion (pinhead to 5 mm in diameter).
20 Bony elevation or prominence.

Down

1 Marked with points or dots.
2 Minute hemorrhagic spots of pinhead to pinpoint size.
3 Circumscribed lesion, a thin surface covering, 1 cm or less in diameter.
5 Any mass of tissue that projects outward or upward.
7 Outer layer, covering, or scab.
8 Depressed lesions representing a loss of continuity of the epithelium.
9 Lesion containing pus more or less than 5 mm in diameter.
12 Shallow, depressed lesion that does not extend through the epithelium.
14 Large lesion (more than 1 cm) filled with fluid
16 Slightly raised lesion with a broad, flat top.

INFOMAP 10-1

ORDER OF EXAMINATION	OBSERVATION	INDICATION AND INFLUENCES ON THE APPOINTMENT
Overall appraisal of patient	Labored breathing	
Face	Evidence of fear or apprehension	
Skin	Multiple light brown macules	
Eyes	Eyeglasses (corrective)	
Nodes	Lymphadenopathy; induration	
Preauricular and postauricular		
Occipital		
Submental; submandibular		
Cervical chain		
Supraclavicular		
Temporomandibular joint	Tenderness; sensitivity; noises (clicking, popping, grating)	
Lips	Blisters, ulcers	
Breath odor	Cigarette odor	
Labial and buccal mucosa	Multiple red nodules on left buccal mucosa	
Tongue	Coating	
Floor of mouth	Limitation or freedom of movement of tongue	
Saliva	Evidences of dry mouth; lip wetting	
Hard palate	Tori	
Soft palate, uvula	Large uvula	
Tonsillar region, throat	Large tonsils	

8. You are working in an oral pathology laboratory and are asked to categorize information found in laboratory reports. Match each category with its description.

LABORATORY REPORT CATEGORY	DESCRIPTION
_____ Class I	A. Normal
_____ Unsatisfactory	B. Uncertain (possible for cancer)
_____ Class V	C. Slide is inadequate for diagnosis
_____ Class II	D. Probable for cancer
_____ Class IV	E. Atypical, but not suggestive of malignant cells
_____ Class III	F. Positive for cancer

9. If the slide is found to be inadequate for diagnosis, explain in your own words why this happened.

_____

_____

_____

10. Using the information in Box 10-1 and Tables 10-1 to 10-4 in the textbook, imagine that your patient presents with the conditions listed in Infomap 10-1 above. Complete the Infomap by identifying the indications and influences on the appointment.

COMPETENCY EXERCISES

1. To prepare for an extraoral examination of each patient, list the steps (in the correct order) you will follow.

_____

_____

_____

_____

_____

_____

2. To prepare for an intraoral examination of each patient, list the steps (in the correct order) you will follow.

_____

_____

_____

_____

_____

_____

3. Your patient, Kurt Bachleim, age 23 years, presents with localized, coalescing multiple lesions on the right buccal mucosa. Mr. Bachleim also has an exostosis extending from tooth 12 to tooth 15 and trismus. Describe what you would expect to see and any possible adaptations you will need to make for the appointment.

_____

_____

_____

_____

_____

_____

4. Your patient Yoon Chang presents with a tiny (about 1 mm) bluish-black lesion on the top right half of her tongue. She said that it wasn't bothering her at all. You palpate the lesion, but do not feel anything unusual. Ms. Chang reports that the same thing had come up on her palate a few weeks ago. As you continue to question her, she mentions that she has had a broken blood vessel or two on her fingers in the past. She had actually forgotten about it until you started asking questions. Dr. Pine is not in the office today, so you document the lesion in the patient record in order to discuss it with him tomorrow and decide appropriate follow-up procedures. (Continued on next page)

Everyday Ethics

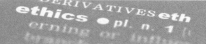

Refer to the Codes of Ethics (Appendices I, II, and III in the textbook) and Framework for Making Decisions (Table 1-2 in the textbook) as you discuss the following scenario with your classmates.

Abby and Sylvia are the two part-time dental hygienists in Dr. Anthony's practice. They work on different days at the office, so they rarely see each other except to attend local dental hygiene association meetings. Most patients know both hygienists and may be scheduled with either depending on available time.

　　Mr. Peters came in for his 3-month maintenance appointment carrying his unlit pipe as usual. This time his appointment was with Abby, and jokes were exchanged about the pipe. During the intraoral examination, Abby found a red lesion on the side of his tongue that was about 4 mm wide. She asked him if he had seen it and his answer was, "Oh yeah, Sylvia mentioned it when I was here last time." Abby glanced at the record and noted that his last date was more than 4 months ago. Nothing could be found in the patient's dental record that mentioned any oral lesions.

Questions for Consideration
1. What ethical issues are involved here?
2. Because Dr. Anthony has never defined a policy for follow-up on such a finding, how should Abby proceed?
3. Privately, Abby is upset, and she is determined that this should be discussed with both Sylvia and Dr. Anthony. Where and how should she approach them, and what recommendations does she need to propose for an office policy?

Factors To Teach The Patient

Aishia Williams presents with a lesion that may be malignant. She has previously been treated for oral cancer and is at risk for recurrence. She has not been evaluated for 18 months. In collaboration with your dentist employer, you have decided to use a toluidine blue. The lesion in Ms. Williams's mouth did not retain the dye after the postrinse solution.

Use the example of a patient conversation in Appendix B of this workbook as a guide to write a statement explaining the need for careful follow-up and frequent evaluation by a dental professional as well as the need for Ms. Williams to perform a regular oral self-examination and to be aware of the warning signs of oral cancer.

Use the conversation you create to role play this situation with a fellow student. If you are the patient in the role play, be sure to ask questions. If you are the dental hygienist, try to anticipate questions and answer them in your explanation.

This scenario is related to the following factors:

- The reasons for a careful extraoral and intraoral examination at each maintenance appointment
- A method for self-examination (The examination should include the face, neck, lips, gingiva, cheeks, tongue, palate, and throat. Any changes should be reported to the dentist and the dental hygienist.)
- The warning signs of oral cancer

Use your institution's guidelines for writing in the patient record and the information in Chapter 10 to describe the lesion on Ms. Chang's tongue in the space below.

Date	Comments	Signature

Study Casts

Chapter Outline

Learning Objectives

Upon successful completion of these exercises, you will be able to:

1. Identify and define key terms and concepts related to making oral study casts.
2. List and discuss the purposes and uses of study casts.

3. Identify the supplies, steps, and procedures involved in taking an impression.
4. List the supplies, steps, and procedures involved in making a study cast.

Word-Search Puzzle

To solve the puzzle, first use the clues to determine the words; then find the words in the grid. Words in the grid can run across, down, or diagonally and can start at the right or left or top or bottom. When you have found all the words, **the first 11 unused letters in the grid will spell out a hidden message.**

Hidden message: Your patients will really appreciate it if you make your clinic a

_____.

C	G	A	O	C	C	L	U	S	A	L	P	L	A	N	E
E	G	F	R	E	E	Z	P	O	N	E	W	K	N	R	T
N	Z	F	H	N	C	M	K	O	N	V	E	G	K	P	L
T	Y	M	D	K	G	N	P	M	L	T	M	J	B	L	L
R	N	F	E	P	M	V	B	Z	A	I	N	T	N	N	D
I	K	L	N	V	M	C	K	N	N	P	S	O	L	E	C
C	X	T	T	B	T	A	I	N	R	T	I	H	N	T	B
O	L	R	A	H	N	G	S	O	G	S	N	T	T	T	T
C	M	K	L	Q	L	W	S	T	S	Y	A	T	Z	Q	X
C	M	N	P	A	T	T	P	E	E	L	N	W	M	F	M
L	J	F	L	L	H	T	R	Z	S	R	X	G	C	Z	X
U	M	Q	A	E	J	P	R	T	M	K	C	Q	L	Y	Y
S	V	R	S	T	M	C	O	C	A	S	T	A	M	B	C
I	R	I	T	I	Q	N	J	V	T	H	D	R	S	Z	R
O	S	D	E	X	E	L	X	D	G	J	B	N	Q	T	W
N	J	H	R	B	X	M	V	M	G	K	R	N	P	Q	

Word-Search Clues

- An aqueous impression material used for recording minimal detail
- A positive life-size reproduction of the teeth and adjacent tissues
- Used to fabricate a dental restoration or prosthesis (two words)
- The usual maximum intercuspation or contact of the teeth of the opposing arches (two words)
- The beta form of calcium sulfate hemihydrate (two words)
- The alpha form of calcium sulfate hemihydrate (two words)
- A negative imprint of an oral structure used to produce a positive replica of the structure
- The average plane established by the incisal and occlusal surfaces of the teeth (two words)
- To make smooth and glossy, usually by friction
- An artificial replacement of an absent part of the human body

KNOWLEDGE EXERCISES

1. Your patient wants to know why you are recommending taking an impression for a study cast and how can study casts be used for different kinds of patients, not just her. In your own words, describe the uses and purposes of study casts.

   _____

   _____

   _____

   _____

   _____

2. You are asked to order all the supplies you will need for taking patient impressions and pouring study casts. List the supplies you will order.

   _____

   _____

   _____

   _____

   _____

3. You have tried in the impression tray for your patient. In checking the width of the tray, you allowed for an adequate thickness of impression material on the facial and lingual surfaces of each tooth to provide _____ and _____ to the impression.

   ■ *Your patient has a tooth in prominent linguoversion, so you allowed for a minimum thickness of _____ to _____ inch.*

   ■ *As you checked the length of the tray, you made sure to allow coverage of the _____ area of the mandible and the _____ of the maxilla.*

4. The steps involved in taking a maxillary impression are listed below. You have already tried in and prepared the tray. Number the list in the correct order (1 = first step; 6 = last step).

   _____ Seat the tray from posterior to anterior.

   _____ Maintain equal pressure on each side of the tray.

   _____ Rinse under cool running water and proceed with disinfection for maxillary cast.

   _____ Insert the tray with a rotary motion.

   _____ Elevate the cheek over the edge of the impression to break the seal, and remove the impression with a sudden jerk.

   _____ Ask the patient to form a tight O with the lips to mold the impression material.

5. Mark each of the following statements **true or false**. If the statement is false, correct it, and write the true statement in the space provided.

   True or False   The material used for the interocclusal record is placed over the occlusal surfaces, and the patient is directed to close in habitual occlusion.

   _____

   _____

   _____

   True or False   When the leftover material on the spatula has lost its surface stickiness, the impression should be held in position in the patient's mouth for 2 minutes more.

   _____

   _____

   _____

   True or False   You stand behind the patient to take a mandibular impression.

   _____

   _____

   _____

   True or False   The patient does not remove an oral prosthesis before the impression is taken.

   _____

   _____

   _____

   True or False   Spatulation for 2 minutes allows the chemical reactions to proceed uniformly.

   _____

   _____

   _____

   True or False   Plaster produces a cast fairly susceptible to breakage.

   _____

   _____

   _____

True or False Ideal gelation time is 7 to 9 minutes when the room temperature is 20° to 21°C (68°–70°F).

_____

_____

_____

True or False The patient is in a supine position when you take an impression.

_____

_____

_____

True or False If alginate powder is left exposed, water condenses on the powder.

_____

_____

_____

True or False To lower the surface tension, the patient should take a deep breath.

_____

_____

_____

True or False The teeth are wet with the air/water syringe before the impression is taken.

_____

_____

_____

True or False The most frequent error in the use of the alginates for impressions is delay in pouring the cast.

_____

_____

_____

True or False You stand at the side and toward the back of the patient to take a maxillary impression.

_____

_____

_____

True or False If you have delayed trimming after separating the impression from the cast, the cast must be thoroughly soaked in water before trimming.

_____

_____

_____

True or False You can wait until you have a break in your schedule before you pour the alginate impression.

_____

_____

_____

True or False The impression tray is seated with a rotary motion.

_____

_____

_____

True or False Dust particles from the alginate impression material can cause serious irritation to the eyes.

_____

_____

_____

True or False Seat the posterior portion of the tray before the anterior portion.

_____

_____

_____

True or False A wax rim around the borders of the tray prevents discomfort.

_____

_____

_____

True or False The maxillary cast is trimmed to a point, and the mandibular cast is rounded.

_____

_____

_____

True or False Rock the impression back and forth to release it.

_____

_____

_____

True or False Precoat vestibular areas, occlusal surfaces, and undercut areas with wax.

_____

_____

_____

True or False Wax is the only material available for obtaining a bite registration.

_____

_____

_____

6. Dental stone is sensitive to changes in the relative humidity of the atmosphere. List some strategies that protect the stone.

_____

_____

_____

7. The steps involved in mixing dental stone are given below. First complete the sentences, and then number the list in the correct order (1 = first step; 6 = last step).

_____ Sift in the powder gradually to _____ _____ and to allow each particle to become _____.

_____ Measure the water and powder according to the manufacturer's specifications. (The ratio of water to powder is _____ mL powder to _____ mL water for _____ g stone.)

_____ Wait briefly until all powder is wet, then vibrate to _____.

_____ Place measured water (which is at _____ temperature) in a clean, dry mixing bowl.

_____ The result is a _____, _____, _____ mix.

_____ Use a vacuum mixer.

8. _____ controls the strength, rigidity, and hardness of the cast.

◼ *Increasing the water to dental stone ratio _____ the strength of the cast.*

◼ *Temperature affects the setting time of the dental stone: _____ water increases it, and _____ water decreases it.*

9. The finished cast has two connected parts: the anatomic portion and the base or art portion. Complete the following sentences to describe the process of pouring the anatomic portion of the cast.

◼ *Shake the_____ out of the impression.*

◼ *Using a vibrator, take a _____ of stone mix on the end of the _____. Start at the most posterior tooth, and allow the mix to flow through the impression. Use _____ amounts and vibrate continually. _____ the impression so the material passes into the indentatious and flows slowly down the side, across the _____ surface or the _____ edge.*

◼ *Air is trapped when the process is hurried or _____.*

◼ *When all tooth indentations are covered, add _____ amounts of mix to _____ the impression.*

10. The base of the cast can be made using a variety of techniques. List the steps for each of the following techniques.

◼ *Rubber model base former*

_____

_____

_____

_____

_____

_____

◼ *Two-step or double pour*

_____

_____

_____

_____

_____

■ *Boxing technique*

_____

_____

_____

_____

_____

_____

11. The exact proportions of the study casts and the steps required to accomplish the trimming and finishing depend on several factors. List these factors.

_____

_____

_____

12. In your own words, describe the features of an acceptable study cast. Use the figures in Chapter 11 of the textbook to help you visualize your descriptions.

_____

_____

_____

_____

_____

_____

13. A completed study cast is finished and polished. Complete the following sentences by circling the correct term or phrase.

■ *Allow casts to dry thoroughly for 2–3 [**days, weeks, months**].*

■ *Smooth the art portion with [**fine, medium, coarse**] sandpaper.*

■ *Soak in heated soap solution for [**15–30, 30–60, 45–60**] minutes.*

■ *Rub with a [**synthetic, wool, chamois or cotton cloth**].*

■ *Talc or baby talcum powder with [**olive, mineral, canola**] oil may be used.*

COMPETENCY EXERCISES

Privesh Doshi is a dental assistant at the dental clinic in which you are practicing. Dr. Pecharo has asked you to teach Privesh how to take an impression (assume that you are in a state or province where it is legal for dental assistants to do impressions). You decide the best way to teach is to make a checklist so Privesh can follow it every time he is taking an impression.

1. Create the checklist.

_____

_____

_____

_____

_____

_____

2. Privesh is concerned about making the patient gag. Give him some suggestions on how to prevent this.

_____

_____

_____

_____

_____

_____

Everyday Ethics

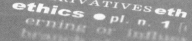

Refer to the Codes of Ethics (Appendices I, II, and III in the textbook) and Framework for Making Decisions (Table 1-2 in the textbook) as you discuss the following scenario with your classmates.

Everyone was rushing around the office trying to finish in time for lunch. Ylena was asked to take the impressions for whitening trays for Mrs. Lattoch. As Ylena places the maxillary tray, the patient begins to gag severely. Mrs. Lattoch pushes Ylena's arm out of the way and attempts to pull the tray out of her mouth. Ylena calls for assistance while forcefully restraining Mrs. Lattoch to keep the tray in until the impression material is set.

Questions for Consideration
1. Describe the ethical principle that best describes the actions of Ylena.
2. By restraining the patient, were the patient's rights violated? Why or why not? Explain the rationale.
3. Professionally, what choices could Ylena have exercised with Mrs. Lattoch to improve the outcome?

Factors To Teach The Patient

You have just seated your patient, Mrs. Lorna Patel. Refer to Appendix D to review her care plan. Before this appointment, Mrs. Patel was unaware of the generalized moderate attrition in her mouth.

   Using the example of a patient conversation in Appendix B as a guide, write a statement explaining to Mrs. Patel the need to take the alginate impression to make study casts so you can document her condition. Be sure to discuss the need to fabricate a night guard and why study casts will help you do that. Compare your conversation with a student colleague to identify any missing information.

This scenario is related to the following factors:

■ Importance and purposes of study casts; reasons for comparative casts after treatment or at a later date
■ Use of the casts of other patients to show effects of treatment or what can happen if the prescribed treatment is not carried out

3. Privesh is concerned about taking the impressions. He needs more information on how to mix the alginate material and wants to know how much time he has to insert the material into the patient's mouth. Explain these procedures.

_____

_____

_____

_____

_____

_____

4. The alginate impression that you took this morning has been sitting on the counter in the laboratory for 4 hours. What are your concerns?

_____

_____

_____

_____

_____

_____

The Gingiva

Chapter Outline

Learning Objectives

Upon successful completion of these exercises, you will be able to:

1. Identify and define key terms and concepts related to the gingiva.
2. Identify the clinical features of the periodontal tissues that must be examined for a complete assessment.

3. List the markers for periodontal infection and classify them by type, degree of severity, and causative factors.
4. Identify gingival landmarks and discuss their significance.

KNOWLEDGE EXERCISES

The Gingiva and Related Structures Crossword Puzzle

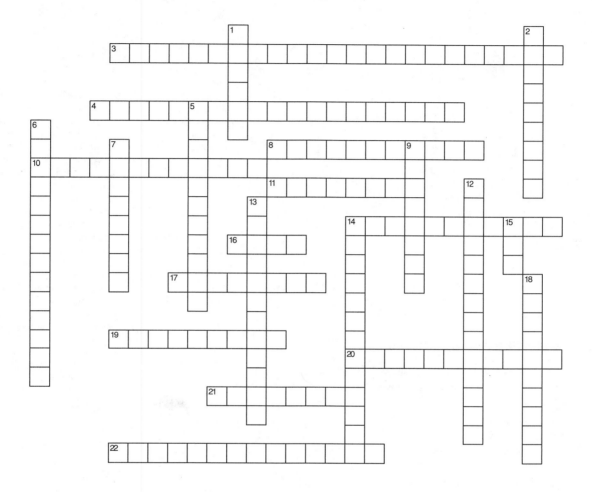

Across

3 The probing depth measured from a fixed point (three words).
4 The cementum, periodontal ligament, and the alveolar bone (two words).
8 Formation of pus.
10 The distance from the gingival margin to the location of the periodontal probe tip inserted for gentle probing at the attachment (two words).
11 Fibers that penetrate connective tissue fibers and attach the tooth to the adjacent alveolar bone.
14 Increase in size of tissue or organ caused by an increase in size of its constituent cells.
16 The type of epithelial tissue that serves as a liner for the intraoral mucosal surfaces.
17 A fibrous change of the mucous membrane as a result of chronic inflammation.
19 The pitted, orange-peel appearance frequently seen on the surface of the attached gingiva.
20 The act of chewing.
21 The type of epithelium that is composed of a layer of flat, scale-like cells; or may be stratified.
22 The type of lining mucosa in which the stratified squamous epithelial cells retain their nuclei and cytoplasm.

Down

1 Identifier; symptoms or signs by which a particular condition can be recognized.
2 Cell junction.
5 Abnormal increase in volume of a tissue or organ caused by formation and growth of new normal cells.
6 Abnormal thickening of the keratin layer (stratum corneum) of the epithelium.
7 A space between two natural teeth.
9 Receptor of taste on tongue and oropharynx (two words).
12 The development of a horny layer of flattened epithelial cells containing keratin.
13 Tissues surrounding and supporting the teeth.
14 Half of a desmosome that forms a site of attachment between junctional epithelial cells and the tooth surface.
15 A fluid product of inflammation that contains leukocytes, degenerated tissue elements, tissue fluids, and microorganisms.
18 Fiber-producing cell of the connective tissue.

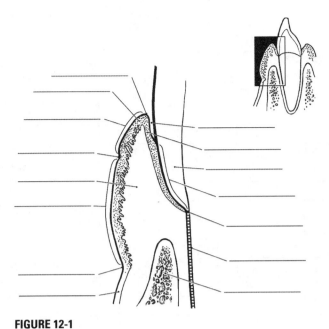

FIGURE 12-1

Terms and Anatomic Structures

1. Use the following terms to label **Figure 12-1** with each of the components of the gingiva and periodontium.

   - ▨ *Alveolar bone*
   - ▨ *Alveolar mucosa*
   - ▨ *Attached gingiva*
   - ▨ *Cementoenamel junction*
   - ▨ *Enamel*
   - ▨ *Free gingiva*
   - ▨ *Free gingival groove*
   - ▨ *Gingival margin*
   - ▨ *Gingival sulcus*
   - ▨ *Junctional epithelium*
   - ▨ *Mucogingival junction*

2. Draw the following gingival fibers in their correct position on the Figure 12-1 diagram. Use colored pencils to help differentiate.

   - ▨ *Alveologingival fibers*
   - ▨ *Circumferential fibers*
   - ▨ *Dentogingival fibers*
   - ▨ *Dentoperiosteal fibers*

3. Draw and label the periodontal ligament in the correct position on Figure 12-1 diagram.

4. Match each term with the appropriate definition.

TERMS RELATED TO THE GINGIVA	DEFINITION
_____ Generalized _____ Marginal _____ Clinical crown _____ Papillary _____ Anatomic root _____ Diffuse _____ Anatomic crown _____ Localized _____ Clinical root	A. A change that is confined to the free or marginal gingiva B. The gingiva is involved about all or nearly all of the teeth throughout the mouth C. A change that involves a papilla but not the rest of the free gingiva around a tooth D. Spread out, dispersed; affects the gingival margin, attached gingiva, and interdental papillae; may extend into alveolar mucosa E. Indicates the gingiva around a single tooth or a specific group of teeth F. The part of the tooth above the attached periodontal tissues; can be considered the part of the tooth where clinical treatment procedures are applied G. The part of the tooth below the base of the gingival sulcus or periodontal pocket; the part of the root to which periodontal fibers are attached H. The part of the tooth covered by enamel I. The part of the tooth covered by cementum

5. Define the following terms in your own words. (*Hint:* You may want to think about location as you define each term.)

   - ▨ *Masticatory mucosa*

   _____

   _____

   _____

   - ▨ *Lining mucosa*

   _____

   _____

   _____

■ *Cementum*

_____

_____

_____

■ *Alveolar bone*

_____

_____

_____

■ *Free gingival groove*

_____

_____

_____

■ *Gingival sulcus (crevice)*

_____

_____

_____

■ *Interdental gingiva*

_____

_____

_____

■ *Col*

_____

_____

_____

6. Use the following terms to label the **Figure 12-2** diagram of teeth and gingiva.

   ■ *Alveolar mucosa*
   ■ *Attached gingiva*
   ■ *Free gingiva*
   ■ *Interdental papilla*
   ■ *Mandibular labial frenum*
   ■ *Maxillary labial frenum*
   ■ *Mucogingival junction*

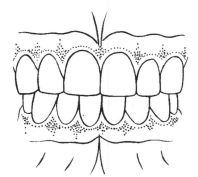

FIGURE 12-2

7. Match the gingival fiber group with the correct location and purpose.

GINGIVAL FIBER GROUP	LOCATION AND PURPOSE
_____ Dentogingival fibers _____ Transseptal fibers _____ Dentoperiosteal fibers _____ Apical fibers _____ Interradicular fibers _____ Circumferential fibers _____ Oblique fibers _____ Alveolar crest fibers _____ Alveologingival fibers _____ Horizontal fibers	A. From the cervical area of one tooth across to an adjacent tooth (on the mesial or distal side only) to provide resistance to separation of teeth B. From the cementum in the cervical region into the free gingiva to give support to the gingiva C. From the root apex to adjacent surrounding bone to resist vertical forces D. From the root above the apical fibers obliquely toward the occlusal to resist vertical and unexpected strong forces E. From the alveolar crest into the free and attached gingiva to provide support F. From the cervical cementum over the alveolar crest to blend with fibers of the periosteum of the bone G. From the cementum in the middle of each root to the adjacent alveolar bone to resist tipping of the tooth H. From the alveolar crest to the cementum just below the cementoenamel junction to resist intrusive forces I. Continuous around the neck of the tooth to help maintain the tooth in position J. From the cementum between the roots of multirooted teeth to the adjacent bone to resist vertical and lateral forces

8. To complete this exercise using Figure 12-2, you will need red, blue, and green pencils.

   ■ *On the left side of the diagram, color the interdental papilla in both the maxillary and mandibular arch in red.*
   ■ *On the right side of the drawing, color the free gingiva in blue.*
   ■ *On the right side of the drawing, color the attached gingiva in green.*

9. You are getting ready to do an examination of Patrice Davis, who is a professional ice skater and is curious about everything. She wants to know exactly how you are going to check her "gum tissues," and she does not want you to "skate over anything." She really wants to have a nice smile for the competitions! Explain the purpose of the examination to Patrice, and list the markers you will use to describe the appearance of her oral tissues.

_____

_____

_____

_____

_____

_____

COMPETENCY EXERCISES

1. Your patient, Tucker McLeimgreen, presents with clinically normal-appearing gingiva. Describe in your own words what you expect to observe as you examine Tucker's gingival tissues both visually and with a probe.

_____

_____

_____

_____

_____

2. Your patient, Xin Singer, is very concerned about the areas of localized, wide, shallow recession she has on teeth 6 and 7 and the narrow, deep (with missing attached gingiva) recession she has on teeth 24 and 25. Using Figures 12-1 and 12-2 from the workbook as a guide, draw a sketch of the recession that is described here. Then identify the points you will discuss with Xin.

_____

_____

_____

_____

_____

3. Your patient Frank Catty presents with gingiva that looks like the tissue that is pictured in Figure 12-10B in the textbook. Based on your understanding of this condition, describe Frank's gingival tissue using the following markers: color, size, shape, consistency, surface texture, position of the gingival margin, and bleeding.

_____

_____

_____

_____

_____

4. You are providing care for Kathleen Gallagher. She is a research scientist particularly interested in inflammation. You have just completed the gingival examination and are planning to discuss the information you have gathered and the causes for the oral changes you have documented. Kathleen has not received dental care for 5 years; she is worried about her "bleeding gums" and wants to know exactly why these changes are occurring. Refer to Table 12-1 in the textbook to help you collect your thoughts and then identify the reasons for each change.

■ *Color: bright red*

_____

_____

■ *Size: enlarged*

_____

_____

■ *Shape: bulbous papillae*

_____

_____

■ *Consistency: soft, spongy (dents readily when pressed with probe)*

_____

_____

■ *Surface texture: smooth, shiny gingiva*

_____

_____

■ *Position of gingival margin: enlarged; higher on the tooth, above normal; pocket deepened*

_____

_____

_____

■ *Position of junctional epithelium: probing is within normal limits*

_____

_____

_____

■ *Bleeding: spontaneous*

_____

_____

_____

■ *Exudate: none on pressure*

_____

_____

_____

5. For some kinds of patient records, you will need to describe a patient's condition in sentence form. In the space provided below, document a brief gingival description that you will include in Kathleen Gallagher's record.

Date	Comments	Signature

Everyday Ethics

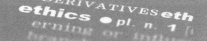

Refer to the Codes of Ethics (Appendices I, II, and III in the textbook) and Framework for Making Decisions (Table 1-2 in the textbook) as you discuss the following scenario with your classmates.

Britain and Nicholas were first-year dental hygiene students just beginning to practice on each other as student partners in the preclinic program. During the oral examination, Britain noticed that Nicholas had some areas of bleeding and changes in the contour of the marginal gingiva. In general, the soft tissue seemed more sponge-like and loose, but Britain was not sure she clearly understood what is considered "normal," remembering that the clinical instructor often referred to a "range" of normal.

　　Britain decided to focus on and document the areas that were pale pink, firm, and pointed in the interproximal areas. She carefully recorded this information with great detail and then signaled for her instructor to verify the

findings. When the instructor sat down and reviewed the examination, she was pleased with Britain's thoroughness. The instructor provided positive feedback and quickly moved on to the next pair of students. Britain began to feel uneasy that she hadn't pointed out the gingival tissues that she thought were possibly inflamed.

Questions for Consideration
1. Explain how the ethical principles of autonomy, benefi-cence, and veracity apply to this situation.
2. Indicate how Nicholas is the center of this dilemma, both from the perspective of Britain, a student, and the clini-cal instructor who finds out from another faculty member that he or she thinks Nicholas has definite signs of peri-odontal disease.
3. Ethically, what alternatives or actions can Britain take at this time to address the 'uneasy' feeling she has about Nicholas's gingival status?

Factors To Teach The Patient

You have just seen Kathleen Gallagher, the patient described in Competency Exercise 4. She is very anxious now that you have told her about all the implications of your findings from the gingival examination.

Working with the data you have collected and the causative factors you have identified, and using the example of a patient conversation in Appendix B as a guide, write a statement explaining what type of tissue changes you would like to see at Kathleen's next appointment.

Use the conversation you create to role play this situation with a fellow student. If you are the patient in the role play, be sure to ask questions. If you are the dental hygienist, try to anticipate questions and answer them in your explanation.

This scenario is related to the following factors:

- Characteristics of normal healthy gingiva
- The significance of bleeding; healthy tissue does not bleed
- Relationship of findings during a gingival examination to the personal daily care procedures for infection control

CHAPTER 13

Examination Instruments and Procedures

Chapter Outline

Learning Objectives

Upon successful completion of these exercises, you will be able to:

1. Identify and define key terms and concepts related to oral examination procedures.

2. Describe the purpose and procedure for the use of each instrument in a basic examination setup.

3. Discuss the implications of various oral findings identified during the examination.

KNOWLEDGE EXERCISES

1. The mouth mirror is made up of three parts: the _____, the _____, and the _____.

2. Describe mirror surfaces in your own words.

_____

_____

_____

3. Identify the purposes and uses of mouth mirrors.

_____

_____

_____

4. Match each term with the correct definition.

EXAMINATION PROCEDURES TERM	DEFINITION
_____ Horizontal bone loss _____ Clinical attachment level _____ Explorer _____ Bifurcation _____ Fremitus _____ Tactile _____ Explorer tip _____ Calibration _____ Probe _____ Probing depth _____ Tactile discrimination	A. A slender instrument, usually round in diameter with a rounded tip, designed for examination of the teeth and soft tissues B. Probing depth as measured from the cementoenamel junction (or other fixed point) to the location of the probe tip at the coronal level of attached periodontal tissues C. Determination of the accuracy of an instrument by measurement of its variation from a standard D. The distance from the gingival margin to the location of the periodontal probe tip at the coronal border of attached periodontal tissues E. A slender stainless-steel instrument with a fine, flexible, sharp point used for examination of the surfaces of the teeth to detect irregularities F. A vibration perceptible by palpation G. Pertaining to touch H. The ability to distinguish relative degrees of roughness and smoothness I. Two roots J. Slender, wire-like, circular in cross-section, and tapering to a fine, sharp point K. When the crest of the bone is parallel with a line between the cementoenamel junctions of two adjacent teeth

5. Air is used to enhance the examination and treatment of a patient. It is believed to improve and facilitate the examination procedures, improve visibility of the treatment area during instrumentation, and prepare teeth and/or gingiva for certain procedures. Give some situational examples to explain these statements.

_____

_____

_____

_____

_____

_____

6. The probe is a slender instrument with a _____, _____ tip designed for the examination of the _____ and the topography of an area. It can be made of steel or plastic. Refer to Table 13-1 and Figure 13-1 in the textbook, and identify the type of probe used at your school. Notice the markings, and be sure you know how to read the probe you are using.

7. Fill in the blanks as you read these facts about pocket characteristics.

   ▪ A pocket is measured from the _____ of the pocket to the _____ margin.

   ▪ The pocket (or sulcus) is _____ around the entire tooth, and the entire sulcus must be measured. _____ probing is inadequate.

   ▪ The _____ varies around an individual tooth, rarely measuring the same all around a tooth or even around one side of a tooth.

   ▪ The _____ of attached tissue assumes a varying position around the tooth.

   ▪ The _____ margin varies in its position on the tooth.

   ▪ Proximal surfaces must be approached by entering from both the _____ and the _____ aspects of the tooth.

   ▪ Gingival and periodontal infections begin in the _____ area more frequently than in other areas.

   ▪ Probing depth may be _____ directly under the contact area because of crater formation in the alveolar bone.

   ▪ Anatomic features of the _____ wall of the pocket influence the direction of probing. Examples are concave surfaces, anomalies, shape of the cervical one third, and position of _____.

8. The probe reading in part A of **Figure 13-1** on the next page is _____ mm. The probe reading in part B of the figure is _____ mm. Given these readings, identify which figure part in Figure 13-1 demonstrates tissue that is within normal limits and which demonstrates periodontal disease.

_____

_____

_____

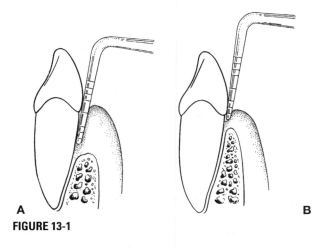

A   **B**

FIGURE 13-1

9. Match the health status of the periodontium with the appropriate location of the probe tip.

PERIODONTAL STATUS	LOCATION OF PROBE TIP
_____ Gingivitis and early periodontitis _____ Normal healthy tissue _____ Advanced periodontitis	A. At the base of the sulcus or crevice, at the coronal end of the junctional epithelium B. Penetrates through the junctional epithelium to reach attached connective tissue fibers C. Within the junctional epithelium

10. The probe is adapted to individual teeth and surfaces. In your own words, describe how to adapt the probe for each of the following structures.

■ *Molars and premolars*

_____

_____

_____

■ *Anterior teeth*

_____

_____

_____

■ *Proximal surfaces*

_____

_____

_____

11. Mark each of the following statements true or false. If the statement is false, correct it.

True or False   When the crest of the bone is parallel with a line between the cementoenamel junctions of two adjacent teeth, the term *vertical bone loss* is used.

_____

_____

_____

True or False   *Attachment level* refers to the position where periodontal tissues are attached, at the base of a sulcus or pocket.

_____

_____

_____

True or False   Radiographs show pockets; soft tissue is seen in a radiograph.

_____

_____

_____

True or False   Clinical attachment level is measured from a changeable point (usually the free gingiva) to the attachment, whereas the probing depth is measured from a fixed point (the crest of the cementoenamel junction) to the point of attachment.

_____

_____

_____

True or False   Stability of attachment is characteristic in health, and treatment procedures may be aimed to obtain an increase in attachment.

_____

_____

_____

True or False   The probing depth is greater than the clinical attachment level when there is visible recession.

_____

_____

True or False   To calculate attachment if the gingival margin is above the cementoenamel junction, subtract the distance (in millimeters) from the cementoenamel junction to the gingival crest from the total probing depth.

_____

_____

_____

True or False A tooth with fremitus has excess contact, possibly related to a premature contact.

_____

_____

_____

True or False Probing depth is greater than the clinical attachment level when the cementoenamel junction is covered by free gingiva.

_____

_____

_____

True or False Inflammation in the periodontal ligament leads to degeneration or destruction of the fibers.

_____

_____

_____

True or False Anatomic variations that complicate furcation examination are fused roots; anomalies, such as extra roots; and low or high furcations.

_____

_____

_____

True or False To examine a furcation, you may use the probe in a diagonal or a horizontal position to examine between roots when there is gingival recession or a flexible, short, soft pocket wall that permits access; or you can use a furcation probe, such as a Nabers 1N or 2N, to examine advanced furcation.

_____

_____

_____

True or False To examine the mucogingival junction, look for blanching at the mucogingival junction while doing the tension test.

_____

_____

True or False Mucogingival involvement is not present when the probe passes through the pocket directly into the alveolar mucosa.

_____

_____

_____

True or False When periodontal disease is not active, pocket formation and migration of the attachment along the cemental surface continue.

_____

_____

_____

True or False Subtract the probing depth from the total gingival measurement to get the width of the attached gingiva.

_____

_____

_____

True or False Whether a shank is straight, curved, or angulated depends on the use and adaptation for which the explorer was designed.

_____

_____

_____

True or False The slender, wire-like working end of an explorer has a degree of flexibility that contributes to decreased tactile sensitivity.

_____

_____

_____

True or False For increased acute tactile sensitivity, a lightweight handle is more effective.

_____

_____

_____

True or False A wide-diameter instrument handle with serrations for friction while grasping can prevent finger cramping from too tight a grasp.

_____

_____

_____

True or False With a lighter grasp, tactile sensitivity can be decreased.

_____

_____

_____

True or False When an explorer tip is sharp and tapered, more pressure is required to increase tactile sensitivity.

_____

_____

_____

True or False The function of each type of explorer is related to its adaptability to specific surfaces of teeth at particular angulations.

_____

_____

_____

True or False Because fremitus depends on tooth-to-tooth contact, determination is made only on the mandibular teeth.

_____

_____

_____

True or False When inflammation is present and a pocket extends to or through the mucogingival junction, a streak of color (red, bluish red) that shows the inflammatory changes from the gingival margin to the mucogingival junction may be apparent.

_____

_____

_____

True or False The periodontal ligament is connective tissue and hence appears in a radiograph as a black radiolucent line next to the root surface.

_____

_____

_____

True or False The development of the ability to use an explorer and a probe is achieved first by learning the anatomic features of each tooth surface and the types of irregularities that may be encountered on the surfaces.

_____

_____

_____

True or False Probes vary in diameter; the thicker types may provide greater tactile sensitivity.

_____

_____

_____

True or False As an explorer or probe moves over the surface of enamel, cementum, a metallic restoration, a plastic restoration, or any irregularity of tooth structure or restoration, a particular surface texture is apparent. With each contact, sound may be created.

_____

_____

_____

True or False The probing depth equals the clinical attachment level when the free gingival margin is level with the cementoenamel junction.

_____

_____

_____

True or False When the probe is used, it is quiet over clean, smooth enamel but is scratchy or noisy on rough cementum or calculus. Sometimes a metallic restoration may cause a squeak or metallic ring. With experience, the clinician can differentiate among surfaces.

_____

_____

_____

True or False A rating of I means the tooth shows severe mobility and may move in all directions, vertically as well as horizontally.

_____

_____

_____

True or False With adequate light, a source of air, proper retraction, and the use of a mouth mirror, dried supragingival calculus can generally be seen as either chalky white or brownish yellow in contrast to the tooth color. A minimum of exploration can confirm the finding.

_____

_____

_____

True or False An intact surface where remineralization may be occurring must be explored vigorously. An aggressive examination can be made by using the side of the explorer's tip.

_____

_____

_____

True or False Calculus deposits may obstruct direct passage of the probe to the base of the pocket. Lift the tip slightly away from the tooth surface and follow over the deposit to proceed to the base of the pocket.

_____

_____

_____

True or False Tactile sensations pass through the instrument to the fingers and hand and to the brain for registration and action.

_____

_____

_____

True or False When probing, you can use a walking stroke in a vertical or diagonal (oblique) direction.

_____

_____

_____

True or False The depth of the stroke used during exploring depends on the skill of the clinician.

_____

_____

_____

True or False In a shallow pocket, the exploring stroke may extend the entire depth, from the base of the pocket to just beneath the gingival margin.

_____

_____

_____

True or False In a deep pocket, controlled strokes 2 to 3 -mm long can provide more acute sensitivity to the surface and allow improved adaptation of the instrument.

_____

_____

_____

True or False A deep pocket should be explored in sections. First explore the apical area next to the base of the pocket, then move up to a higher section, overlapping for full coverage.

_____

_____

_____

True or False Trauma to the gingival margin caused by repeated withdrawal and reinsertion of an instrument can cause the patient posttreatment discomfort.

_____

_____

_____

True or False Roll the explorer instrument handle between the fingers to keep the tip closely adapted as the tooth's contour changes.

_____

_____

_____

True or False Subgingival calculus is most commonly confined to the lingual surfaces of the mandibular anterior teeth and the facial surfaces of the maxillary first and second molars, opposite the openings to the salivary ducts.

_____

_____

_____

True or False To determine the width of the total gingiva, place the probe on the external surface of the gingiva and measure from the mucogingival junction to the gingival margin.

_____

_____

_____

True or False Mobility can be considered abnormal or pathologic when it exceeds normal. Increased mobility can be an important clinical sign of disease.

_____

_____

_____

True or False When a pocket extends into a furcation area, special adaptation of the probe must be made to determine the extent and topography of the furcation involvement.

_____

_____

_____

True or False A double-ended instrument has two working ends, one on each end of a common handle.

_____

_____

_____

True or False A thick explorer usually gives a more acute sense of tactile discrimination to small irregularities than does a fine explorer.

_____

_____

_____

True or False A rating of + means the tooth displays 1° of fremitus; significant vibration can be felt.

_____

_____

_____

True or False On a radiograph, the evidence of health can be identified when the crestal lamina dura is indistinct, irregular, radiolucent, and fuzzy.

_____

_____

_____

True or False Early furcation involvement may appear as a small radiolucent black dot or as a slight thickening of the periodontal ligament space, which can be confirmed by probing.

_____

_____

_____

12. You want to detect the adequacy of the width of the attached gingiva. You decide to conduct a mucogingival examination. Describe the procedure you will use to detect the adequacy of the frenal attachment.

_____

_____

_____

_____

_____

13. Match each tooth with the appropriate anatomic features. There are two answers for each type of tooth.

TYPE OF TOOTH	ANATOMIC FEATURES
_____ and _____ mandibular molars	A. Furcation area is accessible from the mesial and distal aspects under the contact area
_____ and _____ maxillary molars	B. Palatal root and two buccal roots (mesiobuccal and distobuccal); access for probing is from the mesial, buccal, and distal surfaces
_____ and _____ maxillary first premolars	
_____ and _____ maxillary primary molars	
_____ and _____ mandibular primary molars	C. Bifurcation
	D. Widespread roots
	E. Furcation area is accessible from the facial and lingual surfaces
	F. Trifurcation

14. Fill in the blanks to help you learn about the general purposes and uses of the explorer.

   ▓ *An explorer can detect, using _____ sense, the character of the tooth surface and examine the tooth surfaces for _____ and _____ lesions.*

   ▓ *An explorer is used to locate irregularities on the tooth surfaces and _____ of restorations and other irregularities that are not apparent by direct observation.*

   ▓ *An explorer is also used to _____ direct observations. It allows the clinician to define the extent of instrumentation that is needed.*

   ▓ *The explorer is used to _____ the completeness of treatment by identifying a _____ tooth surface or restoration.*

15. Match the tooth surface irregularities with the correct tactile sensation. Each answer is used more than once.

TOOTH SURFACE IRREGULARITY	TACTILE SENSATION
_____ Enamel pearl	A. Normal
_____ Smooth surface of enamel	B. Irregular: increases or elevations in tooth surface
_____ Carious lesion	C. Irregular: depressions, grooves
_____ Anatomic configurations, such as cingula, furcations	
_____ Abrasion	
_____ Root surface that has been planed	
_____ Calculus	
_____ Erosion	
_____ Irregular margins (overhang)	
_____ Pits such as those caused by enamel hypoplasia	
_____ Areas of cemental resorption on the root surface	
_____ Unusually pronounced cementoenamel junction	
_____ Deficient margins	
_____ Overcontoured restoration	
_____ Rough surface of a restoration	

COMPETENCY EXERCISES

1. Your employer, Dr. Harriet Golden, asks you to put together instrument kits for the office and label them "basic setup." Identify the instruments you have placed in the kit, and discuss why you have included each one.

   _____

   _____

   _____

   _____

   _____

   _____

2. Whenever you are using air, you should take care to avoid some very specific situations that may hurt or startle the patient. Identify two situations, and describe how you would avoid them.

   _____

   _____

   _____

   _____

   _____

   _____

3. When your instructor verifies your probing, many differences are found. You are having difficulty and need to look at the factors that affect probe determinations and probing procedures. Knowing the right question to ask yourself is a great way to solve a problem. Develop questions that will help you look at these factors and allow you to critique your own performance.

   _____

   _____

   _____

   _____

4. You are asked to standardize the procedure for periodontal charting in your office. Identify and provide a rationale for each factor to be documented on the periodontal chart.

   _____

   _____

   _____

   _____

   _____

   _____

5. Identify the number on the handle of each explorer in your student kit. Describe each using the following design and use terms.

   ◾ *Working end*

   _____

   _____

   _____

   ◾ *Design (single/paired)*

   _____

   _____

   _____

   ◾ *Handle (weight, diameter)*

   _____

   _____

   _____

   ◾ *Construction (single-ended/double-ended)*

   _____

   _____

   _____

   ◾ *Function*

   _____

   _____

   _____

◾ *Use*

_____

_____

_____

◾ *Adaptability*

_____

_____

◾ *Subgingival effectiveness*

_____

_____

◾ *Sickle or shepherd's hook*

_____

_____

◾ *Pigtail or cowhorn*

_____

_____

◾ *Straight*

_____

_____

_____

Everyday Ethics

Refer to the Codes of Ethics (Appendices I, II, and III in the textbook) and Framework for Making Decisions (Table 1-2 in the textbook) as you discuss the following scenario with your classmates.

Mrs. Claren, a neat-appearing lady in her 50s, was new to the practice. After a careful history recording, Doris, the dental hygienist, started the gingival examination and continued into the routine probing. Many of the probing depths were 3 and 4 mm, and some even 5 mm. Doris could feel subgingival calculus as she probed, and there was bleeding from her gentle probing.

Doris was nearly finished and was recording findings when the patient raised her head and said, "You aren't cleaning my teeth. What is it you are doing?" Suddenly Doris realized that this lady may never have had a complete periodontal examination and was unaware of her moderate to severe chronic periodontitis with generalized subgingival calculus.

Questions for Consideration

1. What ethical responsibility does a dental hygienist have to first-time patients to explain all procedures and educate about observations made while gathering assessment information?
2. When and why (or why not) would a dental hygienist need to obtain informed consent before complete examination and developing a treatment plan?
3. Which of the dental hygiene core values come into play in this scenario between Doris and Mrs. Claren? (For core values, see page 12 and Table II-1. page 20.)

6. Your patient, Tony Wade, presents with both mobility (III on teeth 22–27) and fremitus (+ on teeth 6–11). You note generalized bleeding and probe readings of 5 to 6 mm. The radiographs show horizontal bone loss in all posterior and anterior areas and vertical bone loss on the distal side of tooth 29. The crestal lamina dura is indistinct, irregular, and radiolucent throughout Tony's mouth. There are furcation involvements on teeth 30 and 31. The periodontal ligament spaces are thickened on teeth 28 and 29. Describe how the pocket depth, mobility, and fremitus findings were determined.

_____

_____

_____

7. Label the radiograph in **Figure 13-2** with the following findings.

Findings

■ *Horizontal bone loss*
■ *Vertical bone loss*
■ *Change in crestal lamina dura*
■ *Furcation involvement*
■ *Changes in the periodontal ligament*

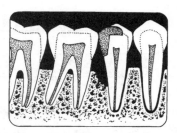

FIGURE 13-2

Factors To Teach The Patient

You have completed assessment procedures for Tony Wade (described in Competency Exercise 6). She is very confused about all the tests you have just performed and what all the information means. She wants you to take the time to explain all the data you have collected and the significance of the information you have identified.

Use the example of a patient conversation in Appendix B as a guide to create a conversation to explain to Tony the need for a careful examination, why bleeding can occur, the relationship of probing depth measurements to normal sulci, and the significance of the mobility. Be sure to refer to the figure you labeled in Competency Exercise 7 to illustrate some of your points. You may find it helpful to draw some pictures when discussing probing depths. *This scenario is related to the following factors:*

■ The need for a careful, thorough examination if treatment is to be complete and effective
■ Information about the instruments and how their use makes the examination complete (e.g., the complete radiographic survey, probing 360° around each tooth, and exploring each subgingival tooth surface)
■ Why bleeding can occur when probing (healthy tissue does not bleed)
■ The relation of probing depth measurements to normal sulci
■ The significance of mobility

CHAPTER 14

Periodontal Disease Development

Chapter Outline

Learning Objectives

Upon successful completion of these exercises, you will be able to:

1. Identify and define key terms and concepts related to the development of periodontal disease.
2. Classify and describe periodontal diseases and conditions.
3. Discuss the development of gingival and periodontal infections.
4. Identify risk factors for development of periodontal disease.

KNOWLEDGE EXERCISES

Terms and Concepts Word Search Puzzle

To solve the puzzle, first solve the clues; then find the answers in the grid. The answers can run across, down, or diagonally and can start at the right or left or top or bottom. When you have found all the words, the **first 40 unused letters in the grid** will spell out a hidden message.

Hidden message: Many factors contribute to the development of oral disease, but

_____

_____

```
D  E  N  T  A  F  L  C  B  I  O  F  I  L  N  M  I  S
T  H  D  G  E  P  O  R  O  I  M  A  R  O  Y  A  E  T
I  O  E  I  L  O  G  O  I  L  C  F  I  A  M  C  T  O
R  X  S  N  R  N  M  C  D  C  L  T  W  E  Z  K  M  G
L  P  Q  G  R  R  G  N  N  I  A  A  D  M  R  K  X  Q
N  E  U  I  H  K  B  X  X  R  M  E  G  X  F  I  K  R
M  R  A  V  M  C  V  H  T  T  Z  P  T  E  R  T  E  F
F  M  M  I  P  Y  M  L  F  I  Q  K  A  T  N  F  D  C
W  E  A  T  P  E  I  N  A  M  K  J  A  C  R  A  B  N
Z  A  T  I  V  F  R  T  D  H  Y  C  K  A  T  K  S  J
R  B  I  S  N  N  R  I  C  L  I  C  C  L  J  I  C  E
X  L  O  I  I  O  A  B  O  C  F  T  J  M  D  Z  O  G
C  E  N  X  G  S  T  H  K  D  O  L  E  S  I  O  N  N
X  Z  O  E  T  X  W  N  V  R  O  T  D  N  W  L  J  J
Z  T  N  E  N  J  F  D  Y  F  Y  N  G  M  N  Q  V  X
N  I  M  Q  C  O  L  L  A  G  E  N  T  P  H  Y  G  R
C  A  X  E  R  O  S  T  O  M  I  A  Y  I  V  C  T  N
H  N  V  P  V  F  L  C  D  G  M  N  K  R  T  Y  Z  T
T  B  A  C  T  E  R  I  A  L  T  O  X  I  N  I  N  N
R  G  E  N  Z  Y  M  E  M  T  N  Y  K  N  M  W  S  T
```

Word-Search Clues

- Any pathologic or traumatic discontinuity of tissue or loss of function of a part; refers to wounds, sores, ulcers, tumors, and any other tissue damage
- Term used to describe a variety of inflammatory and degenerative diseases that affect the supporting structures of the teeth (two words)
- White fibers of the connective tissue
- Poison; protein produced by certain animals, higher plants, and pathogenic bacteria
- Resulting from treatment by a professional healthcare provider
- Shedding of the outer epithelial layer of the stratified squamous epithelium of skin or mucosa
- Accumulation of excessive fluid in cells or tissues
- Not readily responsive to treatment
- Forceful wedging of food into the periodontium by occlusal forces (two words)
- Inflammation of the gingival tissues
- A space or abnormal opening; in dentistry, a space between two adjacent teeth in the same dental arch
- The diffusion or accumulation in a tissue or cells of substances not normal to it or in amounts in excess of normal
- Enzyme that catalyzes the degradation (hydrolysis) of collagen
- Inflammation in the periodontium affecting gingival tissues, periodontal ligament, cementum, and supporting bone
- Protein secreted by body cells that acts as a catalyst to induce chemical changes in other substances but remains unchang*ed itself*
- Permitting passage of a fluid
- Poison produced by bacteria; includes exotoxins, endotoxins, and toxic enzymes (two words)
- Dryness of the mouth from a lack of normal secretions
- Fibrous tissue left after the healing of a wound

Knowledge Exercises

1. Using the information in Table 14-2A in the textbook, describe the types of biofilm-induced gingival diseases.

   _____

   _____

   _____

   _____

   _____

   _____

2. Fill in the blanks to complete the following sentences.

   ▓ _Three bacteria that can lead to gingival lesions are_ _____, _____, _and_ _____.

   ▓ _Gingival diseases of viral origin are_ _____ _infections, primary_ _____ _gingivostomatitis, recurrent_ _____, _and_ _____ _infections._

   ▓ _Gingival diseases of fungal origin can be the result of_ _____ _species infections, such as generalized gingival_ _____, _____ _gingival erythema, and histoplasmosis._

   ▓ _An example of a gingival lesion of genetic origin is hereditary gingival_ _____.

   ▓ _Gingival manifestations of systemic conditions include mucocutaneous disorders such as_ _____, _____, _____, _____, _and_ _____.

   ▓ _Gingival lesions may be caused by allergic reactions to dental restorative materials, such as mercury,_ _____, _and_ _____.

   ▓ _Gingival lesions can be caused by reactions attributable to dental-care products, such as_ _____ _and_ _____, _as well as chewing gum and food_ _____.

   ▓ _The gingiva may suffer from traumatic lesions (factitious, iatrogenic, accidental) caused by_ _____, _____, _or_ _____ _injury or by reactions to_ _____ _bodies._

   ▓ _When all avenues of cause have been investigated without satisfaction, you may need to use the term_ _____.

3. How is the location of chronic and aggressive periodontitis described?

   _____

   _____

4. Periodontitis as a manifestation of systemic disease can be associated with hematologic disorders. Name some conditions in which you may find this association may be found.

   _____

   _____

   _____

5. Periodontitis can be associated with genetic disorders. Name some conditions in which this association may be found.

   _____

   _____

   _____

   _____

   _____

   _____

   _____

6. Name the necrotizing periodontal diseases.

   _____

   _____

   _____

7. List types of abscesses of the periodontium.

   _____

   _____

   _____

8. You may find periodontitis associated with endodontic lesions. These are referred to as

   _____

9. Periodontitis as a manifestation of systemic disease can be associated with _____ or acquired deformities and conditions.

10. Localized tooth-related factors that modify or predispose the area to biofilm-induced gingival diseases/periodontitis include tooth anatomic factors, dental _____, root fractures, cervical _____ resorption, and cemental tears.

11. Mucogingival deformities and conditions around the teeth that are manifestations of systemic disease include gingival _____, lack of _____ gingiva, _____ vestibular depth, aberrant frenum/muscle position, and gingival excess.

12. Occlusal trauma is classified as _____ or _____ and is noted as a manifestation of periodontitis associated with systemic disease.

13. Match each descriptive statement with the appropriate stage of development of gingivitis and periodontal disease. Each answer may be used more than once.

DEVELOPMENTAL STAGE	DESCRIPTION
A. Initial lesion B. Early lesion C. Established lesion D. Advanced lesion	_____ Inflammation spreads through the bone marrow and out into the periodontal ligament _____ Inflammatory response to biofilm occurs within 2–4 days _____ Fluid and leukocyte migration into tissues and sulcus increase; plasma cells are related to areas of chronic inflammation _____ Pocket formation, mobility, bone loss as signs of periodontitis _____ Biofilm becomes older and thicker (7–14 days; time reflects individual differences) _____ Exposed cementum where Sharpey fibers were attached becomes altered by inflammatory products of bacteria and the sulcus fluid _____ Clear evidence of inflammation is present, with marginal redness, bleeding on probing, and spongy marginal gingiva; later, chronic fibrosis develops _____ Periods of inactivity alternating with periods of activity can be expected _____ Proliferation of the junctional and sulcular epithelium continues in an attempt to wall out the inflammation _____ Migration and infiltration of white blood cells into the junctional epithelium and gingival sulcus _____ Inflammation spreads through the loose connective tissue along (beside) the blood vessels to the alveolar bone _____ Signs of gingivitis become apparent with slight gingival enlargement

_____ Connective tissue fibers below the junctional epithelium are destroyed; the epithelium migrates along the root surface

_____ No clinical evidence of change

_____ Alveolar bone destruction

_____ Infiltration of fluid, lymphocytes, and neutrophils with a few plasma cells into the connective tissue

_____ Bacteria from supragingival biofilm enter the sulcus and provide the source for subgingival biofilm

_____ The gingivitis is reversible when biofilm is controlled and inflammation is reduced; healthy tissue may be restored

_____ Progression to early periodontal lesion may occur, or some established lesions may remain stable for extended periods of time

_____ Diseased cementum contains a thin superficial layer of endotoxins from the bacterial breakdown

_____ Formation of pocket epithelium

_____ Increased flow of gingival sulcus fluid

_____ Without treatment, the pocket becomes progressively deepened

14. In your own words, define and describe a periodontal pocket. Include the following in your description:

   ■ *What distinguishes a pocket from a sulcus?*
   ■ *Describe the walls and the base of a pocket.*
   ■ *Compare the histology of a healthy pocket and the histiopathology of a diseased pocket.*

   _____

   _____

   _____

   _____

   _____

   _____

15. Use the following terms to label **Figure 14-1** on the next page, which illustrates types of periodontal pockets.

   ■ *Normal relationship*
   ■ *Gingival pocket*
   ■ *Periodontal pocket*
   ■ *Suprabony*

- Intrabony
- Cementoenamel junction
- Enamel
- Cementum
- Alveolar bone
- Gingival tissue
- Calculus

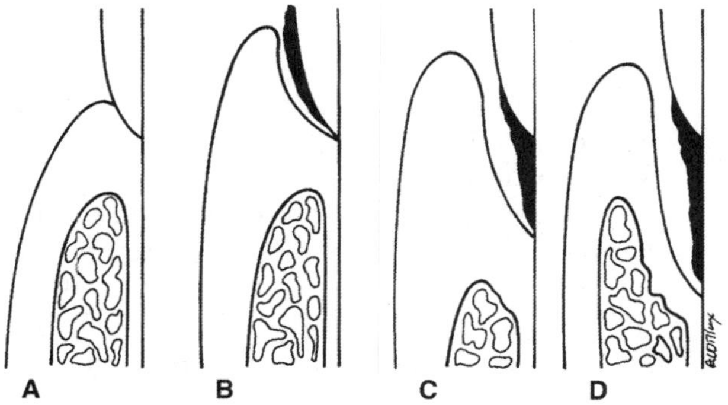

A   **B**   **C**   **D**

FIGURE 14-1

16. Fill in the blanks to complete the following sentences about **gingival** pockets.

- A gingival pocket is a pocket formed by gingival _____ without apical migration of the _____.

- The margin of the gingiva has moved toward the _____ or _____ direction, without the deeper periodontal structures becoming involved.

- The tooth wall is _____. During eruption, the base of the _____ is at various levels along the wall.

- The base of the sulcus of a fully erupted tooth is near the _____ junction.

- All gingival pockets are _____—that is, the base of the pocket is coronal to the crest of the alveolar bone.

17. Fill in the blanks to complete the following sentences about **periodontal** pockets.

- A periodontal pocket is formed as a result of disease or degeneration that caused the _____ to migrate apically along the _____.

- The periodontal deeper structures (attachment apparatus) involved in periodontal pocketing are the _____, _____ ligament, and _____.

- The tooth wall is _____ or partly _____ and partly enamel.

- The _____ of the pocket is on cementum at the level of the attached periodontal tissue.

- Periodontal pockets may be _____ or intrabony.

- When the base of the pocket is coronal to the crest of the alveolar bone, the pocket is _____.

- When the base of the pocket is below or apical to the crest of the alveolar bone, the pocket is _____.

18. Match each of the following definitions with the correct term.

FACTOR	DEFINITION
A. Etiologic factor B. Predisposing factor C. Risk factor D. Contributing factor E. Local factor F. Systemic factor	_____ A factor that lends assistance to, supplements, or adds to a condition or disease _____ A factor that results from or is influenced by a general physical or mental disease or condition _____ A factor that is the actual cause of a disease or condition _____ A factor in the immediate environment of the oral cavity or specifically in the environment of the teeth or periodontium _____ A factor that renders a person susceptible to a disease or condition _____ An exposure that increases the probability that disease will occur

19. In your own words, describe the sequence of natural self-cleansing mechanisms that happen during and after mastication.

_____

_____

_____

_____

_____

_____

_____

_____

_____

_____

_____

_____

COMPETENCY EXERCISES

1. After probing, you determine that disease is limited to the gingiva. Discuss the care-planning objectives and some questions you may have for your patient.

   _____

   _____

   _____

   _____

   _____

   _____

2. Your next patient presents with apical positioning of the periodontal attachment, with alveolar bone loss and other indications of periodontitis. List some questions, concerns, and general guidelines you consider as you start to plan treatment for this patient.

   _____

   _____

   _____

   _____

   _____

   _____

3. As you assess your patient Chu His, you observe that clear evidence of inflammation is present, with marginal redness, bleeding on probing, and spongy marginal gingival. He has a history of diabetes, _Candidiasis_ infections, and an allergy to dental restorative materials. Describe the disease classification you would use for this patient.

   _____

   _____

   _____

4. You detect a class II furcation on tooth 30 and a class III furcation involvement on tooth 31 as you collect data for your 10:00 patient, Woody Green. Woody asks many questions and wants to understand what these terms mean. Explain the terms to him, and use drawings of the teeth to help describe the conditions.

   _____

   _____

   _____

5. You are asked to develop patient education materials for the practice you are in. You decide to focus on local contributing factors in disease development and to take a checklist approach to enable the staff to provide specific information to each patient when they are providing oral health education. Develop a checklist that identifies all the potential factors that contribute to oral disease.

   ▪ _Tooth surface irregularities_

   _____

   _____

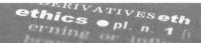

Everyday Ethics

Refer to the Codes of Ethics (Appendices I, II, and III in the textbook) and Framework for Making Decisions (Table 1-2 in the textbook) as you discuss the following scenario with your classmates.

Holly found it interesting that even after practicing dental hygiene for 5 years full-time, the "lightbulb" connecting certain conditions in the mouth with causative factors went on. While listening to Mr. Zajek complain about food impaction, Holly noted the poor contours of crowns in the premolar area lacking proximal contact, as well as loss of both mandibular first molars.

   Ideally, Mr. Zajek needed teeth to be repositioned and occlusal deviations to be corrected through orthodontic treatment. Holly hesitated to even mention it to Mr. Zajek because he was 55 years old. However, she found herself thinking that if Mr. Zajek was 25 years old, she wouldn't hesitate to recommend a referral to address these contributing factors.

Questions for Consideration
1. Is age alone a factor in this scenario that precludes the hygienist from presenting an "optimal" dental hygiene diagnosis and care plan? Explain why or why not.
2. Using the step-approach decision model, consider Mr. Zajek's existing oral findings and prioritize options for treatment that Holly can reference when developing a self-care plan for him.
3. Morally, is Holly obligated to spend extra appointment time convincing Mr. Zajek that he should seek referrals in another specialty dental office? Respond based on the duties and rights of both Holly and Mr. Zajek in the provider-patient relationship.

_____

_____

_____

_____

■ *Tooth contour factors*

_____

_____

_____

_____

_____

■ *Tooth position factors*

_____

_____

_____

_____

_____

■ *Dental prostheses factors*

_____

_____

_____

_____

_____

_____

■ *Gingival factors*

_____

_____

_____

_____

Factors To Teach The Patient

During data collection for your patient, Maria Manuela Rodriguez, you note the following:

■ She smokes two packs of cigarettes per day.
■ She takes 10 mg Fosamax (alendronate) per day to prevent/control osteoporosis.
■ There is a family history of diabetes.
■ She is overweight.
■ She takes 10 mg Procardia three times per day to treat her high blood pressure and ventricular arrhythmia (this is nifedipine, which is a calcium channel blocker).
■ She tends to have a soft diet.

Use the example of a patient conversation in Appendix B as a guide to write a statement explaining Maria's risk factors for periodontal disease.

Use the conversation you created to educate a patient or friend, and then modify it based on what you learned. *This scenario is related to following factors:*

■ Factors that contribute to disease development and progression
■ What a risk factor is and the importance of planning personal and professional care to include risk factor problems

_____

_____

■ *Personal factors*

_____

_____

_____

_____

_____

_____

15 CHAPTER

The Teeth

Chapter Outline

Learning Objectives

Upon successful completion of these exercises, you will be able to:

1. Identify and define key terms and concepts related to the teeth.
2. Discuss various types of dental caries in terms of classification, development, and detection.
3. Describe noncarious dental lesions and their causes and appearance.
4. Describe a clinical examination of the teeth.
5. Detail the development and eruption of permanent teeth.
6. Identify various strategies for the recognition of carious lesions and describe tests for vitality.

KNOWLEDGE EXERCISES

Terminology Crossword Puzzle

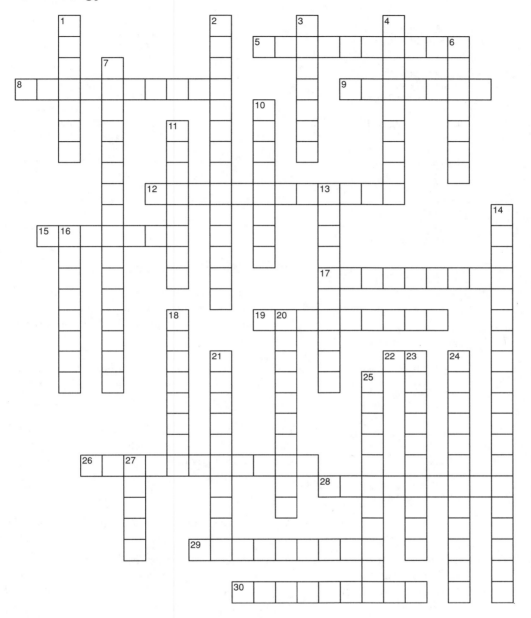

Across

5 Conducive to dental caries.
8 A calcified spherical body, composed of cementum, lying free within the periodontal ligament, attached to the cementum or imbedded within the cementum.
9 One of the terms used to refer to the first teeth; normally will be shed and replaced by permanent teeth.
12 Disease of the mineralized structures of the teeth characterized by demineralization of the hard components and dissolution of

the organic matrix (two words).
15 This term is used to describe the widespread formation of chalky white areas and incipient carious lesions that may increase in size over a comparatively short time.
17 Term used to refer to dental caries that occur on a surface adjacent to a restoration; may be a continuation of the original lesion; also called secondary caries.
19 The natural teeth in the dental arch.

22 The symbol of hydrogen ion concentration expressed in numbers corresponding to the acidity or alkalinity of an aqueous solution; the range is from 14 (pure base) to 0 (pure acid); neutral is at 7.0.
26 Loss of primary teeth following physiologic resorption of root structure.
28 A term that is used to refer to adult dentition; the natural 32 teeth that serve throughout life.
29 Refers to a secondary canal that extends from the pulp to the surface of

the root; frequently found near the apex of a root but may occur higher and provide a connection to a periodontal pocket.
30 Beginning; coming into existence.

Down

1 Term used to refer to dental caries that occur on a surface not previously affected; also called initial caries; early lesion may be referred to as incipient caries.
2 Combination of primary and permanent teeth

between ages 6 and 12 when primary teeth are being replaced; starts with the eruption of the first permanent tooth (two words).
3 An oral habit of grinding, clenching, or clamping the teeth; involuntary, rhythmic, or spasmodic movements outside the chewing range; may damage teeth and attachment apparatus.
4 One of the terms used to refer to the first teeth; normally will be shed and replaced by permanent teeth.
6 Used to define a carious lesion.
7 Incomplete or defective formation of the enamel of either primary or permanent teeth. The result may be an irregularity of tooth form, color, or surface (two words).
10 The science or study of the cause of a disease or disorder.
11 The term used to refer to a carious lesion that has become stationary and does not show a tendency to progress further; frequently has a hard surface and takes on a dark brown or reddish-brown color.
13 Removal of bone or tooth structure; gradual dissolution of the mineralized tissue; may be internal or external; occurs during exfoliation of a primary tooth and from the pressure of orthodontic treatment.
14 Refers to a patient when some, but not all, teeth are missing (two words).
16 The tearing away or forcible separation of a structure or part. Tooth avulsion is the traumatic separation of a tooth from the alveolus.
18 Refers to the pH at which demineralization occurs; for enamel, pH 4.5 to 5.5; for cementum, pH 6.0 to 6.7.
20 Without teeth.
21 Denoting a condition of unknown cause.
23 Incomplete development or underdevelopment of a tissue or organ.
24 Production and development of enamel.
25 A conductor; a substance that, in solution, dissociates into electrically charged particles (ions) and thus is capable of conducting an electric current.
27 A small flattened surface on a tooth that results from attrition or repeated parafunctional contact.

Matching Questions

1. Match the description with the correct term. Each term may be used more than once.

TERMINOLOGY	DESCRIPTION
A. Simple cavity B. Compound cavity C. Complex cavity D. Pit and fissure caries E. Smooth surface caries	_____ Covers mesio-occlusal-distal surfaces _____ Involves more than two tooth surfaces _____ Occlusal surfaces of molars _____ Covering two surfaces _____ Closure of the enamel plates is imperfect _____ Occurs in proximal tooth surfaces _____ Referred to as an M-O-D cavity _____ Mesio-occlusal cavity, for example _____ Occurs at the endings of grooves _____ Involves one tooth surface _____ and _____ The buccal groove of a mandibular molar, for example _____ Occurs on the cervical third of teeth _____ Referred to as a D-O cavity _____ and _____ Irregularity occurs where three or more lobes of the developing tooth join _____ Caries that begins in an area where there is no pit, groove, or other fault

2. The standard method for classifying dental caries was developed by Dr. G. V. Black. Match the description with the correct classification. Each classification may be used more than once.

G. V. BLACK CLASSIFICATIONS	DESCRIPTION
A. Class I B. Class II C. Class III D. Class IV E. Class V F. Class VI	_____ Cavities in pits or fissures _____ Cavities in the cervical third of facial or lingual surfaces (not pit or fissure) _____ Radiographs not useful for detection _____ Cavities in proximal surfaces of incisors or canines that involve the incisal angle

_____ Lingual surfaces of maxillary incisors
_____ Cavities in proximal surfaces of premolars
_____ and _____ Transillumination is useful for detection
_____ Facial and lingual surfaces of molars
_____ and _____ Early caries detected by radiographs
_____ Cavities in proximal surfaces of incisors and canines that do not involve the incisal angle
_____ Cavities on incisal edges of anterior teeth and cusp tips of posterior teeth
_____ Occlusal surfaces of premolars and molars

Fill-in-the-Blank Exercises

1. As you examine your next patient, you note a defect that occurs as a result of a disturbance in the formation of the organic enamel matrix. This condition is referred to as _____.

2. The condition you identified in question 1 is hereditary. This is defined as the enamel being partly or _____ missing. An example is _____.

3. Factors that may contribute to enamel hypoplasia during tooth development include _____ deficiency, particularly rickets, and fever-producing diseases, such as _____, chickenpox, and _____.

4. A visual examination can be used to identify dental caries.

   ■ _Initially, you should dry each tooth or group of teeth with _____ air and carefully inspect each surface._

   ■ _Characteristic changes in the _____ and _____ of tooth structure may be observed._

   ■ _Such changes are either _____ signs of dental caries progress or may lead the examiner _____ to dental caries, which can then be checked further with an explorer._

   ■ _Variations in color and translucency include _____ white areas of demineralization or _____ discoloration of marginal ridges caused by dental caries of the _____ surface underneath._

   ■ _Grayish white color spreading from the margins of _____ is caused by the lesions of secondary dental caries._

- In relation to an amalgam restoration, dental caries appears _____ in the outer portion and white or _____ adjacent to the amalgam.
- Open carious lesions may vary in color from _____ to _____.
- Discoloration is generally less severe when dental caries progresses _____ than when it progresses _____.
- Dull, flat, white _____ areas under direct light indicate loss of _____.
- A dark shadow on a proximal surface may be observed by using _____.
- This type of observation is especially useful for _____ teeth and unrestored posterior teeth.

5. An exploratory examination can be used to identify dental caries.
   - When exploring for smooth surface caries, the clinician adapts the side of the _____ of the explorer closely to the tooth surface.
   - Examine for _____ versus softness, for _____ versus smoothness, and for _____ of the tooth surface.
   - Do not use pressure or attempt to _____ the surface when checking for dental caries.
   - Follow the margins of all restorations around with an _____.
   - Overhanging margins may or may not appear in the radiographs because of overlapping or _____.
   - Chart irregularities of existing restorations. When a _____ or _____ is discolored, it is not possible to determine visually whether dental caries is present, except when a large obvious cavity can be seen.
   - An _____ should not be explored.

6. During the clinical examination, information revealed by radiographs is used for supplementation and confirmation.
   - Neither clinical nor radiographic examination is _____ without the other.
   - A few principal items to be seen in a radiographic examination of the teeth are _____, _____, _____, internal and root _____, dental caries, and _____ radiolucencies.
   - Periapical radiographs usually provide sufficient information concerning the teeth, but _____, _____, or _____ radiographs may be needed for detecting additional anomalies and pathologic lesions outside their scope.

- _____ or periapical radiographs made by a paralleling technique with no _____ are most satisfactory for dental caries detection.
- Mounted radiographs displayed on an adequately _____ view box are a necessity during _____ and treatment procedures.
- For the detection of early carious lesions on radiographs, a handheld _____ can be of invaluable assistance.

7. During the examination, it is important to remember the following.
   - Radiographs are not needed for _____, _____, or occlusal carious lesions because these lesions are accessible and best observed by _____ and _____ vision. Furthermore, because of superimposition of other parts of the tooth, these carious lesions need to be fairly well advanced before they are _____ in a radiograph.
   - _____ surface lesions may be missed if radiographs are not used.
   - Clinical skills for caries discernment need to be perfected to prevent excess patient exposure to unnecessary _____.
   - Properly angulated radiographs with no _____ are required for the detection of small lesions that involve the enamel or extend slightly into the dentin.
   - Dental caries under an overhanging filling may be present, even if none can be seen in the radiograph because of _____.
   - An explorer must be passed around the complete _____ of the filling to confirm dental caries.
   - Most _____ caries lesions occur in the vicinity of and just beneath the cementoenamel junction. These lesions appear as _____-shaped lesions in a radiograph.
   - Root caries may appear to _____ the enamel or may be located beneath an _____ filling.

Short-Answer Questions

1. Describe the appearance of various types of hypoplasia.

   _____

   _____

   _____

   _____

   _____

   _____

   _____

INFOMAP 15-1					
CONDITION	**DEFINITION**	**OCCURRENCE**	**ETIOLOGY**	**PREDISPOSING FACTORS**	**APPEARANCE**
ATTRITION					
EROSION					
ABRASION					

2. List the teeth most frequently affected by enamel hypoplasia. Why are these teeth affected?

_____

_____

_____

3. Complete Infomap 15-1 above to help you differentiate among attrition, erosion, and abrasion.

4. Your 10:30 patient, Radnor Davis, has presented with a fistula on tooth 9 that opens into the oral cavity. You take a radiograph and discover an apical radiolucency. There is a large carious lesion on the mesial surface. You use an electric pulp tester to perform a vitality test. For each possible test result, make a determination of the possible findings.

RESULT OF VITALITY TEST	**FINDING**
No response	_____
Lingering pain after removal of stimulus	_____
Pain subsides promptly	_____

5. List and describe the types of thermal tests you could perform.

_____

_____

_____

_____

_____

6. List and describe the factors that could be influencing Radnor's response or reaction to the thermal tests.

_____

_____

_____

_____

_____

_____

COMPETENCY EXERCISES

1. Your patient presents with both Class II and V dental caries. Describe how you detected each of these lesions.

_____

_____

_____

2. Your patient, Oliver Summerlin, uses a hard toothbrush and an abrasive nonfluoride-containing dentifrice. He wears a partial denture on the mandible and takes a medication that causes xerostomia. You note abrasion in all four quadrants and root caries on the facial surfaces of teeth 27 to 30. Differentiate abrasion from root caries, and discuss the prevention of both root caries and abrasion.

_____

_____

_____

_____

_____

3. Your patient at 3:00 is Paulo Jacoby. He is 16 years old, is an avid basketball player, and never wears a mouthguard. Describe potential oral injuries.

_____

_____

Everyday Ethics

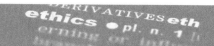

Refer to the Codes of Ethics (Appendices I, II, and III in the textbook) and Framework for Making Decisions (Table 1-2 in the textbook) as you discuss the following scenario with your classmates.

Barbara, the dental hygienist, has just finished a thorough review of oral hygiene instruction with Mrs. Canavan when she is called out of the treatment room. In today's examination, Barbara had charted two possible carious lesions that will need to be restored. Barbara wanted Mrs. Canavan to realize all the things she could do to prevent dental caries. Her 9-year-old daughter, Millie, had several restorations today at her appointment with the dentist in another treatment room, had finished first, and was waiting for her mom.

When Barbara returned, she could overhear Mrs. Canavan talking with her daughter and explaining how she got all the cavities. She described biofilm as painful and how "that's what happens when you eat a lot of candy and drink a lot of soft drinks instead of milk. "Barbara stopped to watch quietly. Apparently Millie seemed to understand that it is the biofilm that causes all her cavities, but she was not getting accurate information on the mechanism of action. Mrs. Canavan seemed to be threatening her daughter.

Questions for Consideration

1. Would it be ethical for Barbara to join the conversation and attempt to clarify for both of them? Could she help them both understand the real prevention plan?
2. Describe the positive and negative effects that may occur if Barbara should correct the mother in front of the daughter, or instead, if she asks the daughter to go back to the reception room, and then tries to discuss daily biofilm removal again with Mrs. Canavan.
3. Which of the core values or principles of ethical behavior come into play in patient education efforts such as described in this scenario?

4. Review the data collection forms that are used in your dental hygiene program. What form will you use to document each of the examination features that are listed in Table 15-4 in the textbook?

5. Clive Williams is 10 years old. He wants to know if he will get "more grown-up teeth." Explain to him the formative stages that his remaining teeth are in and the age at which most children can expect more permanent teeth to erupt.

 Factors To Teach The Patient

Andrea Carfagno has arrived in the reception area of the clinic. She is holding her 26-month-old daughter, Nicole, and her 9-month-old twin boys are in a stroller. Nicole is your patient today. The girl is holding a baby bottle filled with fruit punch. She is a happy, attentive youngster who is anxious to please.

Use the example of a patient conversation in Appendix B as a guide to write a statement explaining the need to have Nicole switch from a bottle to a cup. Be sure to address the use of fruit juices in a bottle and to explain early childhood caries. These issues pertain to both Nicole and her brothers.

Use the conversation you create to role play this situation with a fellow student. If you are the patient in the role play, be sure to ask questions. If you are the dental hygienist, try to anticipate questions and answer them in your explanation.

This scenario is related to the following factors:

■ The cause and process of enamel or root caries formation and development for the patients at risk
■ Methods for prevention of dental caries, such as fluorides, biofilm prevention and control, and control of cariogenic foods in the diet
■ Methods for prevention of early childhood caries (Nothing but plain water should be used in bedtime or nap-time nursing bottles. Avoid the use of a sweetener on a pacifier. Use of a cup for milk or juice by the baby's first birthday.)

6. Clive's cousin Jamal is 5 years old. He and Clive have a bet as to who still has the most teeth to erupt. Who will win the bet and why?

_____

_____

_____

7. Jamal's sister wants to get in on the bet. She is 15 years old and says she will not have any more teeth erupt because all of her teeth are in and she is a grown-up. She has never had any teeth extracted. Who will win the bet and why?

_____

_____

_____

The Occlusion

Learning Objectives

Upon successful completion of these exercises, you will be able to:

1. Identify and define key terms and concepts related to occlusion.
2. Classify malocclusions for both adult and child patients.
3. Discuss functional occlusion in terms of occlusal and proximal contacts.
4. Identify the types of trauma from occlusion, including clinical and radiographic findings.

KNOWLEDGE EXERCISES

1. Fill in the blanks in the following statements concerning facial profiles.

   ■ *Your patient presents with a prominent maxilla and a mandible posterior to its normal relationship.*
   ▪ *This is known as a convex, or _____, profile.*
   ■ *This patient's cousin has slightly protruded jaws, which give the facial outline a relatively flat appearance. This is known as a straight, or _____, profile.*
   ■ *The father of your patient is waiting in the reception area. He has a prominent, protruded mandible and a normal maxilla. This is known as a concave, or _____, profile.*

2. Match the following definitions with the correct term.

DEFINITION	TERMS
_____ Head-holding instrument used to obtain cephalometric radiographs	A. Centric relation
_____ Any deviation from the physiologically acceptable relationship of the maxillary arch and/or teeth to the mandibular arch and/or teeth	B. Trauma from occlusion
_____ Space between two adjacent teeth in the same arch	C. Centric occlusion
_____ All teeth in the maxillary arch are in maximum contact with all teeth in mandibular arch in a definite pattern; maxillary teeth slightly overlap the mandibular teeth on the facial surfaces	D. Parafunctional
_____ Migration with a healthy periodontium	E. Dental ankylosis
_____ Abnormal or deviated function	F. Orthodontic and dentofacial orthopedics
_____ Specialty area of dentistry concerned with the diagnosis, supervision, guidance, and treatment of the growing and mature dentofacial structures	G. Cephalostat
_____ Shiny, flat, worn spot on the surface of a tooth, frequently on the side of a cusp	H. Occlusal guard
_____ Orienting device for positioning the head for radiographic examination and measurement	I. Cephalometer
_____ Diastema, or gap, in the tooth row occasionally observed in the human primary dentition	J. Ankylosis
_____ Process of evaluating dental and skeletal relationships by way of measurements obtained directly from the head or from cephalometric radiographs and tracings made from the radiographs	K. Pathologic migration
_____ Occurs when disease is present	L. Cephalometric analysis
_____ Rigid fixation of a tooth to the surrounding alveolus as a result of ossification of the periodontal ligament; prevents eruption and orthodontic movement	M. Diastema
_____ Correction of abnormal form or relationship of bone structures	N. Occlusal prematurity
_____ Injury to the periodontium that results from occlusal forces in excess of the reparative capacity of the attachment apparatus	O. Orthopedics
_____ Removable dental appliance usually made of plastic that covers a dental arch and is designed to minimize the damaging effects of bruxism and other oral habits	P. Tongue thrust
_____ Any contact of opposing teeth that occurs before the desirable intercuspation	Q. Static occlusion
_____ Seen when jaws are closed in centric relation	R. Normal occlusion
_____ Consists of all contacts during chewing, swallowing, or other normal action	S. Malocclusion
_____ Most unstrained, retruded physiologic relation of the mandible to the maxilla from which lateral movements can be made	T. Functional occlusion
_____ Movement of a tooth out of its natural position as a result of periodontal infection; contrasts with mesial migration	U. Primate space
_____ Maximum intercuspation or contact of the teeth of the opposing arches; also called habitual occlusion	V. Facet
_____ Infantile pattern of suckle–swallow movement in which the tongue is placed between the incisor teeth or alveolar ridges	W. Pathologic migration
_____ Union or consolidation of two similar or dissimilar hard tissues previously adjacent but not attached	X. Drifting

3. Label each of the following figures (**Figures 16-1** to **16-15**) with the condition illustrated; then write a short description of that condition.

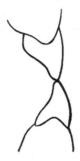

FIGURE 16-1

_____

_____

_____

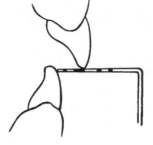

FIGURE 16-2

_____

_____

_____

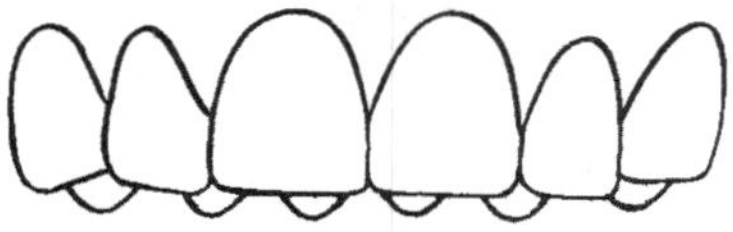

FIGURE 16-3

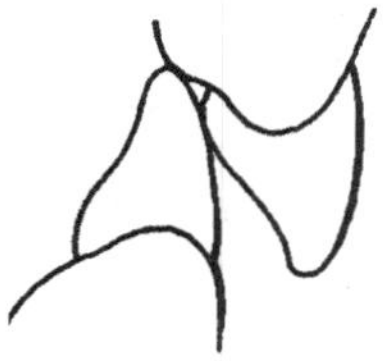

_____

_____

_____

FIGURE 16-7

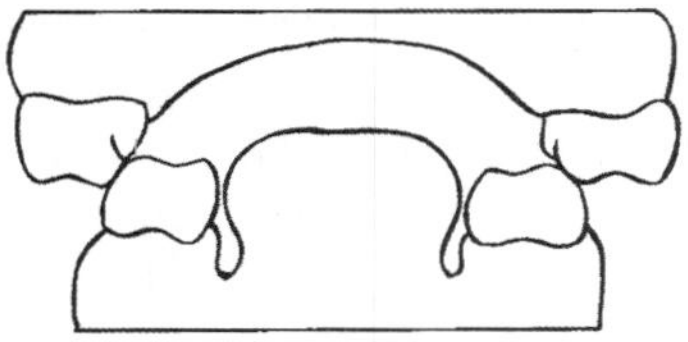

_____

_____

_____

FIGURE 16-4

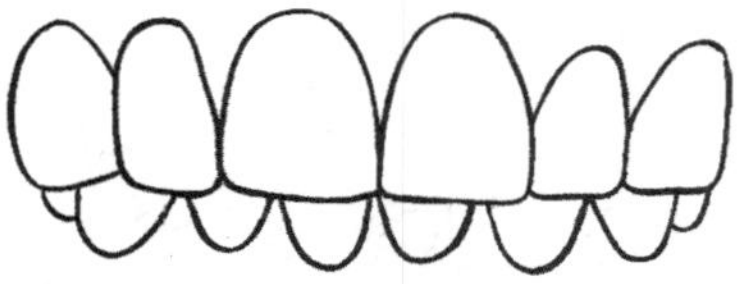

_____

_____

_____

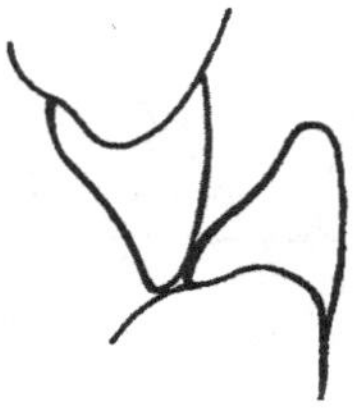

FIGURE 16-8

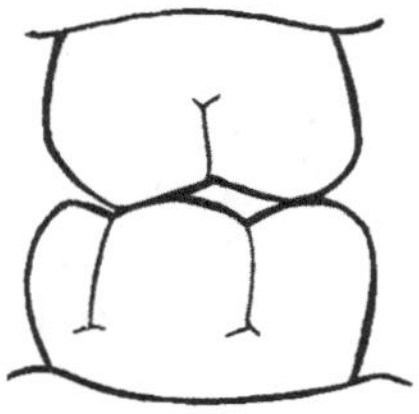

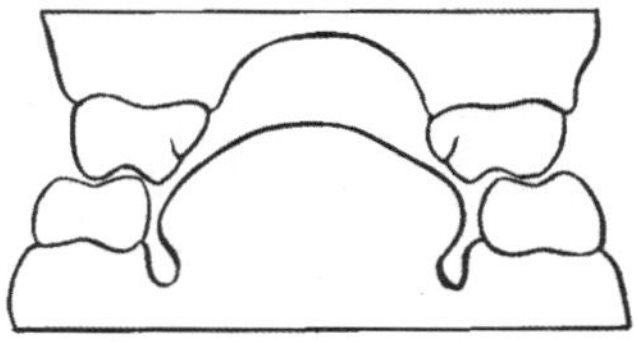

_____

_____

_____

FIGURE 16-5

_____

_____

_____

FIGURE 16-9

_____

_____

_____

FIGURE 16-6

_____

_____

_____

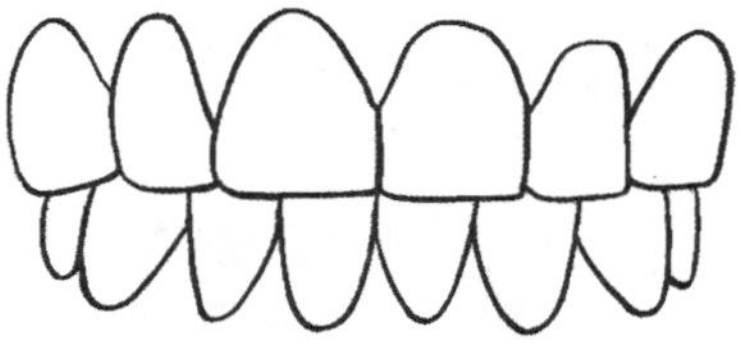

FIGURE 16-10

_____

_____

_____

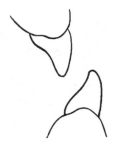

FIGURE 16-11

_____
_____
_____

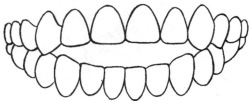

FIGURE 16-12

_____
_____
_____

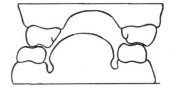

FIGURE 16-13

_____
_____
_____

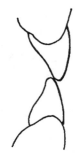

FIGURE 16-15

_____
_____
_____

4. Fill in the blanks as you think about the occlusion of the primary teeth.

■ _The primary canine relation is _____ the permanent dentition._

■ _When a patient has primate spaces in the _____ arch, you see these between the canine and first molar._

■ _In the _____ arch, you see primate spaces between the lateral incisor and canine._

■ _You can expect the second primary molar relation to appear as the _____ cusp of the maxillary second primary molar occluding with the _____ groove of the mandibular second primary molar._

■ _There can be variations in distal surface relationships called terminal steps. An example is when the _____ surface of the mandibular primary molar is _____ to that of the maxillary, thereby forming a mesial step._

■ _Although there can be morphologic variation in molar size, maxillary and mandibular primary molars are approximately the same in _____ width._

■ _When a patient has a terminal step, the first permanent molar erupts directly into _____ occlusion._

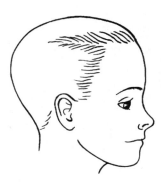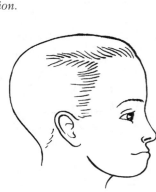

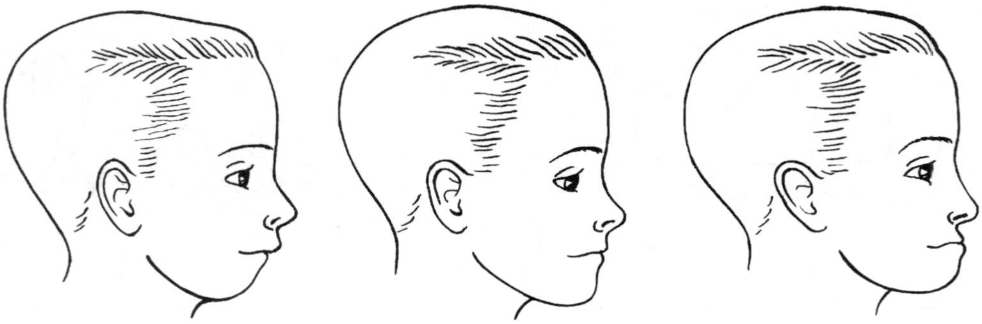

_____   _____   _____

FIGURE 16-14

■ *A terminal plane occurs when the _____ surfaces of the maxillary and mandibular primary _____ are on same _____ plane.*

■ *The maxillary molar is _____ mesiodistally than the mandibular molar.*

■ *When a patient has a terminal plane, the first permanent molars erupt _____ to _____.*

■ *Primate spaces affect the eruption of the first permanent molars. When there is a _____ primate space, an _____ mesial shift of the _____ molars into the primate space occurs, and the permanent mandibular molar shifts into proper occlusion.*

■ *When there are no primate spaces, a _____ mesial shift of the permanent mandibular molar into proper occlusion occurs after exfoliation of the _____ primary molar.*

■ *Malocclusions of primary teeth are _____ the permanent dentition.*

5. Functional occlusion consists of all contacts during chewing, swallowing, and other normal action. Functional occlusion is associated with performance. List some reasons why normal functional occlusion benefits the patient.

_____

_____

_____

6. Match each definition with the correct term. Each term is used more than once.

TERM	DEFINITION
A. Functional contact	____Made outside the normal range of function
B. Parafunctional contact	____When contact is lost, teeth can drift into spaces created by unreplaced missing teeth
C. Proximal contact	____This results from occlusal habits and neuroses
	____Normal contact that is made between the maxillary teeth and the mandibular teeth during chewing and swallowing
	____This is potentially injurious to the periodontal supporting structures, but only in the presence of bacterial plaque and inflammatory factors
	____Attrition or wear of the teeth occurs at this type of contact

____This creates wear facets and attrition on the teeth

____Each contact is momentary, so the total contact time is only a few minutes each day

____Tooth-to-tooth contact; bruxism, clenching, tapping

____This serves to stabilize the position of teeth in the dental arches and to prevent food impaction between the teeth

____Tooth-to-hard-object contact; nail biting, occupational use (tacks or pins), use of smoking equipment (pipestem or hard cigarette holder)

____Tooth-to-oral-tissues contact; lip or cheek biting

____Pathologic migration

7. Refer to Figure 16-16 below when answering the following questions.

■ *Using a red pencil, mark the teeth you will evaluate to determine this patient's occlusal classification.*

■ *Describe the tooth relationships that will influence your decision about the patient's occlusal classification.*

_____

_____

_____

■ *What is this patient's occlusal classification?*

_____

_____

_____

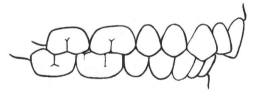

FIGURE 16-16

8. Refer to Figure 16-17 when answering the following questions.

■ *Using a red pencil, mark the teeth you will evaluate to determine this patient's occlusal classification.*

■ *Describe the tooth relationships that will influence your decision about the patient's occlusal classification.*

_____

_____

_____

■ *What is this patient's occlusal classification?*

_____

_____

_____

_____

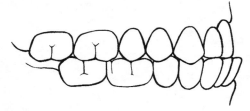

FIGURE 16-17

9. Refer to Figure 16-18 below when answering the following questions.

■ *Using a red pencil, mark the teeth you will evaluate to determine this patient's occlusal classification.*

■ *Describe the tooth relationships that will influence your decision about the patient's occlusal classification.*

_____

_____

■ *What is this patient's occlusal classification?*

_____

_____

_____

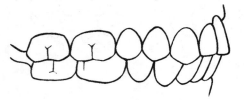

FIGURE 16-18

10. Refer to Figure 16-19 below when answering the following questions.

■ *Using a red pencil, mark the teeth you will evaluate to determine this patient's occlusal classification.*

■ *Describe the tooth relationships that will influence your decision about the patient's occlusal classification.*

_____

_____

_____

■ *What is this patient's occlusal classification?*

_____

_____

_____

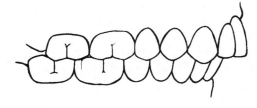

FIGURE 16-19

COMPETENCY EXERCISES

1. You are performing an examination to determine if your patient has an overbite. Describe the strategies you will use and how you will describe your findings. Which figures from Knowledge Exercises question 3 will help you explain an overbite to your patient?

_____

_____

_____

_____

_____

_____

2. You are asked to explain an overjet. Which figure from Knowledge Exercises question 3 will help you do this? Describe the procedure for evaluating an overjet, then go back to the figure from the

Everyday Ethics

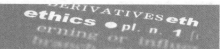

Refer to the Codes of Ethics (Appendices I, II, and III the textbook) and Framework for Making Decisions (Table 1-2 in the textbook) as you discuss the following scenario with your classmates.

Many of the first-year dental hygiene students struggled to learn the specific classifications of malocclusion and how to recognize them in their patients.

    The problem was often a locker room discussion item, and it was agreed that they noticed that the instructors didn't always look for the details of a patient's occlusion when the record was checked.

    One clinic day Roxanne was confused, and she decided to just write anything down on the patient's chart.

When the instructor came to check the oral examination, she questioned why Roxanne had the classification documented as a Class II (distoclusion). The student just shrugged her shoulders and said, "I don't know."

Questions for Consideration

1. What are the issues with Roxanne's apparent lack of knowledge about occlusion and saying "I don't know" to her teacher?
2. What should Roxanne do to be more accurate with her clinical charting and documentation?
3. Can Roxanne "justify" her actions to the patient and to the instructor? Give a rationale.

Knowledge Exercises and measure the overjet reading for this patient.

_____

_____

_____

3. Your patient Song Yee presents with chronic, generalized, moderate periodontal disease. Song just had new restorations placed on teeth 30 and 3. You are concerned about her occlusion, because you have seen evidence of both primary and secondary trauma in her mouth. She wants to understand the term you used and to understand these concepts by being given an example of what you saw in her mouth. Explain to Song the clinical and radiographic findings that you have evaluated to determine that her occlusion is a factor in her periodontal disease.

_____

_____

_____

_____

_____

_____

Factors To Teach The Patient

Your patient, Placido Perez, is a 35-year-old insurance salesman. He is overweight and reports that he can eat only soft foods because of the way he bites. Although Placido admires that famous late-night talk show host that everyone tells him he looks like, he is unhappy with his appearance. He presents with a class III malocclusion.

    Use the example of a patient conversation in Appendix B as a guide to write a statement explaining the figures in Knowledge Exercises questions 7 to 10 to show Placido what you see in his mouth and what ideal occlusion looks like. Explain why referral to an orthodontist may be recommended.

    Use the conversation you create to role play this situation with a fellow student. If you are the patient in the role play, be sure to ask questions. If you are the dental hygienist, try to anticipate questions and answer them in your explanation.

This scenario is related to the following factors:

- Interpretation of the general purposes of orthodontic care (function and aesthetics) to patients referred by the dentist to an orthodontist
- Dependence of masticatory efficiency on the occlusion of the teeth
- Influence of masticatory efficiency on food selection in the diet
- Influence of masticatory efficiency and diet on the nutritional status of the body and oral health

17 | CHAPTER

Dental Biofilm and Other Soft Deposits

Chapter Outline

Learning Objectives

Upon successful completion of these exercises, you will be able to:

1. Identify and define key terms and concepts related to oral soft deposits.
2. Differentiate dental biofilm from pellicle, materia alba, and food debris in terms of composition, significance, and detection.
3. Discuss the implications of dental biofilm in terms of periodontal disease and caries.
4. Describe the essentials for dental caries as well as other contributing factors.

KNOWLEDGE EXERCISES

Biofilm Terms Crossword Puzzle

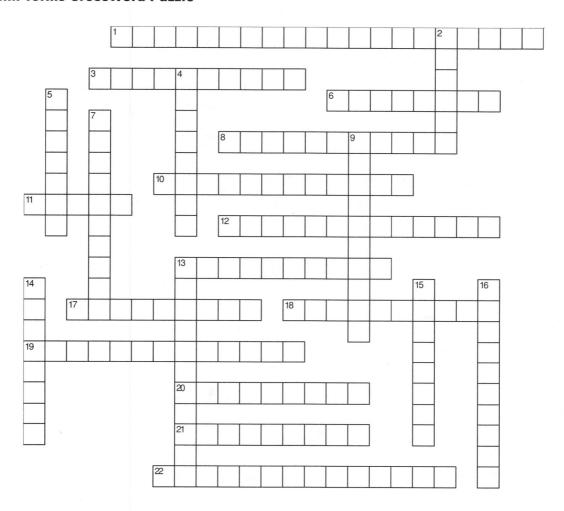

Across

1 Material present between bacteria in dental biofilm; derived from saliva and gingival exudate. (two words).
3 Any organism, such as bacteria, that lives upon dead or decaying organic matter.
6 Heterotrophic microorganism that lives and grows in complete (or almost complete) absence of oxygen; some are obligate, others facultative.
8 Able to live under more than one specific set of environmental conditions; contrast with obligate.
10 Development of dental caries.
11 The collective organisms of a given locale.
12 Minute living organisms, usually microscopic; includes bacteria, rickettsiae, viruses, fungi, and protozoa.
13 The microscopic living organisms of a region.
17 Invasion and multiplication of a microorganism in body tissues.
18 Pleomorphic, gram-negative bacteria that lack cell walls; many are regular oral cavity residents; some are pathogenic.
19 Not self-sustaining; feeding on others.
20 Not made up of or containing cells.
21 White blood corpuscle capable of ameboid movement; functions to protect the body against infection and disease.
22 Formation of calculus.

Down

2 Heterotrophic microorganism that can live and grow in the presence of free oxygen; some are obligate, others facultative.
4 Ability to survive only in a particular environment; opposite of facultative.
5 Matrix-enclosed bacterial populations adherent to each other and/or to surfaces or interfaces.
7 Stage or process of attaining maximal development; become mature.
9 Attachment of one substance to the surface of another; the action of a substance in attracting and holding other materials or particles on its surface
13 White or cream-colored cheesy mass that can collect over dental biofilm on unclean, neglected teeth (two words).
14 Disease-producing agent or microorganism.
15 Plant or animal that lives on or within another living organism and draws its nourishment therefrom; may be obligate or facultative.
16 Adjective to indicate a conduciveness to the initiation of dental caries.

Biofilm Knowledge Exercises

1. List and describe the various types of nonmineralized tooth deposits. Be sure to identify the derivation of each.

_____

_____

_____

2. Make a drawing of each of these bacteria.
   - ▇ *Bacillus*
   - ▇ *Coccobacilli*
   - ▇ *Diplococci*
   - ▇ *Filamentous bacilli*
   - ▇ *Fusiform bacilli*
   - ▇ *Sarcina*
   - ▇ *Spirochetes*
   - ▇ *Staphylococci*
   - ▇ *Streptococci*
   - ▇ *Vibrios*

3. Label **Figure 17-1** to identify the bacteria present. To the right of the figure, indicate the time frame for the development of the observed changes in the bacteria when the teeth are not cleaned.

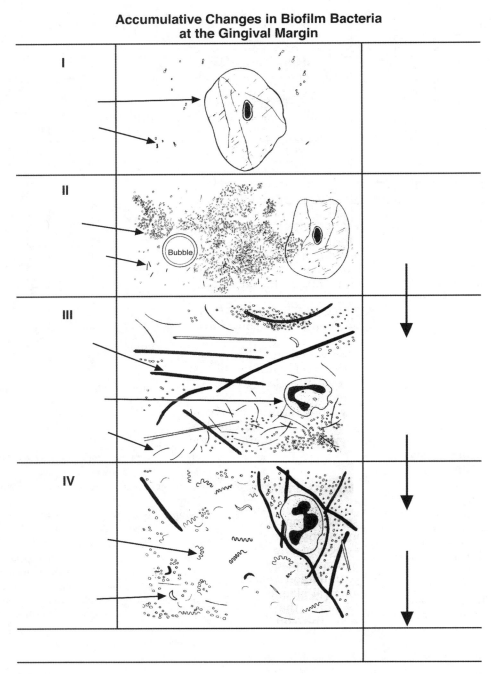

Accumulative Changes in Biofilm Bacteria at the Gingival Margin

FIGURE 17-1

4. Why is acquired pellicle significant?

   _____

   _____

   _____

5. The interactions involved in the formation of biofilm are listed below. Number the list in the correct order (1 = first interaction; 5 = last interaction).

   _____ Matrix formation

   _____ Formation of a pellicle

   _____ Biofilm growth and maturation

   _____ Bacterial multiplication and colonization

   _____ Bacteria attach to the pellicle

6. Mark each of the following statements as true or false. If the statement printed here is false, correct it.

   True or False _____ Dental caries and gingival and periodontal infections are not caused by microorganisms in microbial or dental biofilms.

   _____

   _____

   _____

   True or False _____ Cleansing of debris from about fixed prostheses and orthodontic appliances is an important part of oral sanitation.

   _____

   _____

   _____

   True or False _____ The hard deposits are acquired pellicle or cuticle, dental biofilm, materia alba, and food debris.

   _____

   _____

   _____

   True or False _____ The soft deposits on teeth are dental calculus.

   _____

   _____

   _____

   True or False _____ The incipient carious lesion begins as visible demineralization.

   _____

   _____

   True or False _____ Acquired pellicle is composed primarily of glycoproteins from the saliva, which are selectively adsorbed by the hydroxyapatite of the tooth surface.

   _____

   _____

   _____

   True or False _____ The unstained pellicle is readily visible.

   _____

   _____

   _____

   True or False _____ The probability of the development of dental caries and/or gingivitis increases as the number of microorganisms decreases.

   _____

   _____

   _____

   True or False _____ Gingivitis develops in 2 to 3 days when biofilm is left undisturbed on the tooth surfaces.

   _____

   _____

   _____

   True or False _____ Subgingival biofilm results from the apical proliferation of microorganisms from supragingival biofilm.

   _____

   _____

   _____

   True or False _____ The flora of the subgingival biofilm does not differ from that of the supragingival biofilm.

   _____

   _____

   _____

   True or False _____ The biofilm attached to the tooth surface is associated with calculus formation, root caries, and root resorption.

   _____

   _____

   _____

True or False _____ Between the layers of attached biofilm are many motile, gram-negative organisms. These are considered part of the attached biofilm.

_____

_____

_____

True or False _____ Loosely attached to the pocket epithelium are many gram-negative microorganisms and numerous white blood cells. These make up the epithelium-associated biofilm.

_____

_____

_____

True or False _____ Biofilm is composed of microorganisms and intermicrobial matrix. Organic and inorganic solids constitute approximately 80%, and water accounts for 20%. Microorganisms make up at least 20–30% of the solid matter, which is higher in subgingival biofilm than in the supragingival form.

_____

_____

_____

True or False _____ Microbial biofilm plays a major role in the initiation and progression of both dental caries and periodontal diseases.

_____

_____

_____

True or False _____ Surface pellicle is continuous with subsurface pellicle, which is embedded in the tooth structure, particularly where the tooth surface is partially demineralized.

_____

_____

_____

True or False _____ The concentration of calcium, phosphorus, magnesium, and fluoride is higher in biofilm than in saliva.

_____

_____

_____

True or False _____ Biofilm on the lingual surfaces of the maxillary anterior teeth contains a higher concentration of calcium and phosphate than does biofilm on the other teeth, and the concentration of these minerals is even higher in heavy calculus formers.

_____

_____

_____

True or False _____ When stained with a disclosing agent, unstained pellicle appears thin, with a pale staining that contrasts with the thicker, darker staining of dental biofilm.

_____

_____

_____

True or False _____ The concentration of fluoride in biofilm is higher when fluoridated water is used, and it increases after professional topical applications of fluoride and the use of fluoride-containing dentifrices and mouth rinses.

_____

_____

_____

True or False _____ Carbohydrates contribute to the adherence of the microorganisms to each other and the teeth.

_____

_____

_____

True or False _____ The acquired pellicle begins to form within hours after all external material has been removed from the tooth surfaces with an abrasive.

_____

_____

_____

True or False _____ Subgingival biofilm contains proteins from gingival sulcus fluid.

_____

_____

_____

True or False _____ General oral cleanliness is not influenced by the removal of dental biofilm deposits.

_____

_____

True or False _____ Dental caries is a disease of the dental calcified structures (enamel, dentin, and cementum) that is characterized by demineralization of the mineral components and dissolution of the organic matrix.

_____

_____

_____

True or False _____ Most gingivitis is irreversible, and even when the gingiva is treated by biofilm removal procedures, the gingiva will not return to health.

_____

_____

7. Match the following descriptions of biofilm with the correct type. Each type is used more than once.

TYPE OF BIOFILM	DESCRIPTION
A. Supragingival biofilm B. Subgingival biofilm	_____ Shape and size are affected by the friction of tongue, cheeks, and lips
	_____ The main source of nutrients for bacterial proliferation is gingival sulcus fluid
	_____ Coronal to the margin of the free gingiva
	_____ May become thicker as the diseased pocket wall becomes less tight
	_____ Early biofilm; primarily gram-positive cocci
	_____ Heaviest collection on areas not cleaned daily by patient
	_____ Found on the cervical third, especially facial surfaces, the lingual mandibular molars, and proximal surfaces
	_____ Down growth of bacteria from supragingival biofilm
	_____ Diseased pocket; primarily gram-negative, motile, spirochetes, rods
	_____ Sources of nutrients for bacterial proliferation are saliva and ingested food
	_____ Made up of three layers
	_____ The structure is an adherent, densely packed microbial layer over pellicle on the tooth surface

8. The sequence of events for demineralization and dental caries follows a predictable pattern. Number the list of events in the correct order (1 = first event; 5 = last event).

_____ Demineralization occurs

_____ Acid forms immediately

_____ Cariogenic food stuff eaten

_____ Biofilm in the oral cavity

_____ White spot lesions; incipient lesions formed

_____ Frequent exposure of tooth surface to acid

_____ Fermentable carbohydrate taken into biofilm

_____ Caries process initiated

_____ pH of biofilm drops

_____ Dental caries occurs

COMPETENCY EXERCISES

1. Your patient, Daron Horwitz, is curious about how to remove the soft deposits in his mouth. He presents with biofilm, materia alba, and food debris. Discuss patient instructions for the removal of all three deposits.

_____

_____

_____

_____

_____

_____

2. As you evaluate Mrs. Eltheia Shore, you note that she presents with a significant amount of supragingival, subgingival, gingival, and fissure biofilm. Educate her about the factors that can contribute to biofilm accumulation and the surfaces most commonly affected. Describe the strategies used for detection of biofilm.

_____

_____

_____

_____

_____

_____

Everyday Ethics

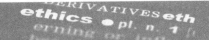

Refer to the Codes of Ethics (Appendices I, II, and III in the textbook) and Framework for Making Decisions (Table 1-2 in the textbook) as you discuss the following scenario with your classmates.

Daria was particularly excited to begin her patient schedule today because a student from the local community college was coming to observe her. Daria had graduated from the same dental hygiene program 4 years earlier and had volunteered to participate in the program for students to observe practitioners.

Roland, a second-year student, presented promptly at the receptionist's window 15 minutes before the first patient. Daria was already busily preparing her treatment room, and she quickly introduced herself to the student. She invited Roland to ask her any questions but not in front of a patient. She said she would introduce him to the patient at the beginning of each appointment and would request verbal approval from the patient for his presence in the treatment room. Roland was impressed with Daria's professionalism.

After the first appointment was completed, Roland asked Daria why she was still using the term *plaque* during patient instruction instead of *biofilm* and why she didn't disclose the teeth before the selective polishing procedures. "Oh," Daria replied, "Is this something new you learned in school? I've only been to one continuing education course since I left school, but I didn't hear anything about—what is it? Biofilm?".

Questions for Consideration

1. Role play the dialogue that might take place regarding use of the term *plaque* versus *biofilm,* which was a new concept for Daria.
2. Ethically, how is Daria violating/not violating any ethical principles relative to beneficent care by not using disclosing agent to identify the biofilm?
3. What ethical elements of the provider-patient relationship can Daria impress upon this student as a practicing hygienist?

---

3. You are providing patient education for Alison Alverez and her 10-year-old son, Juan. Juan has multiple carious lesions, and his mother is very interested in preventing more from occurring. Juan drinks soda daily. He purchases a 32-oz. bottle on his way to school and sips the soda every chance he gets. Juan's mother remembers hearing something about acids in the mouth and wants to know more about this.

_____

_____

_____

_____

_____

_____

_____

4. Your patient is Nguyen Tho Phan, a 58-year-old research microbiologist. Her area of research is disease prevention, and she wants to understand the major pathogens that are identified in destructive periodontal disease and caries. If Nguyen presents with *Mutans streptococci,* what disease is she most at risk for? Her brother has periodontal disease, and

Factors To Teach The Patient

You have just seated your patient, Mrs. Lorna Patel. Refer to her care plan in Appendix D to review the assessment findings, concentrating on her dental history and dental findings.

Use the example of a patient conversation in Appendix B as a guide to write a statement explaining to Mrs. Patel the appearance of acute gingivitis and the impact of effective brushing and flossing after a specified period of time. You may also want to refer to the figure in Knowledge Exercise 4 when writing your statement. Compare your conversation with a student colleague to identify any missing information.

This scenario is related to the following factors:

■ Location, composition, and properties of dental biofilm with emphasis on its role in dental caries and periodontal infections
■ Effects of personal oral care procedures in the prevention of dental biofilm
■ Biofilm control procedures with special adaptations for individual needs

Nguyen want to know if he would have the same bacteria in his mouth.

_____

_____

_____

_____

_____

5. Specific microorganisms, a susceptible tooth surface, and a diet high in cariogenic foods are essential for caries to develop. Discuss recommendations you can provide for an adult patient for prevention of dental caries.

_____

_____

_____

Calculus

Chapter Outline

Learning Objectives

Upon successful completion of these exercises, you will be able to:

1. Identify and define key terms and concepts related to dental calculus.
2. Describe calculus in terms of type, location, distribution, occurrence, appearance, and consistency.

3. Describe calculus formation, composition, and attachment.
4. Discuss the significance of calculus.

KNOWLEDGE EXERCISES

1. What is the main objective for removing calculus from the surfaces of teeth?

   _____

   _____

   _____

2. Fill in the blanks as you learn about supragingival calculus.

   Supragingival calculus is located on the _____ crown _____ to the margin of the gingiva. It is found most frequently on the _____ surfaces of _____ anterior teeth and the _____ surfaces of _____ first and second _____, opposite the openings of the _____ of the _____ glands; _____ of teeth out of occlusion; _____ teeth; and teeth that are _____ during daily biofilm removal (toothbrushing, flossing, or other personal care). It can also be found on surfaces of _____ and barbells worn in tongue piercings.

3. Supragingival calculus may be referred to by other names. List some of these other terms.

   _____

   _____

   _____

4. Match each term with its definition.

TERMS RELATED TO CALCULUS	DEFINITION
_____ Pyrophosphate _____ Amorphous _____ Germ free _____ Matrix _____ Calculus _____ Nidus _____ Apatite _____ Saturated _____ Denture calculus _____ Supersaturated _____ Ectopic oral calcification _____ Mineralization _____ Ectopic	A. Mineralized biofilm covered on the external surface with vital, tightly adherent, nonmineralized biofilm B. Without definite shape or visible differentiation in structure C. Intercellular or intermicrobial substance of a tissue or the tissue from which a structure develops, gains support, and is held together D. Nucleus; focus; point of origin E. Free from microorganisms F. Crystalline mineral component of bones and teeth that contains calcium and phosphate G. Abnormal concretion composed of mineral salts H. Examples are pulp stones, denticles, and salivary calculi I. Out of place; arising or produced at an abnormal site or in a tissue where it is not normally found J. Addition of mineral elements, such as calcium and phosphorus, to the body or a part thereof with resulting hardening of the tissue K. Inhibitor of calcification that occurs in parotid saliva of humans in variable amounts; anticalculus component of tartar-control dentifrices L. Holding all of a substance (solute) that can be dissolved in the solution M. A solution containing more of an ingredient than can be held in solution permanently

5. List the agents that can be used as active ingredients in "tartar control" mouth rinses and dentifrices.

_____

_____

_____

6. Match the description with the type of calculus deposit. Each type of deposit is used more than once.

TYPE OF CALCULUS DEPOSIT	DESCRIPTION
A. Supragingival calculus B. Subgingival calculus	_____ Light to dark brown, dark green, or black _____ May be stained by tobacco, food, or other pigments _____ Crusty, spiny, or nodular _____ Shape of calculus mass is determined by the anatomy of teeth; contour of gingival margin; and pressure of tongue, lips, and cheeks _____ Thin, smooth veneers _____ Amorphous, bulky _____ Increased amount in tobacco smokers _____ Newest deposits near bottom of pocket are less dense and hard _____ White, creamy yellow, or gray _____ Brittle, flint-like _____ Finger- and fern-like _____ Slight deposits may be invisible until dried with compressed air _____ Flattened to conform with pressure from the pocket wall _____ Moderately hard _____ Stains derived from blood pigments from diseased pocket _____ Newer deposits less dense and hard

7. Fill in the blanks as you read about subgingival calculus.

Subgingival calculus is located on the _____ crown apical to the _____ of the gingiva. It extends nearly to the _____ of the pocket. As the pocket is deepened by _____, calculus forms on the _____ root surface. This deposit may be generalized or _____ on _____ teeth or a group of teeth. _____ deposits are found on the proximal surfaces.

8. Subgingival calculus may be referred to by other names. List some of these terms.

_____

_____

_____

9. You are exploring to detect supragingival and sub-gingival calculus. Identify some strategies that will help you find calculus in your patient's mouth.

_____

_____

_____

_____

_____

_____

10. Calculus formation occurs in three basic steps: (1) _____, (2) _____, (3) _____.

11. Mark each of the following statements true or false. If the statement is false, correct it.

    True or False   The control of biofilm deposits by the patient, supplemented by complete professional calculus removal, can reduce or eliminate gingival inflammation.

    _____

    _____

    _____

    True or False   Calculus is a predisposing factor in pocket development because it provides a haven for the collection of bacterial masses on the deposit's rough surface.

    _____

    _____

    _____

    True or False   Dental calculus is classified by its location on a tooth surface as related to the cemented-enamel junction—that is, supragingival or subgingival.

    _____

    _____

    _____

    True or False   With its rough surface, permeable structure, and porosity, calculus can act as a reservoir for endotoxins and tissue breakdown products.

    _____

    _____

True or False   Calculus occurs only on the permanent teeth and in patients older than 12 years.

_____

_____

True or False   Subgingival calculus is always covered by masses of active biofilm. The bacterial mass is in contact with the diseased pocket epithelium and promotes gingivitis and periodontitis.

_____

_____

_____

True or False   Subgingival deposits may be seen directly or indirectly, using a mouth mirror.

_____

_____

_____

True or False   Irritation to the pocket lining stimulates greater flow of gingival sulcus fluid, which contains minerals for supragingival calculus formation.

_____

_____

_____

True or False   A gentle air blast can deflect the gingival margin from the tooth for access into the pocket.

_____

_____

_____

True or False   Subgingival calculus does not develop by direct extension from supragingival calculus. Subgingival biofilm forms by extension of supragingival biofilm. Each biofilm mineralizes separately.

_____

_____

_____

True or False Mineralization of supragingival and subgingival calculus is essentially the same; even the source of the elements for mineralization is the same.

True or False The location of supragingival calculus is related to the openings of the salivary gland ducts, especially the facial surface of mandibular molars and the facial surface of mandibular anterior teeth.

True or False Pellicle begins to form within hours after all deposits have been removed from the tooth surface.

True or False The source of elements for formation of subgingival calculus is the saliva.

True or False The gingival sulcus fluid and the inflammatory exudate supply the minerals for the supragingival deposits.

True or False Pyrophosphate is an inhibitor of calcification and is used in anticalculus dentifrices.

True or False Subgingival biofilm contains pathogenic bacteria that cause inflammation and destruction of the gingival tissue and lead to loss of attachment to the tooth surface and development and deepening of the pocket.

True or False Dental enamel is the most highly calcified tissue in the body and contains 96% inorganic salts; dentin contains 65%, and cementum and bone contain 45% to 50%.

True or False Current research studies point to the probability that calcification of calculus may involve the same phenomena as other ectopic calcifications (e.g., urinary or renal calculi) and may be similar to normal calcification of bone, cartilage, enamel, and dentin.

True or False The biofilm on the calculus surface contains nonviable organisms.

True or False The surface of a calculus mass is rough and can be detected by use of an explorer. As observed by electron microscope, the surface roughness appears as depressions, ridges, and ledges.

True or False The ease or difficulty of removal can be related to the manner of attachment of the calculus to the tooth surface.

True or False　Heavy calculus formers have higher levels of parotid pyrophosphate than do light calculus formers.

_____

_____

_____

True or False　Calculus is primarily made up of organic components and water.

_____

_____

_____

True or False　Inorganic components of calculus are mainly calcium (Ca), phosphorus (P), carbonate (CO_3), sodium (Na), magnesium (Mg), and potassium (K).

_____

_____

_____

True or False　The concentration of fluoride in calculus varies and is influenced by the amount of fluoride received from drinking water, topical application, dentifrices, or any form that is received by contact with the external surface of the calculus.

_____

_____

_____

True or False　The surface of the enamel is more permeable than the surface of the cementum and thus has a higher fluoride content.

_____

_____

_____

True or False　At least two thirds of the inorganic matter of calculus is crystalline, principally apatite. Pyrophosphate, which is the same crystal present in enamel, dentin, cementum, and bone, is predominant.

_____

_____

True or False　The organic proportion of calculus consists of various types of nonvital microorganisms, desquamated epithelial cells, leukocytes, and mucin from the blood.

_____

_____

_____

True or False　The microorganisms in early biofilm are predominantly filamentous. After 5 days, cocci and rod-shaped organisms are found.

_____

_____

_____

True or False　Most of the organisms within calculus are considered viable.

_____

_____

_____

True or False　Small amounts of calculus that have not been stained are frequently more visible when they are wet with saliva.

_____

_____

_____

True or False　With increased pocket depth, greater amounts of biofilm can accumulate, with increased numbers of pathogenic organisms.

_____

_____

_____

True or False　The incidence of calculus decreases with age.

_____

_____

_____

True or False　Although the proportion varies, depending on the age and hardness of a deposit and the location from which the sample for analysis is taken, mature calculus usually contains between

75% and 85% inorganic components; the rest is organic components and water.

_____

_____

_____

True or False Calculus is mineralized biofilm. The biofilm next to the tooth surface is mineralized last.

_____

_____

_____

True or False Various trace elements have been identified in inorganic calculus. These include chlorine (Cl), zinc (Zn), strontium (Sr), bromine (Br), copper (Cu), manganese (Mn), tungsten (W), gold (Au), aluminum (Al), silicon (Si), iron (Fe), and fluorine (F).

_____

_____

_____

True or False Agents used in "tartar control" dentifrices and mouth rinse act only on calculus and have no effect on oral tissues.

_____

_____

_____

COMPETENCY EXERCISES

1. Compare and contrast the distribution of supragingival and subgingival calculus. Discuss how the distribution affects your detection strategies.

_____

_____

_____

_____

_____

_____

2. Discuss calculus formation in your own words. Be sure to address pellicle formation and biofilm maturation. Concentrate on mineralization.

_____

_____

_____

_____

_____

3. Your patient John Weston is wondering about calculus formation. He is trying to understand exact time frame of the process. Help him understand calculus formation by defining calculus and discussing the influencing factors. Make a list that

Everyday Ethics

Refer to the Codes of Ethics (Appendices I, II, and III in the textbook) and Framework for Making Decisions (Table 1-2 in the textbook) as you discuss the following scenario with your classmates.

Coronal polishing legislation had just been passed at the state level. Certified dental assistants (CDA) were now eligible to take a course and then begin polishing procedures on a patient after the dentist or the dental hygienist removes all calculus deposits. Mindy, the CDA in the office, completed the course and was ready to polish. As the hygienist in the office, Hilary was basically unaffected by the change in the dental practice act and continued to treat her patients in all aspects of the preventive protocol.

However, Dr. Bell found that additional services could be offered to his patients at the time of their restorative

appointment by removing the calculus and then having Mindy finish with the polish. One day, as Hilary was on her way to find Dr. Bell to check her patient, she saw Mindy using a curet to remove what she stated as, "slight subgingival deposits that didn't come off with the polishing cup."

Questions for Consideration
1. Would you consider what the hygienist observed the dental assistant doing an ethical issue or dilemma? Explain your answer.
2. Is it necessary for the CDA to understand the attachment, maturation, and structure of calculus to provide "beneficent" care to the patient? Why or why not?
3. If Dr. Bell dismisses the fact that Mindy was using instruments to remove calculus, what choices of action could Hilary pursue?

Factors To Teach The Patient

Louisa Gregory, a 53-year-old first-grade teacher, is busy with her two daughters, aged 12 and 14. She does not take time for herself and has come to the dental hygiene clinic after a 5-year absence. She uses any type of toothpaste that is on sale, and her current dentifrice is in a decorative dispenser; she does not know anything else about it except that it matches her bathroom perfectly! As you examine Louisa's mouth you see generalized heavy supragingival and subgingival calculus. She wants to know what to do about "all this hard stuff" on her teeth.

Use the example of a patient conversation in Appendix B as a guide to create a conversation to educate Louisa about the impact of good oral hygiene and frequent professional care for complete scaling on the levels of supragingival and subgingival calculus. Be sure to address product selection criteria and the need for the use of an anticalculus toothpaste.

Use the conversation you create to role play this situation with a fellow student. If you are the patient in the role play, be sure to ask questions. If you are the dental hygienist, try to anticipate questions and answer them in your explanation.

This scenario is related to the following factors:

- That good oral hygiene and frequent professional care for complete scaling are consistent with low levels of supragingival and subgingival calculus
- The effect of calculus on the health of the periodontal tissues and, therefore, on the general health of the oral cavity
- What to expect from use of an anticalculus dentifrice
- The importance of selecting products with an ADA Seal of Approval

describes calculus formation in terms of minutes, hours, and days.

_____

_____

_____

_____

_____

_____

4. While scaling in the mandibular right quadrant, you are having varying degrees of difficulty detecting and removing the calculus. Describe the three modes of calculus attachment. Explain how each mode affects detection and removal.

_____

_____

_____

_____

_____

_____

Dental Stains and Discolorations

Learning Objectives

Upon successful completion of these exercises, you will be able to:

1. Identify and define key terms and concepts related to dental stains and discolorations.

2. Classify various stains as to their location and source.

KNOWLEDGE EXERCISES

1. Match the following terms with the correct definition.

TERM	DESCRIPTION
A. Chlorophyll B. Endogenous C. Chronologic D. Chromogenic E. Dentinogenesis imperfecta F. Amelogenesis imperfecta G. Hypoplasia	_____ Incomplete development or underdevelopment of an organ or a tissue _____ Producing color or pigment _____ Imperfect formation of enamel; hereditary condition in which the ameloblasts fail to lay down the enamel matrix properly or at all

H. Intrinsic I. Exogenous J. Extrinsic	_____ Originating outside or caused by factors outside _____ Hereditary disorder of dentin formation in which the odontoblasts lay down an abnormal matrix; can occur in both primary and permanent dentitions _____ Produced within or caused by factors within _____ Situated entirely within _____ Green plant pigment essential to photosynthesis _____ Arranged in order of time _____ Derived from or situated on the outside; external

2. Stains are classified by location and source.
   ▪ *List examples of extrinsic exogenous stains.*

   _____

   _____

   _____

   ▪ *List examples of intrinsic endogenous stains.*

   _____

   _____

   _____

   ▪ *List examples of intrinsic exogenous stains.*

   _____

   _____

3. Complete Infomap 19-1 below to help you organize information on extrinsic stains.

4. Your patient presents with a stained pulpless tooth. Describe the clinical appearance of the stain and how it was formed. The patient is scheduled for endodontic treatment on another tooth and wants to know if that tooth will also stain. What would you tell this patient?

   _____

   _____

   _____

   _____

   _____

   _____

5. Clinically you observe enamel that is partially or completely missing because of a generalized disturbance of the ameloblasts. Teeth are yellowish brown or gray-brown. What is this condition is called?

   _____

   _____

   _____

6. Your patient was born with erythroblastosis fetalis (Rh incompatibility). This condition may a leave the teeth with a _____ hue.

INFOMAP 19-1					
TYPE OF STAIN	**APPEARANCE**	**DISTRIBUTION**	**OCCURRENCE**	**CAUSE/ORIGIN**	**CLINICAL ISSUES**
Yellow					
Green					
Other green					
Black line					
Tobacco					
Other brown					
Orange and red					
Metallic—industrial					
Metallic—drugs					

Everyday Ethics

Refer to the Codes of Ethics (Appendices I, II, and III in the textbook) and Framework for Making Decisions (Table 1-2 in the textbook) as you discuss the following scenario with your classmates.

Daniel returned to the dental office of Dr. Windum after 3 years of working on the East Coast. At the age of 32, Daniel was exhibiting signs of gingival inflammation and increased subgingival calculus. Ruthie, the dental hygienist, immediately began talking to Daniel about biofilm and suggesting improvements for his personal daily brushing and flossing. After she completed a quadrant of scaling with local anesthesia, she suggested that rinsing with chlorhexidine after brushing before going to bed would help the healing.

Dr. Windum confirmed Ruthie's recommendation and wrote the prescription. Daniel left the office only to call a

few days later to report the "awful brown stain on his teeth and horrible taste of the mouthrinse." He further indicated that he had stopped using the product and wanted to come in and have the stain removed immediately.

Questions for Consideration

1. Was Ruthie unethical? It seems that she did not completely inform Daniel about the side effects of prescribed rinses. Use ethical principles to support your answer.
2. Daniel seems to be more concerned about the staining that has occurred than the condition of his periodontium. How can Ruthie respect Daniel's feelings while helping him understand the potential outcomes of his daily personal oral care?
3. How could Ruthie and Dr. Windum "justify" the stain that results from the product while making Daniel "value" his gingival condition?

COMPETENCY EXERCISES

1. Your patient, Betty Cohen, presents with a dark brown stain on the lingual surfaces of her maxillary posterior teeth. As you observe the oral cavity, you describe the stain as a continuous unerupted line, following the gingival crest. The gingiva is firm with little or no tendency to bleed. What do you determine this stain to be?

   _____

   _____

   _____

2. Your 1:30 patient, Fawez Sadarage, 47 years old, presents with stain on his maxillary anterior teeth caused by tetracycline. Describe the stain that you see and list some follow-up questions you will ask Mr. Sadarage. About how old was Mr. Sadarage when he took this antibiotic?

   _____

   _____

   _____

   _____

   _____

   _____

3. Several strategies will help you recognize and identify stains in the oral cavity. Provide examples of

Factors To Teach The Patient

Your patient, Shaneeka Harris, is a 21-year-old college student. She has recently started to smoke cigarettes and marijuana and drink a lot of coffee and tea. Her last blood test showed that she was anemic, and her physician has prescribed daily oral doses of iron. Shaneeka is finding college overwhelming and very stressful. The reason she made an appointment in the dental hygiene clinic is because she has noticed that her teeth have a brown and gray-green stain, and she is really unhappy with how they look. She does not remember having all these stains before.

Use the example of a patient conversation in Appendix B as a guide to write a statement to help Shaneeka understand the factors affecting stain accumulation and the removal and prevention strategies.

Use the conversation you create to role play this situation with a fellow student. If you are the patient in the role play, be sure to ask questions. If you are the dental hygienist, try to anticipate questions and answer them in your explanation.

This scenario is related to the following factors:

- Predisposing factors that contribute to stain accumulation
- Personal care procedures that can aid in the prevention or reduction of stains
- Advantages of starting a smoking-cessation program
- Reasons for not using an abrasive dentifrice with vigorous brushing strokes to lessen or remove stain accumulation
- The need to avoid tobacco, coffee, tea, and other beverages or foodstuffs that can stain to prevent discoloration of new restorations

stains (color and cause) that can be detected by each of the strategies listed below.

■ *Medical history*

_____

_____

_____

■ *Questions about industrial occupation*

_____

_____

_____

■ *Questions about dietary habits*

_____

_____

_____

■ *Dental history*

_____

_____

■ *Dental charting (e.g., endodontic therapy, restorative materials)*

_____

_____

_____

Indices and Scoring Methods

Learning Objectives

Upon successful completion of these exercises, you will be able to:

1. Identify and define key terms and concepts related to dental indices and scoring methods.
2. Identify the purpose, criteria for measurement, scoring methods, range of scores, and reference or interpretation scales for a variety of dental indices.
3. Select and calculate dental indices for a use in a specific patient or community situation.

Dental Indices Terms and Concepts Crossword Puzzle

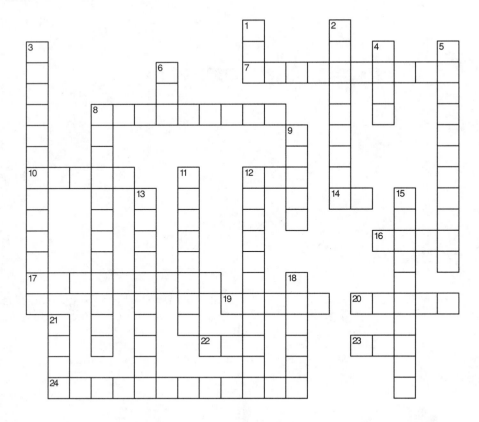

Across

7 An index that measures a condition that can be changed and no evidence of the condition will remain; example is dental biofilm.

8 Refers to the number of new cases of a disease that occur during a certain period of time.

10 An expression of clinical observations in numerical values.

12 Periodontal screening index that monitors individual or group periodontal treatment needs.

14 A sweeping motion of the dental probe determines one aspect of gingival health when this gingival/periodontal index is used.

16 Determines caries experience in adult dentition.

17 A factor that is measured and analyzed to describe health status.

19 Measures what it is intended to measure.

20 An index that measures fluorosis using five categories.

22 Uses unwaxed dental floss to determine areas of interproximal gingival bleeding.

23 Assesses thickness of dental biofilm at the gingival area.

24 The systematic collection of oral health data for use in planning public health programs.

Down

1 Periodontal screening index used for individual patients.

2 Refers to a brief initial exam for an individual or an assessment of many individuals to determine a certain characteristic in a population.

3 Dental indices are used to collect data for this type of a study.

4 Uses a triangular wooden interdental cleaner to identify areas of interproximal bleeding.

5 Consistency of measurement; enhanced by calibration of examiners.

6 Uses standardized gentle probing technique to locate areas of gingival bleeding.

8 An index that measures conditions that are not able to be changed; in other words, evidence of the condition will remain even after treatment; example is dental caries.

9 Combines a debris score and a calculus score using specific surfaces of six teeth.

11 Refers to teeth nos. 3, 9, 12, 19, 25, and 28; teeth used for classic epidemiologic studies of periodontal disease.

12 A determination of accuracy and consistency between examiners; affects the reliability of data collection.

13 The total number of cases of some disease or condition in a given population.

15 An index that measures all the evidence of a condition, past and present.

18 A category of indices that measures only the presence or absence of a condition.

21 A more sensitive index that measures dental caries experience on the surfaces of adult teeth.

KNOWLEDGE EXERCISE

Dental Indices Infomaps

Infomaps are tables that place related information about different factors of one topic on a single page. This method of organizing not only allows you to learn information as you transfer key points from the textbook but also provides a study guide that lets you visually compare and contrast the different dental indices easily and effectively.

Transfer enough basic information about each index from the textbook to the appropriate Infomap so that you can use the collected data to complete the Competency Exercises for this chapter. The blank Infomaps, 20-1 to 20-5, are located on the next few pages.

COMPETENCY EXERCISES

Answer the following questions based on this community case scenario.

You, several student colleagues, and some of the faculty members at your school are asked to be part of a statewide, community-based oral health surveillance project conducted by your local Department of Community Health. The project requires that you collect data during the local Toothtown Activity Center Health Fair for young adults ages 17–25.

You are excited that you will be participating in calibration exercises, collecting data with other members of your school team, and then actually calculating and interpreting the results of your own data collection. What a great way to learn about the dental indices you have just been studying!

1. Determine the index (or identify a group of indices) that will provide the most comprehensive information about this population. What are the advantages or disadvantages of the indices you have selected?

   _____

   _____

   _____

   _____

   _____

   _____

2. The Department of Community Health has decided to use the DMFT index to collect data about the caries experience of the group of individuals at the activity center. Discuss the advantages and disadvantages of using this index instead of the DMFS index for community screening.

   _____

   _____

   _____

   _____

   _____

   _____

INFOMAP 20-1	ORAL HYGIENE STATUS INDICES				
INDEX	**WHAT IS MEASURED?**	**TEETH AND/OR SURFACES SCORED**	**CRITERIA USED FOR MEASUREMENT**	**SCORING/ CALCULATION OF INDEX**	**REFERENCE SCALES, RANGE OF SCORES, AND ADDITIONAL INFORMATION**
PL I					
"Plaque-Control Record"					
"Plaque-Free Score"					
PHP					
OHI-S					

INFOMAP 20-2	GINGIVAL HEALTH INDICES				
INDEX	WHAT IS MEASURED?	TEETH AND/OR SURFACES SCORED	CRITERIA USED FOR MEASUREMENT	SCORING/ CALCULATION OF INDEX	REFERENCE SCALES, RANGE OF SCORES, AND ADDITIONAL INFORMATION
SBI					
GBI					
EIBI					
GI					

INFOMAP 20-3	INDIVIDUAL AND COMMUNITY PERIODONTAL INDICES				
INDEX	WHAT IS MEASURED?	TEETH AND/OR SURFACES SCORED	CRITERIA USED FOR MEASUREMENT	SCORING/ CALCULATION OF INDEX	REFERENCE SCALES, RANGE OF SCORES, AND ADDITIONAL INFORMATION
PSR					
CPI					

INFOMAP 20-4	DENTAL CARIES INDICES				
INDEX (AND AUTHOR)	WHAT IS MEASURED?	TEETH AND/OR SURFACES SCORED	CRITERIA USED FOR MEASUREMENT	SCORING/ CALCULATION OF INDEX	ADDITIONAL INFORMATION
DMFT					
DMFS					
dft and dfs					
deft and defs					
dmft and dmfs					
ECC and S-ECC					
RCI					

INFOMAP 20-5	FLUOROSIS INDICES				
INDEX (AND AUTHOR)	**WHAT IS MEASURED?**	**TEETH AND/OR SURFACES SCORED**	**CRITERIA USED FOR MEASUREMENT**	**SCORING/ CALCULATION OF INDEX**	**ADDITIONAL INFORMATION**
Dean's Fluorosis Index					
TSIF					

3. After participating in the screening day at the Tooth-town Activity Center, you feel quite confident about using the DMFT index and OHI-S to score individuals as well as the GI that your team decided to use. Now it is time to calculate the results and practice interpreting your findings.

   Using the information in Table 20-1 below, calculate the individual DMFs, the total group DMF, and the group average DMF.

   _____

   _____

   _____

4. Using the data in Table 20-1, calculate the percentage of DMF teeth in this group that currently have decay.

   _____

   _____

   _____

5. Using the data in Table 20-1, calculate the percentage of DMF teeth that have been restored.

   _____

   _____

   _____

6. Using the data in Table 20-1, calculate the percentage of individuals in this group who have at least one decayed tooth.

   _____

   _____

   _____

7. Using the data in Table 20-1, calculate the percentage of individuals in this group who have treatment needs.

   _____

   _____

   _____

8. Use Tables 20-2 and 20-3 on the next page to calculate a gingival index (GI) score for Grace and an average GI score for all the individuals in the group.

9. What does Grace's GI score mean?

   _____

   _____

   _____

TABLE 20-1	CALCULATING DMF DATA			
INDIVIDUAL	**D**	**M**	**F**	**INDIVIDUAL DMF**
Abbe	12	0	14	
Bill	0	0	6	
Charlie	4	2	0	
David	1	0	6	
Edwin	3	0	0	
Frank	0	1	1	
Grace	4	0	6	
Harry	6	0	7	
Ida	18	2	0	
Joe	2	0	5	
Total				
Group Average DMF				

TABLE 20-2	CALCULATING GI DATA: AREA SCORES FOR GRACE		
TOOTH	**M**	**F**	**D**	**L**
3 (16)	2	0	2	0
9 (21)	0	0	0	0
12 (24)	1	0	1	0
19 (36)	2	0	2	0
25 (41)	0	0	0	0
28 (44)	1	0	1	0
Total				
GI score				

10. What is your interpretation of the average gingival health of the group?

_____

_____

_____

11. Imagine that you have calculated GI scores for more than 150 individuals who were screened at the Activity Center Health Fair. You calculate that this group's average score is 2.78. How can you use this group average score as baseline data to evaluate the

effect of oral hygiene presentations that you and your students will provide at a later time?

In other words, explain how you will use this baseline average GI score to determine whether the people in this community were motivated to better oral health because of your education project.

_____

_____

_____

_____

_____

_____

12. Use Table 20-4 below to calculate a DI score, a CI score, and an OHI-S score for Bill.

13. Use Table 20-5 below to calculate a group OHI-S score. Make sure to include Bill's score.

14. What does each individual person's score indicate about his or her oral cleanliness? What does the average group score indicate?

_____

_____

_____

15. You and your classmates had so much fun and learned so much at the Toothtown Activity Center screening that you want to do some more community-based screenings. You find out that the Department of

TABLE 20-3	CALCULATING THE GROUP AVERAGE GI SCORE
NAME	**GI SCORE**
Charlie	2.9
Harry	1.0
Ida	1.7
Joe	2.6
Grace	
Total	
Group Average GI	

TABLE 20-4	OHI-S DATA FOR BILL	
TOOTH	**DI**	**CI**
3 (16)	3	0
8 (11)	3	0
14 (26)	3	2
19 (36)	3	0
24 (31)	3	0
30 (46)	2	0
Total		
Scores		
OHI-S score		

TABLE 20-5	CALCULATING GROUP OHI-S DATA
INDIVIDUAL	**OHI-S SCORE**
Abbe	4.33
Bill	
Charlie	1.20
David	1.03
Edwin	1.00
Group OHI-S	

Community Health is planning to set up a mobile clinic to provide dental services for a group of 3000 homeless individuals in your city. There is not enough money to offer all possible services for this group of people, but the health department is hoping to provide enough care to meet most of the people's needs.

Your class decides to visit with the director of community health to explain how the results of a basic screening survey that you and your classmates plan to conduct can help to identify and prioritize the oral health services that are needed by this population. Present your ideas for class discussion and compare them with the ideas of your other classmates.

_____

_____

_____

_____

_____

_____

16. As part of the screening you conduct among the homeless population, you also provide individualized oral hygiene instructions and free oral health products to everyone who agrees to participate in the screening. One person, Mrs. Combs, is missing teeth 1, 2, 16, 17, and 32. The others are present. When you disclose her teeth before providing oral hygiene instructions, you note that there is significant biofilm on every single proximal surface, the facial surfaces of 3 and 4, and the lingual surfaces of all four mandibular molars.

Use the patient biofilm recording form that your clinic recommends (or make up one of your own using the models provided in the textbook) and color in all the areas with biofilm with a red pen or pencil.

Everyday Ethics

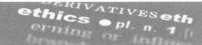

Refer to the Codes of Ethics (Appendices I, II, and III in the textbook) and Framework for Making Decisions (Table 1-2 in the textbook) as you discuss the following scenario with your classmates.

Susanna began practicing in the team clinic at the dental school and found the work to be very challenging. As a hygienist, she was not only performing preventive treatment on maintenance patients but was also responsible for data collection for several research projects. Suddenly, the importance of understanding and calculating the various indices became critical. In particular, Susanna found herself reviewing the procedures for the OHI-S, bleeding indices, and the DMFT.

Susanna had always enjoyed her clinical interactions with patients, but now scoring and recording information on each and every tooth was beginning to cause her some stress. Generally Susanna worked without an assistant and found it difficult to do both examining and recording. Near the end of one day when she was organizing the day's work for Dr. Lowe's caries study, she discovered that she had omitted several surfaces in one quadrant. This was the patient's final visit to the dental school. Susanna contemplated what to do when she realized the data was missing.

Questions for Consideration
1. Discuss how ADHA's roles for dental hygienists apply to Susanna's daily duties.
2. Can Susanna defend her actions to Dr. Lowe by submitting the data she does have on the patient? Explain your rationale.
3. Which of the core values or principles of ethical behavior come into play in collecting research data such as described in this scenario?

Factors To Teach The Patient

As you are marking the areas of biofilm on the patient form, Mrs. Combs (from Competency Exercise 16) asks why dental hygienists always bother to do all that "extra work" just to provide oral hygiene instructions. Apparently no one had ever explained it to her before.

Using the example of a patient conversation in Appendix B as a guide, write a statement explaining these dental indices to your patient.

Use the conversation you create to role play this situation with a fellow student. If you are the patient in the role play, be sure to ask questions. If you are the dental hygienist, try to anticipate questions and answer them in your explanation.

This scenario is related to the following factors:

- How an index is used and calculated and what the scores mean
- Correlation of index scores with current oral health practices and procedures
- Procedures to follow to improve index scores and bring the oral tissues to health

Using the information from this form, calculate *both* the plaque-control record and the plaque-free scores for biofilm on Mrs. Combs's teeth.

- *"Plaque-control record score"*

_____

- *"Plaque-free score"*

_____

DISCOVERY EXERCISES

Explore the Association of State and Territorial Dental Directors Web site (http://www.astdd.org) to locate information about the *Basic Screening Surveys: An Approach to Monitoring Community Oral Health* community data collection system. Many states in the U.S. use this system to gather oral health surveillance data. Download and study all of the components that are available on the Web site to help you learn about how this oral health surveillance system works. Consider purchasing the training videotape so you and your classmates can be trained to use the system in a future community screening.

Assessment

■ Chapters 6–20

COMPETENCY EXERCISES

1. Create a step-by-step list that you can use to help you keep on track and on task so that you don't miss any important data collection procedures during your patient's dental hygiene assessment appointment. Include information from all the chapters in this section that is relevant to the particular clinical situation at your school. Include items such as the following:

   ■ *The order in which specific data collection procedures are performed in your clinic*

   ■ *The type and location of equipment and materials you need for patient assessment*

   ■ *Specific dental indices and data collection techniques that you are required to use when you assess each patient*

   Compare the list you created with those created by your student colleagues. Refine your own aid based on the comparison and then laminate the final version to use as a procedure manual when you first start providing patient care in your school clinic.

2. Select one or more of the patient assessment summary examples in Appendix D. For each patient you select, write a paragraph describing the specific data collection methods and techniques that were used to complete each component of the significant findings column of the assessment summary.

3. Are any of the dental indices discussed in Chapter 20 used to collect assessment data in your school clinic? One example might be the index you use to document the amount of dental biofilm on your patient's teeth before you provide oral hygiene instruction. Will you have any opportunities at your school to use dental indices to collect community health status information? An example would be participating in a dental screening at a community-based health fair. Identify the indices in Chapter 20 that are used, or are similar to assessment data collection methods used, at your school.

4. Identify some of the Factors to Teach the Patient from each chapter of the textbook that were not addressed in chapter exercises in this workbook. Using the example of a patient conversation in Appendix B as a guide, role play one or more of these patient-education situations with a student colleague. If you are the patient in the role play, be sure to ask questions. If you are the dental hygienist, try to anticipate questions and answer them in your explanation.

   Some examples of factors that were not addressed in the chapter exercises are listed here, but there are many others throughout the chapters in the textbook.

   ■ *Assurance that all information received is completely confidential and that the records are locked when the office is closed (Chapter 6)*

   ■ *The educational features in dental radiographs (Chapter 9)*

   ■ *How the method of brushing, stiffness of toothbrush filaments, abrasiveness of a dentifrice, and pressure applied during brushing can be factors in gingival recession (Chapter 12)*

5. Mr. Yukas, 45 years old, is scheduled later today for a new patient examination. Yesterday, you received a package in the mail from Mr. Yukas's previous dentist in another city. The package contained a recent set of full-mouth radiographs and a set of study casts of Mr. Yukas's teeth. You set them up on the counter in your treatment room as you wait for Mr. Yukas to arrive. Unfortunately, Mr. Yukas has car trouble and calls at the last minute to cancel his appointment. As you are putting the radiographs and study casts away, you decide to spend the extra time you have examining them.

   ■ *What assessment data can you determine just from examining Mr. Yukas's radiographs and study casts?*

■ *What assessment information would still be missing until you meet with Mr. Yukas in person to collect the data?*

6. Gather and record complete oral assessment data for either a student colleague or a patient in your school clinic. Make a copy of the assessment findings section of the patient-specific care plan template (in Appendix C) and use the template to create a patient assessment summary that is similar to those in Appendix D in this workbook.

DISCOVERY EXERCISES

1. Collect samples of the worksheets that are used for patient assessment record keeping from several dental practices in your community. Compare these systems with those used in your school clinic. Discuss the advantages and disadvantages of each system with your student colleagues.

2. Many patients you provide dental hygiene care for will not speak English (or the language that most people in your country speak) as their first language. Those patients can often have a more difficult time accurately completing health history information. Investigate to discover health history forms that are translated into other languages. A fine place to start is at the MetDental.com Web site (*www.metdental.com/prov/execute/Content*). This Web page includes a link leading you to a site where you can download and print health history forms in a variety of languages. Follow the links to the RESOURCE CENTER and then to PATIENT RESOURCES.

3. There are also patient-education materials available for non-English–speaking patients at the Proctor and Gamble *Dental Resource Net Patient Education* Web page (*www.dentalcare.com/drn.htm*). Just for fun, explore the Internet to see what else you can find that will assist your patients whose native language is different from your own.

4. Look through the scientific literature to find periodontal disease studies that use some of the dental indices you learned about in Chapter 20 to collect data on periodontal disease status.

5. Check out the data in the Healthy People 2010 Oral Health Objectives (Chapter 21) to see if you can figure out which indices have been used to collect some of the caries experience or gingival and periodontal health assessment data that are included in this important document. You can find the Healthy People 2010 document online at *www.healthypeople.gov*.

FOR YOUR PORTFOLIO

1. Include your personal written responses to the questions in the Everyday Ethics section from any of the chapters.

2. Explore the Internet to find oral health surveillance statistics for your community, state, or country. Analyze the statistics to describe the oral health status, and write a description of specific ways in which the oral health status of the population in your community might be improved by community-based dental hygiene interventions.

3. Include the patient assessment summary you developed in Competency Exercise 6 above. Write a short description of how the assessment data collection methods you used are linked to each component of patient information that is listed on the care plan template.

4. Demonstrate your interest and the development of your skills in providing culturally competent care by including any patient data collection or patient education materials that you discover for patients who are culturally different from yourself or most of your other patients. Include a discussion of how you have used these materials to enhance the quality of dental hygiene care you provide for your patients.

Dental Hygiene Diagnosis and Care Planning

Chapter 21-22

■ SECTION IV LEARNING OBJECTIVES

Completing the exercises in this section of the workbook will prepare you to:

1. Use assessment data to write dental hygiene diagnostic statements.
2. Use Evidence Based Decision Making (EBDM) steps to locate and evaluate current scientific evidence related to dental hygiene interventions.
3. Write a formal dental hygiene care plan based on the dental hygiene diagnosis that sequences evidence-based dental hygiene interventions in order to address identified patient needs.
4. Identify and apply procedures for obtaining informed consent.

■ COMPETENCIES FOR THE DENTAL HYGIENIST (APPENDIX A)

The following ADEA competencies are supported by the learning in Section IV.

Core Competencies: C3, C4, C5, C8, C9, C10, C11

Health Promotion and Disease Prevention Competencies: HP1, HP2, HP4, HP5, HP6

Patient/Client Care Competencies: PC1, PC2, PC3, PC5

Planning for Dental Hygiene Care

Learning Objectives

Upon successful completion of these exercises, you will be able to:

1. Identify and define key terms and concepts related to planning dental hygiene care.
2. Identify and explain assessment findings and individual patient factors that affect patient care.

3. Identify additional factors that can influence planning for dental hygiene care.
4. Apply the evidence-based decision-making process to determine patient care recommendations.

KNOWLEDGE EXERCISES

1. Supply the term or concept that matches each of the following descriptions:

   A. Measure of ability to perform self-care.

   _____

   B. A measure that integrates a combination of physical and cognitive ability.

   _____

   C. Statements that identify a problem.

   _____

   D. Identifies a problem within the dental hygiene scope of practice.

   _____

   E. An outcome that can be expressed as "excellent," "poor," or "guarded."

   _____

F. A diagnostic model that uses the phrase *related to* to link identified patient problems with risk factors or etiology.

_____

_____

G. Systemic conditions, behavioral factors, or environmental factors that can lead to increased probability of oral disease.

_____

_____

2. List the factors that determine prognosis after dental hygiene interventions.

_____

_____

_____

3. In your own words, define *anticipatory guidance*.

_____

_____

_____

4. List potential positive outcomes that might be expected following dental hygiene interventions.

_____

_____

_____

5. Identify and briefly describe the issues indicated by the mnemonic OSCAR.

O _____

S _____

C _____

A _____

R _____

6. Your patient's clinical diagnosis, provided by the periodontist, is chronic periodontitis. List the therapeutic goals of treatment for this patient.

_____

_____

_____

_____

_____

COMPETENCY EXERCISES

1. List three examples of *modifiable* risk factors for poor response to periodontal therapy.

_____

_____

_____

2. Mr. Diamond (Patient Assessment Summary #7, Appendix D) has numerous posterior teeth that present with significant bone loss, generalized mobility, and class II or III furcations. Moreover, he is not particularly compliant with your recommendations for self-care for those furcation areas. What is the prognosis for those teeth that you will discuss with Mr. Diamond when you are providing patient education?

3. For each patient description given below:
   - ◼ Circle the OSCAR issue(s) identified by the description.
   - ◼ Circle the American Society of Anesthesiologists (ASA) classification you might assign when assessing the patient during planning of dental hygiene care.
   - ◼ Write a justification for your selection.

A. Mrs. Kujath is 90 years old and in very good physical and mental health. She has chronic arthritis that is managed quite well with daily pain medication and has only minor problems with mobility, including sitting still for a long period of time. She doesn't really like the way her old denture looks and she wants a new one. She states that there is no problem about having the money to pay for the new denture.

O	S	C	A	R	
ASA:	I	II	III	IV	V

_____

_____

_____

B. Mr. Diamond (Patient Assessment Summary #7, Appendix D) has type 1 diabetes. His blood sugar levels indicate that his diabetes is not well controlled.

O	S	C	A	R	
ASA:	I	II	III	IV	V

_____

_____

_____

C. Mrs. Abdul must make a decision about treatment options for several teeth with severe periodontal involvement. Her health history indicates mild hypertension, well controlled by medication. It has been many years since she has been to the dentist because of an extremely unpleasant dental experience she had as a child.

She squirmed and protested when you measured her probing depths and, in general, had a very difficult time cooperating during the collection of assessment data. She says that she must talk with her son, as he will be bringing her for her appointments and will be paying for whatever treatment is decided on.

O   S   C   A   R
ASA: I   II   III   IV   V

_____

_____

D. Ms. Anitha Jones (Patient Assessment Summary #5, Appendix D) has cerebral palsy. She arrives at the dental office in a wheelchair and is accompanied by an attendant. Owing to extreme muscle spasticity caused by her condition, her arms and legs are in constant motion, sometimes lashing out unexpectedly, and she must have a variety of pads and restraints to maintain her position and safety in her wheelchair. You and her caregiver plan to transfer her from her wheelchair to the dental chair for treatment. Her health history indicates that she is *not* mentally disabled.

O   S   C   A   R
ASA: I   II   III   IV   V

_____

_____

4. Consider the periodontal diagnosis and assessment findings documented in the Patient Assessment Summary #7 for Mr. Diamond (Appendix D, page ____). Use the information in Table 21-4 of the textbook to identify treatment considerations for planning initial therapy dental hygiene care for this patient.

_____

_____

5. What is the plan for continuing care if Mr. Diamond's initial therapy outcomes are not optimal?

_____

_____

DISCOVERY EXERCISES

Before you begin, take some time to read the Primer on Evidence-Based Decision Making (EBDM) at the front of the workbook. Remember that finding current evidence to support your dental hygiene interventions is a skill that you will practice many times before you become proficient. This exercise is only a beginning.

Use the Patient Assessment Summary #1 for Christopher Michaels (Appendix D of this workbook) as a case study for this exercise. Your dental hygiene care plan, after Christopher's chief symptom has been resolved, will probably contain a recommendation for fluoride therapy. Apply the steps for evidence-based decision making to help you determine the best fluoride therapy regimen for this patient.

1. Develop a PICO question related to determining the best **fluoride regimen** to recommend for Christopher Michael's case.

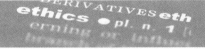

Everyday Ethics

Refer to the Codes of Ethics (Appendices I, II, and III in the textbook) and the Framework for Making Decisions (Table 1-2 in the textbook) as you discuss the following scenario with your classmates.

Victoria, a dental hygienist, is discussing the assessment findings for her patient Mr. Rush with the rest of the dental team. Mr. Rush has stated that he has already been told at his general dental office that he has extensive active periodontal disease. He was referred to this practice because he wants all of the most compromised teeth extracted and dental implants placed.

Mr. Rush has a number of risk factors, such as poorly controlled diabetes and smoking. Because his dental insurance is running out in 3 months, everyone is in a rush

to get the treatment started, and the potential for a poor prognosis has not been discussed. In fact, Victoria's concerns about the patient's risk factors are being pushed aside.

Questions for Consideration
1. What is Victoria's obligation (duty) to make sure that Mr. Rush understands how his risk factors compromise the prognosis of his treatment plan?
2. What action can Victoria take if her concerns continue to be ignored and treatment progresses without interventions that address the risk factors involved in Mr. Rush's case?
3. How should Victoria proceed to obtain informed consent from Mr. Rush and ensure that his rights to optimal care are maintained?

Factors To Teach The Patient

Your next patient, Jonathon Meyers, is a 26-year-old graduate student. He has not seen a dentist since he was a child. When his girlfriend told him about his bad breath, he decided to take advantage of the services offered at the dental clinic.

He presents with an aggressive periodontal condition in the lower anterior sextant of his mouth. Because he was not exposed to much dental education in his life, Jon has a low dental IQ and doesn't understand the cause and progression of dental disease. He smokes, demonstrates poor biofilm control, and states that he wants you to just "fix him up" with your treatments.

Using the example of a patient conversation from Appendix B as a guide, write a statement explaining why disease control measures must happen before and in conjunction with scaling. Explain *his role* in attaining and maintaining oral health.

Use the conversation you create to role play this situation with a fellow student. If you are the patient in the role play, be sure to ask questions. If you are the dental hygienist, try to anticipate questions and answer them in your explanation.

This scenario is related to the following factors:

- Why disease control measures are learned before and in conjunction with scaling
- Facts of oral disease prevention and oral health promotion relevant to the patient's current level of healthcare knowledge and individual risk factors

2. Type the components of your PICO question into the EviDents search engine (*http://medinformatics.uthscsa.edu/EviDents*). How many article citations did you receive? If necessary, go back to the EviDents search engine to explore ways to either limit or expand your search for articles.

3. Select two or three current articles from your literature search that seem as if they would be useful for helping you decide which fluoride therapies you will recommend for Christopher. Either go to the library to find the paper journal or use online full-text sources to read the articles you have selected. Read the articles and evaluate the strength and usefulness of the information that is in them.

4. Explore the Cochrane Collaboration Web site (*www.cochrane.org*) to discover how the site works. Explore the site to find and read abstracts or plain language summaries for the Cochrane Collaboration Systematic Review articles about fluoride.

The Dental Hygiene Care Plan

Chapter Outline

Learning Objectives

Upon successful completion of these exercises, you will be able to:

1. Identify and define key terms and concepts related to the written dental hygiene care plan.
2. Identify the components of a dental hygiene care plan.
3. Write dental hygiene diagnostic statements based on assessment findings.
4. Prepare a written dental hygiene care plan.
5. Apply procedures for discussing a care plan with the dentist and the patient.
6. Identify and apply procedures for obtaining informed consent.

KNOWLEDGE EXERCISES

1. Define the following terms in your own words.

   A. Dental hygiene intervention

   _____

   _____

   _____

   B. Informed consent

   _____

   _____

   _____

   C. Implied consent

   _____

   _____

   _____

   D. Informed refusal

   _____

   _____

   _____

2. Identify and define the three parts of a dental hygiene care plan.

_____

_____

_____

_____

_____

_____

3. List the components of a written care plan.

_____

_____

_____

4. List three individual patient requirements that can significantly influence the way in which a care plan is written.

_____

_____

_____

5. What is the purpose for explaining the entire treatment plan to the patient?

_____

_____

_____

6. What are some important points to consider when explaining the dental hygiene care plan to the patient?

_____

_____

_____

_____

_____

7. Identify five areas of information that you will discuss with the patient when you are obtaining informed consent.

_____

_____

_____

8. Which of the following is a factor that might affect the quadrant scaling and root planing sequence in a dental hygiene care plan?
   A. Availability of a power-driven scaler
   B. A periodontal abscess
   C. The amount of calculus in the lower anterior sextant
   D. Chronic systemic disease

COMPETENCY EXERCISES

1. Explain the role of the patient in prioritizing the patient's needs.

_____

_____

_____

_____

2. Explain the relationship between the master treatment plan and the dental hygiene care plan.

_____

_____

_____

_____

_____

3. Why are medical, personal, and clinical findings linked to actual or potential risk factors in the assessment findings section of a written dental hygiene care plan?

_____

_____

_____

_____

_____

4. Using your institution's guidelines for writing in patient records, document that the dental hygiene care plan was explained to the patient and informed consent was obtained.

Date	Comments	Signature

5. Using your institution's guidelines for case presentations, write a paragraph summarizing assessment findings for Mr. Harold Wilmot (Patient Assessment Summary #6, Appendix D) to present to the supervising dentist.

_____

_____

_____

_____

_____

_____

6. Select at least one risk factor or origin/cause from the list below that is related to each problem in the dental hygiene diagnostic statements below.

PROBLEM	CAUSE (RISK FACTORS AND ETIOLOGY)

Rampant caries related to _____

Plaque related to _____

At-risk pregnancy related to _____

Poor treatment prognosis related to _____

A. Inadequate daily care
B. Periodontal infection
C. Dietary factors
D. Tobacco use

7. Use the following information from the case of Jonathon Meyers, the 26-year-old graduate student you met in Chapter 21 of this workbook, to answer the questions below. Jon has not seen a dentist since he was a child. When his girlfriend told him about his bad breath, he decided to take advantage of the services offered at the dental clinic.

Jon presents with an aggressive periodontal condition in the lower anterior sextant of his mouth. He has a low dental IQ and doesn't understand the cause and progression of dental disease. He smokes, demonstrates poor biofilm control, and states that he wants you to just "fix him up" with your treatments.

A. Write a dental hygiene diagnosis statement using the assessment data on Jonathon Meyers.

Problem _____

Related to _____

B. What interventions will you plan to target the problem you identified?

_____

_____

_____

C. Write a goal for the problem you identified. Include a time frame for meeting the goal. How will you measure whether Jon met the goal?

Goal _____

Evaluation method _____

Time frame _____

DISCOVERY EXERCISES

Before you begin, take some time to again read the Primer on Evidence-Based Decision Making (EBDM), at the front of the workbook. Remember that finding and using current evidence to support your dental hygiene interven-

Everyday Ethics

Refer to the Codes of Ethics (Appendices I, II, and III in the textbook) and the Framework for Making Decisions (Table 1-2 in the textbook) as you discuss the following scenario with your classmates.

Ellen is responsible for explaining two alternative treatment plans to Mrs. Kwan, who is new to the practice. Mrs. Kwan must decide between several extractions, which would require expensive crown and bridge replacement, and treatment of periodontally involved teeth with poor prognosis. The decision must be made today if she is to begin treatment early next week, when there are several open appointments that must be filled.

English is not Mrs. Kwan's first language, and no one in the office speaks her language. Ellen has explained the information carefully, using pictures and patient-appropriate words, and has gone over both treatment alternatives several times. When Ellen asks Mrs. Kwan to summarize her understanding of the care plan, the patient just nods her head, smiles, and says, "I'll sign whatever you say."

Questions for Consideration
1. Does it appear that Mrs. Kwan understands her treatment alternatives and is informed sufficiently to give consent? How can voluntary informed consent be ensured?
2. What is Ellen's responsibility, as the knowledgeable professional, in selecting the choice of treatments while ensuring Mrs. Kwan's autonomy?
3. In what ways does the pressure of making a timely decision reflect paternalistic treatment of Mrs. Kwan by the dental office?

Factors To Teach The Patient

Using the example of a patient conversation from Appendix B as a guide, write a statement explaining to Mrs. Kwan, the patient in the Everyday Ethics scenario, what informed consent means.
This scenario is related to the following factors:

- Why patient input into the final care plan is important
- The patient's rights and responsibilities regarding informed consent

tions is a skill that you will practice many times before you become proficient. This exercise is only a beginning.

1. Use the scientific evidence you located in the Discovery Exercises for Chapter 21 to write a patient-specific dental hygiene care plan for Christopher Michaels that includes an evidence-based regimen for fluoride therapy.

2. What factors might influence how Christopher or his parents comply with the recommendations in your care plan? How will you adapt your care plan (or educate your patient) if you suspect that there will be problems with compliance?

Dental Hygiene Diagnosis and Care Planning

■ Chapters 21-22

COMPETENCY EXERCISES

1. Using the template provided in Appendix C or the care plan form that you use in your dental hygiene program, develop a comprehensive dental hygiene care plan using assessment data from one of the patient cases provided in Appendix D of this workbook.

2. Write an outline of important points to address when obtaining informed consent for the care plan you developed in Exercise 1 above. Adapt this outline to use in clinic when you are discussing a care plan with a patient.

3. Practice documenting informed consent for a patient record.

DISCOVERY EXERCISES

1. Type the phrase *evidence based* into your favorite Internet search engine. Explore some of the Web sites listed in the results of the search to discover resources available to support an evidence-based approach to health care. Are there any resources that are specific to the dental profession? Which ones contain oral health information?

2. Remember Jonathon Meyers, the graduate student from the exercises in Chapters 21 and 22? Imagine that you have now completed his initial therapy plan and are evaluating the results. He has reached most of the goals you set together in the plan, and his oral health status has much improved.

   You recommend a 3-month periodontal maintenance interval, but he wants to wait at least 6 months before coming to see you again. He cites recent toothpaste television commercials that recommend seeing a dentist every 6 months. You know that patients with a history of periodontal infection need to be seen more often.

   Conduct a brief review of recent literature to determine what scientific evidence supports a shorter periodontal maintenance interval. Explain to Jon why those research findings influence your recommendations for his continuing care plan.

QUESTIONS PATIENTS ASK

"I saw something on the Internet recently about new research that proves that a certain new kind of treatment is more effective than the recommendations you have made in my dental hygiene care plan. Can we change my dental hygiene care plan?"
Points to consider when you answer:
■ First conduct a literature search to identify the research study that the patient is talking about. Find out if there are more studies that substantiate the efficacy of the new treatment. Take time to evaluate the information in the articles according to the principles of EBDM.
■ Assure your patient that the recommendations in his care plan are based on multiple factors identified in the evidence-based decision-making model and not just on one new research study.
■ Discuss the way in which the level of evidence available about this new treatment will affect your determination of how valuable and useful the information is in making recommendations for patient care.

FOR YOUR PORTFOLIO

1. Using the patient-specific dental hygiene care plan template in Appendix C or the care-plan format used in your dental hygiene program, complete comprehensive dental hygiene care plans for a variety of patients you have assessed in your school clinic. Demonstrate your ability to plan for a diverse selection of patients by selecting care plans prepared for patients with a variety of systemic conditions, risk factors, and levels of dental disease.

2. Include a care plan prepared at the beginning of your education and one for a similar patient prepared near the end of your education. Provide a written statement that reflects on and analyzes the ways in which a comparison of the two care plans demonstrates what you have learned about planning patient care.

Implementation: Prevention

■ SECTION V LEARNING OBJECTIVES

Completing the exercises in this section of the workbook will prepare you to:
1. Educate patients regarding the prevention of oral disease.
2. Promote patient behaviors and practices that enhance oral health.
3. Select patient-specific dental hygiene interventions that will prevent oral disease and promote oral health.

■ COMPETENCIES FOR THE DENTAL HYGIENIST (APPENDIX A)

The following ADEA competencies are supported by the learning in Section V.
Core Competencies: C3, C4, C5, C6, C8, C9, C10,C11
Health Promotion and Disease Prevention Competencies: HP1, HP2, HP4, HP5
Patient/Client Care Competencies: PC1, PC2, PC3, PC5

CHAPTER 23

Health Promotion and Disease Prevention

Chapter Outline

Learning Objectives

Upon successful completion of these exercises, you will be able to:

1. Identify and define key terms and concepts related to health promotion and disease prevention.
2. List and describe the steps in a preventive program.
3. Describe key factors and procedures that enhance successful patient learning and motivation.
4. Identify and describe disclosing agents.
5. Identify the causes, effects, and management of xerostomia and halitosis.

KNOWLEDGE EXERCISES

1. Your skills in communication and marketing will have an effect on patient motivation and compliance with oral health recommendations. In your own words, define these concepts.

   ◼ *Communication*

   _____

   _____

   _____

   ◼ *Marketing*

   _____

   _____

   _____

   ◼ *Motivation*

   _____

   _____

   _____

■ *Compliance*

_____

_____

_____

2. In your own words, define *behavior modification*.

_____

_____

_____

3. Patients who desire to attain and maintain their own oral health will often increase their knowledge or skills in all three learning domains. Identify and describe the three domains of learning.

_____

_____

_____

4. Read the definitions of *dental health education, health education, health promotion,* and *preventive dental hygiene* in Box 23-1 in the textbook. Combine these definitions to define your role as a health educator during each patient's dental hygiene appointment.

_____

_____

_____

5. In your own words, briefly describe each of the steps in a preventive program.

_____

_____

_____

_____

_____

6. In your own words, briefly summarize or restate the principles of learning.

_____

_____

_____

_____

_____

7. Why is it important to provide initial oral hygiene instructions for your patient before any clinical treatment is started?

_____

_____

_____

8. Patient education is not provided in a rote, unchanging manner but rather is adapted to individual patient needs and current health status. Oral disease prevention programs are usually more successful if a series of lessons are planned and coordinated to build and reinforce patient knowledge and skills. State the objective and briefly describe what is included in each lesson of a series of patient-education sessions in biofilm control.

■ *Lesson 1*

_____

_____

_____

■ *Lesson 2*

_____

_____

_____

■ *Additional lessons*

_____

_____

_____

9. Identify the general characteristics that determine the value of teaching aids and health-education reading materials that you select for patient education.

_____

_____

_____

10. Models and toothbrushes are commonly used to teach brushing methods to patients. What factors limit this method of teaching oral hygiene measures for individual patients?

_____

_____

_____

11. In what ways does a disclosing agent help you provide patient instruction?

_____

_____

_____

12. List the properties of an acceptable disclosing agent.

_____

_____

_____

13. Identify the major types of disclosing agents that are available for use. Be sure to ask your instructor how much detail you will be expected to know about the composition of each formula.

_____

_____

_____

_____

_____

_____

14. List the steps for direct application of a disclosing agent.

_____

_____

_____

_____

_____

_____

15. What steps will you take after you have applied the disclosing solution to your patient's teeth?

_____

_____

_____

16. The best prevention programs help your patients increase their knowledge about all aspects of their oral health. During oral hygiene instructions, you will teach your patients much more about oral disease prevention than just biofilm removal. For example, saliva has numerous functions relating to the maintenance of oral health. List the functions of saliva that help protect your patients' oral health.

_____

_____

_____

17. What are the oral effects of xerostomia?

_____

_____

_____

18. Dental hygienists are often the first to recognize or hear patient reports of oral dryness. What recommendations can you make to help your patient overcome the effects of xerostomia?

_____

_____

_____

19. Halitosis can be described as the _organoleptic_ recognition of _putrefaction_ or _volatile sulfur compounds._ Use the definitions of the italicized terms to explain halitosis (see Box 23-1 in the textbook).

_____

_____

_____

20. Identify the oral and nonoral factors that you will investigate if your patient reports halitosis.

▪ _Oral factors_

_____

_____

▪ _Nonoral factors_

_____

_____

_____

COMPETENCY EXERCISES

1. Describe how the steps in a preventive program (listed at the beginning of the textbook chapter) are integrated with the dental hygiene process of care; in other words, compare these two concepts.

_____

_____

_____

2. When you complete your assessment for Patrick Callaghan, who has presented for a 6-month maintenance appointment, you conclude that overall he has very good oral hygiene and periodontal health. You notice only very slight biofilm and slightly

enlarged and reddened interproximal papilla in the maxillary right molar area. You note a slight coating on his tongue and think that this may be related to his comment that he sometimes feels like he has bad breath, especially in the morning when he wakes up.

Write a dental hygiene diagnosis statement for Mr. Callaghan's care plan.

Problem	Cause (risk factors and origin)
_____ *related to* _____	

3. You decide Mr. Callaghan needs very little reinforcement for his toothbrushing techniques, as his biofilm levels are very low. You spend the available patient-education time concentrating on his flossing technique in the upper right side of his mouth, where you noticed the biofilm on the proximal surfaces. You also spend a few minutes demonstrating tongue cleaning with a scraper to help him learn how to remove the biofilm accumulating there. Using your institution's guidelines for writing in patient records, document your oral hygiene instructions for Mr. Callaghan.

Date	Comments	Signature

4. It has been slightly more than 1 year since you last saw Melina, age 15, for a dental hygiene maintenance appointment. As you update her health history, Melina impresses you with a description of her school science fair project, which focuses on the effects of different diseases on the quality of life. She talks to you for a long time about her discovery, from reading the surgeon general's *Report on Oral Health* and other documents, that the effects of oral diseases, especially dental caries and periodontal infections, can cause children and adults to miss millions of hours of work and school. She accurately discusses the concept that oral diseases are directly related to general health status. She excitedly gives you examples of how oral diseases are completely preventable by limiting sucrose in the diet, taking adequate oral hygiene measures, using

Everyday Ethics

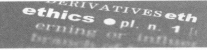

Refer to the Codes of Ethics (Appendices I, II, and III in the textbook) and Framework for Making Decisions (Table 1-2 in the textbook) as you discuss the following scenario with your classmates.

Jeremy was a favorite patient in the dental office. Jeremy had undergone extensive restorative work as a young child because he had collided on a swing set with an older sibling, which resulted in trauma to both maxillary and mandibular incisors and permanent tooth buds. Now 15 years old, Jeremy seemed to grow 2 or 3 inches each time he came for his maintenance appointments.

Tressa, the dental hygienist, always commented on what a handsome young man Jeremy was becoming. He received a "fair plus" on his oral home-care report card the last few visits, but this time something was different. Tressa noticed more biofilm on Jeremy's teeth, and a distinct unpleasant odor. Tressa made a mental note to let him smell the dental floss she used in his mouth as part of her personal home-care review.

Questions for Consideration
1. Professionally, was the dental hygienist approaching Jeremy according to his needs while developing a realistic dental hygiene treatment plan for educating him?
2. Was Tressa's assumption that Jeremy had halitosis as a result of poor oral hygiene correct? What other factors could have been considered or communicated to Jeremy?
3. Suggest which of the core values apply in this scenario. Is this something Tressa should keep confidential from Jeremy's parents? Why or why not?

fluorides, and having regular access to preventive dental services.

When you collect intraoral assessment data for Melina, you discover that her own daily brushing and flossing are inadequate for biofilm removal and, like many other teenagers, she often drinks carbonated beverages and juice several times during the day.

Where is Melina on the learning ladder for attaining and maintaining oral health?

_____

_____

_____

5. How can you plan care and education interventions for Melina, during this and subsequent dental hygiene appointments, that will help her climb each remaining step of the learning ladder?

_____

_____

_____

Factors To Teach The Patient

Mr. Callaghan (presented in Competency Exercise question 2) compliments you on your oral hygiene instructions and says he remembers that the other dental hygienist, Patty, whom he saw 6 months ago, told him exactly the same things. He wonders if you two have a memorized script that you each simply repeat every time a patient comes in.

Use the example of a patient conversation in Appendix B as a guide to write a statement explaining your patient-education procedures to Mr. Callaghan.
This scenario is related to the following factors:

- The relationship between preventive measures and clinical services
- Why particular preventive measures are selected for a particular patient

24 CHAPTER

Protocols for Prevention and Control of Dental Caries

Chapter Outline

Learning Objectives

Upon successful completion of these exercises, you will be able to:

1. Identify and define key terms and concepts related to dental caries.

2. Identify the stages of dental caries and describe the caries process.
3. Plan protocols for prevention, remineralization, and maintenance based on individualized assessment of risk factors for dental caries.

KNOWLEDGE EXERCISES

Key Words and Terms Crossword Puzzle

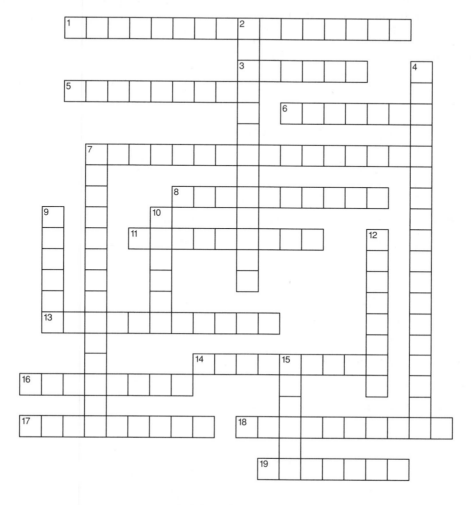

Across

1 Dissolution of enamel or cementum and dentin caused by acid-producing bacteria.
3 Professional term meaning cavities or dental decay.
5 Another term for secondary caries.
6 Describes rapidly progressing caries in many teeth; an acute condition as opposed to a chronic condition.
7 Aided by sufficient saliva and by the action of topical fluorides.
8 The final stage in the process of caries formation.
11 The science and study of dental decay.
13 Habits, behaviors, lifestyles, or conditions that increase the probability of a disease occurring (two words).
14 A term that refers to diagnosis of dental caries.
16 Describes the caries process that has been halted.
17 This lesion gives evidence of subsurface demineralization (two words).
18 Refers to bacteria that are capable of turning fermentable carbohydrates into acid.
19 Ingredient in chewing gum that reduces levels of *Streptococcus mutans* and promotes remineralization.

Down

2 Another species of bacteria that are more active in the later stages (progression) of decay.
4 Refers to types of bacteria that predominate in the initial stages of the caries process.
7 Determination of a patient's risk factors (two words).
9 One function (action) of saliva; helps to increase the amount of acid necessary to produce a change in pH that initiates the demineralization process.
10 Buffers acids in the mouth and supplies minerals to replace the calcium and phosphate ions dissolved during demineralization.
12 Type of radiograph that can reveal caries on proximal surfaces of teeth.
15 A hole; in dentistry, another word for dental caries.

Control of Dental Caries

1. In your own words, describe how the metabolic action of *Streptococcus mutans* and *Lactobacillus* bacteria contributes to the destruction of tooth structure and causes dental caries.

   _____

   _____

   _____

2. A child can be at risk for dental caries as soon as tooth eruption begins. Why?

   _____

   _____

   _____

3. List the types of fermentable carbohydrates.

   _____

   _____

   _____

4. Identify the acids produced during the metabolic process of the bacteria in dental biofilm.

   _____

   _____

   _____

5. The _____ of carbohydrate ingestion in your patient's diet has a strong influence on the amount of acid produced and the extent of tooth destruction.

6. In what ways does the presence of adequate saliva protect your patient against dental decay?

   _____

   _____

   _____

7. In your own words, describe how fluoride protects your patient against dental decay.

   _____

   _____

   _____

8. Although the incidence of dental caries in the general population has declined in recent years, dental caries is still a major problem that affects the health and welfare of adults and children alike. The dental hygienist's focus in caries detection has changed from identifying only end-stage dental caries that require restoration to identifying patient risk factors and the earliest stages of dental caries. At this point, dental hygiene interventions can help remineralize the natural tooth structure. What tools will you use to identify dental caries at very early stages during an oral examination of your patient?

   _____

   _____

   _____

9. In your own words, describe what you will observe during a visual examination at each of the stages of dental caries on a tooth surface.

   ▆ *Initial infection*

   _____

   _____

   ▆ *Early subsurface infection*

   _____

   _____

   ▆ *Early white spot lesion*

   _____

   _____

   ▆ *Later white spot lesion*

   _____

   _____

   ▆ *Cavitation*

   _____

   _____

   ▆ *Radiographic (proximal surface) early dental caries*

   _____

   _____

   ▆ *Large proximal surface dental caries*

   _____

   _____

10. In your own words, outline the dental hygienist's role (objectives and interventions) in planning patient care for caries management.

_____

_____

_____

_____

_____

_____

11. What is the purpose of discussing individualized caries risk assessment with each patient?

_____

_____

_____

12. How can you best gather data to assess your patient's individual caries risk factors?

_____

_____

_____

_____

_____

_____

13. Outline a protocol for remineralization that you can initiate when your patient has evidence of early carious lesions that do not yet require restorative treatment.

_____

_____

_____

_____

_____

COMPETENCY EXERCISES

1. Seventeen-year-old Tren Nguyen emigrated to the United States with his family about 6 years ago. Since he arrived, Tren has embraced all things American and spends his free time playing computer games, snacking on fast food, and hanging out with friends. Tren's history of dental visits has been infrequent. He has been seen in your office only twice before—right after he arrived in the United States and then again about 3 years ago for a prophylaxis. No significant dental findings were charted at either of those visits. He has no history of previous dental restorations. He came to the clinic today because a dental checkup is required as part of his physical examination to play sports when he goes off to college next fall.

   When you examine Tren's mouth today, you find significant early and late white spot lesions on the facial surfaces of almost all of his teeth. It is interesting that there are no observable caries in the pits and fissures on the occlusal surfaces of any of his teeth and the surfaces are not deeply grooved. Make a list of the questions you will ask Tren as you gather caries risk-assessment data before you write his dental hygiene care plan.

   _____

   _____

   _____

   _____

   _____

   _____

2. Now comes the fun part. You don't usually get to make up answers for all the questions that you ask your patients, but this time we can't go any further with these exercises unless we have some data. In the interest of your own learning, make up reasonable-sounding answers for each of the questions you asked Tren during your discussion of caries risk factors.

   Using the data you have collected from Tren's caries risk assessment, write two dental hygiene diagnosis statements for his care plan.

   Problem   **Cause (risk factors and origin)**

   _____ *related to* _____

   _____ *related to* _____

3. List the dental hygiene interventions you will plan to help Tren *arrest or control* disease and *regenerate, restore, or maintain* his oral health.

   ■ *Clinical interventions*

   _____

   _____

   _____

◼ *Education/counseling*

_____

_____

◼ *Oral hygiene instructions/home care*

_____

_____

_____

_____

4. Write a goal for each problem identified in the dental hygiene diagnosis statements (question 2) you wrote for Tren's care plan. Include a time frame for meeting each goal. How will you measure whether your patient met each goal?

Goal 1

_____

_____

◼ *Evaluation method*

_____

_____

_____

◼ *Time frame*

_____

_____

_____

Goal 2

_____

_____

_____

◼ *Evaluation method*

_____

_____

_____

◼ *Time frame*

_____

_____

Goal 3

_____

_____

_____

Everyday Ethics

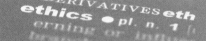

Refer to the Codes of Ethics (Appendices I, II, and III in the textbook) and Framework for Making Decisions (Table 1-2 in the textbook) as you discuss the following scenario with your classmates.

Sophie and Helen were two sisters who had been Dr. Newbury's patients for the past 30 years. Now in their 70s, they were experiencing new concerns with restorations and crowns that showed signs of occlusal wear and recurrent caries. Many margins of amalgam restorations had catches with the explorer upon examination.

Ken, the dental hygienist, continued to stress the importance of more frequent maintenance visits, but Sophie curtly reminded him that she "has been coming to the dentist since before he was born!" Ken suspected they did not want to hear about crowns that should be replaced or make decisions about the restorations that needed replacement.

A progress note in Helen's chart read, "the patient was not open to new home-care education techniques or interested in a proposed treatment plan to replace amalgam restorations in teeth nos. 15, 18, 19, 30, and 31."

Questions for Consideration
1. What possible errors in judgment have Dr. Newbury and Ken made in discussing the current oral condition of Sophie's and Helen's restorative needs?
2. Is the entry in the patient's chart appropriate? Why or why not? Explain your rationale using ethical principles to defend your documentation.
3. What role can prevention play in the patient/provider relationship depicted in this scenario?

■ *Evaluation method*

_____

_____

_____

■ *Time frame*

_____

_____

_____

Factors To Teach The Patient

Use the example of a patient conversation in Appendix B as a guide to write a conversation explaining the components of Tren's care plan to him in such a way that you will motivate him to comply with your recommendations. (This patient was introduced in the Competency Exercises.) *This scenario is related to the following factors:*

■ What causes cavities and how they develop
■ That early dental caries is not a cavity; what demineralization means
■ How remineralization can be accomplished using fluoride toothpaste and drinking fluoridated water daily
■ That the use of fluorides is necessary throughout life

Oral Infection Control: Toothbrushes and Toothbrushing

Chapter Outline

Learning Objectives

Upon successful completion of these exercises, you will be able to:

1. Identify and define key terms and concepts related to toothbrushes and toothbrushing.
2. Describe the characteristics, factors influencing selection, and proper care of manual toothbrushes.
3. Describe indications, procedures, and limitations for a variety of toothbrushing methods and select appropriate toothbrushing methods for individual patients.
4. Discuss indications for use of power toothbrushes and identify important design, technique, and patient instruction factors.
5. Identify indications and methods for supplemental brushing.
6. Select toothbrushing techniques for special conditions.

KNOWLEDGE EXERCISES

There's a Method to Our Madness

There are a variety of different toothbrushing methods you can teach your patients. Some are better than others for maximizing plaque removal and minimizing damage to oral tissues. But all of them are included in this word search puzzle.

To solve the puzzle, find the words in the grid. Words in the grid can run across, down, or diagonally and can start at the right or left or top or bottom. When you have found all the words, the first 24 unused letters in the grid will complete the hidden message.

Hidden message: When you provide oral hygiene instructions to your patient,

_____

_____

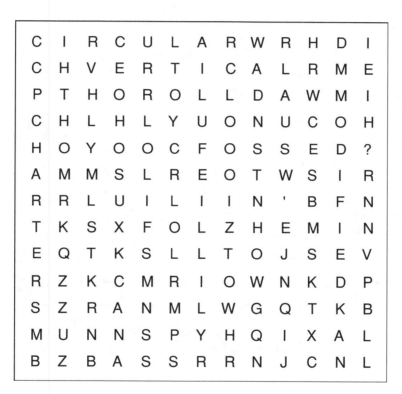

```
C  I  R  C  U  L  A  R  W  R  H  D  I
C  H  V  E  R  T  I  C  A  L  R  M  E
P  T  H  O  R  O  L  L  D  A  W  M  I
C  H  L  H  L  Y  U  O  N  U  C  O  H
H  O  Y  O  O  C  F  O  S  S  E  D  ?
A  M  M  S  L  R  E  O  T  W  S  I  R
R  R  L  U  I  L  I  N  '  B  F  N
T  K  S  X  F  O  L  Z  H  E  M  I  N
E  Q  T  K  S  L  L  T  O  J  S  E  V
R  Z  K  C  M  R  I  O  W  N  K  D  P
S  Z  R  A  N  M  L  W  G  Q  T  K  B
M  U  N  N  S  P  Y  H  Q  I  X  A  L
B  Z  B  A  S  S  R  R  N  J  C  N  L
```

Word Search Words

Bass	Leonard	Smith's
Charters	Modified	Stillman
Circular	Physiologic	Sulcular
Fones	Roll	Vertical
Horizontal	Scrub	

Techniques and Equipment

1. Define *toothbrush abrasion*.

   _____

   _____

   _____

2. In your own words, describe an effective toothbrush handle.

   _____

   _____

   _____

3. Describe a tuft in the head of a toothbrush.

   _____

   _____

   _____

4. List four factors that affect the stiffness or firmness of toothbrush filaments.

   _____

   _____

   _____

5. List four factors that influence the type of toothbrush selected for an individual patient.

   _____

   _____

   _____

6. In your own words, describe the procedure for holding a toothbrush and positioning it in the mouth for effective removal of dental biofilm.

   _____

   _____

   _____

7. Identify three methods for timing patient brushing to enhance effectiveness.

   _____

   _____

   _____

8. The Bass method of brushing is widely taught by dental hygienists to enhance effectiveness of their patients' oral cleaning. What problems are some-times encountered as patients try to learn this technique?

   _____

   _____

   _____

9. Which two methods of toothbrushing are some-times taught to young children when they have difficulty mastering a sulcular brushing technique?

   _____

   _____

   _____

10. Describe the procedure for the modified Stillman method of toothbrushing.

    _____

    _____

    _____

11. Which toothbrushing methods instruct the patient to direct the brush filaments at a 45° angle toward the gingival margin?

    _____

    _____

    _____

12. Which toothbrushing method instructs the patient to direct the brush filaments at a 45° angle toward the occlusal plane?

    _____

    _____

    _____

13. What are the problems with biofilm removal when the patient uses the method identified in question 12?

    _____

    _____

    _____

14. What three factors in toothbrushing are most likely to contribute to gingival recession or tooth abrasion?

    _____

    _____

    _____

15. List two methods for brushing occlusal surfaces.

_____

_____

_____

16. What two anatomic features contribute to retention of dental biofilm on a patient's tongue?

_____

_____

_____

17. Identify two methods for cleaning the tongue.

_____

_____

_____

18. List two alterations in the appearance of gingival tissues that require you to teach a different toothbrushing technique to correct or reduce gingival damage.

_____

_____

_____

19. Identify three special circumstances in which the use of a powered toothbrush can enhance the removal of bacterial biofilm.

_____

_____

_____

20. In your own words, describe the motion of an oscillating power toothbrush head. (*Hint:* Use your hand to demonstrate the motion described in Table 25-3 in the textbook.)

_____

_____

_____

COMPETENCY EXERCISES

1. Nicholas Bean, a 12-year-old who is your first patient of the day, is going right from his prophylaxis appointment to the orthodontist's office, where they will be placing full-mouth bands and brackets on his teeth. You know that the best toothbrush to recommend for him to use is a bilevel-orthodontic toothbrush, but you do not happen to have a sample to give him. You decide to tell his mother what it looks like so she can get one. Using terminology from Figure 25-1 in the textbook and the pictures from Figure 25-2 in the textbook, write a brief description of this type of toothbrush trim profile.

_____

_____

_____

2. Mr. Gabriel Chin is one of your favorite patients, and he loves to share stories of his travels around the world. Today when he presents for his recall appointment, he shows you some toothbrushes that he recently brought back from a trip to visit relatives in his native country. The toothbrush, he states proudly, is the type his family has been using for many years and is made from the hairs of wild boars. You want to educate him without belittling his enthusiasm for his family's history. To help him understand about a better alternative, list three reasons why nylon or synthetic filaments are used today for toothbrushes instead of natural bristles.

_____

_____

_____

3. Mrs. Janette Evans has been diagnosed with active periodontal disease. You will be working closely with her once a week for the next 2 months to control oral disease and obtain periodontal health because she will soon be going into the hospital for open-heart surgery. What important information should you give her about how to care for her toothbrush?

_____

_____

_____

4. As you are providing oral hygiene instructions using the Bass method for Mrs. Evans, she asks you how much time she should spend brushing her teeth in order to thoroughly remove all of the biofilm, as you are recommending. Explain one of the methods she can use to monitor her toothbrushing.

_____

_____

_____

_____

_____

_____

5. When you are showing Mrs. Evans how to brush, you note that she needs some extra help with the distal surfaces of tooth 19, the most posterior tooth in that arch. Explain how she should position her toothbrush.

_____

_____

_____

6. How can Mrs. Evans effectively use her toothbrush to clean the mesial surface of tooth 7, which is extremely rotated and tilted in a labial direction?

_____

_____

_____

7. Using your institution's guidelines for writing in patient records, document the oral hygiene instructions you provided for Mrs. Evans. Be sure to include enough detail so that you can use the comments at a subsequent visit to reinforce the information you provided.

Date   **Comments**   **Signature**

_____

_____

8. When you see Mrs. Evans a week later, her biofilm scores are a bit lower but still not up to the levels you would like to see after your extensive oral hygiene instructions. When you do your intraoral examination, you notice a scuffed epithelial surface, several red pinpoint spots, and some generalized redness along the lingual gingival margin of teeth 13–15 and the facial margins of teeth 29–31. You determine that these acute lesions may be the result of toothbrushing activity during the previous week. Identify three possible precipitating factors, and explain measures you or Mrs. Evans should take to eliminate the problems.

_____

_____

_____

Everyday Ethics

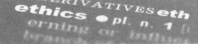

Refer to the Codes of Ethics (Appendices I, II, and III in the textbook) and Framework for Making Decisions (Table 1-2 in the textbook) as you discuss the following scenario with your classmates.

RJ is 19 years old and works in the sterilization center of a local hospital. In the past 6 months, his work schedule was changed from a day shift to a shift that requires him to work at night. At his maintenance appointment, Brandi, the dental hygienist, reviewed the patient's history and noted that everything seemed the same except that RJ had developed the habit of drinking many cups of coffee to help stay awake at work.

RJ has noticed more staining on his teeth and tongue than ever before, and he reports a bad taste in his mouth. Brandi plans to recommend a power toothbrush and a tongue cleaner.

Questions for Consideration

1. Is it ethical for the dental hygienist to address RJ's consumption of coffee before reviewing brushing techniques? From what role or perspective would this be appropriate?

2. RJ interprets his change in oral health to be a result of working at night because he is not following his normal routine of brushing. What suggestions can Brandi offer RJ that would facilitate a regular routine of brushing?

3. The office in which Brandi practices provides a specific brand of power brush to their patients as a part of the maintenance visit. Brandi has never used the product, and neither has she read any research or literature about the product. She is basing her recommendation of the brush on the fact that she has seen some good results in other patients. Is there an ethical problem in recommending a product about which Brandi knows very little? What types of questions might Brandi's patients have that she would not be able to answer? Why is it the responsibility of a dental hygienist to know about a variety of over-the-counter products?

9. What are some reasons you might recommend a power toothbrush for Mrs. Evans instead of the manual toothbrushing technique you originally taught her?

_____

_____

_____

DISCOVERY EXERCISES

Collaborate with your classmates to gather samples of a variety of different power toothbrushes. (*Hint:* Contacting dental product companies is one way to do this, or you can use models that you, your classmates, or your faculty already own.)

1. For each brand or model of power toothbrush, determine the following information:
   - *Motion*
   - *Brush head shape*
   - *Filaments*
   - *Handle size and shape*
   - *Overall weight*
   - *Power source*
   - *Speed*

2. Discuss which model would be best for a variety of situations—for example, which one would you recommend for a child? for a caregiver to use when brushing someone else's teeth? Think of other situations and types of patients.

3. Is there any research evidence to support the recommendation of any of these types of power toothbrushes for your patients?

QUESTIONS PATIENTS ASK

"What toothbrush is right for me?" "Is a power toothbrush really worth buying? Will it help keep my teeth

Factors To Teach The Patient

Thomas Raveli, 18, is home for the holiday from his first term at college, and his mother has insisted that he keep his appointment with you for his regular 6-month cleaning. As you collect assessment data before providing dental hygiene care, you become very aware that his overall oral status is not the same as it has been at previous visits. You note generalized bleeding on probing and overall red and inflamed gingiva. Fortunately, there is no radiographic evidence of bone level changes.

Further questioning reveals that his overall home-care routine has not been adequate and his eating patterns include frequent snacking because he doesn't particularly like the regular meals served in his dorm. He tells you about how hard it is to keep a regular schedule when he is so stressed by his college workload. He comments that it has been especially tough during the last several weeks when he was writing final exams. That's when he started noticing that his gums were bleeding every time he brushed his teeth! It hurt to brush, so he admits that he has been neglectful of his daily oral care.

Use the example of the patient conversation Guidelines for Teaching Toothbrushing in Appendix B to write a statement explaining how using the proper brushing techniques can help prevent future problems for Thomas.

Use the conversation you create to role play this situation with a fellow student. If you are the patient in the role play, be sure to ask questions. If you are the dental hygienist, try to anticipate questions and provide evidence-based answers for them in your explanation.

cleaner and my gums healthier?" How do you know that the toothbrushing method you are teaching me is right for me?" You will hear these types of questions from your patients many, many times.

What sources of information can you identify that will help you answer your patient's questions in this scenario? How will you use the evidence-based decision-making methods you learned from reading the EBDM Primer in the front of this workbook to help answer these questions for each specific patient?

Interdental Care

Chapter Outline

Learning Objectives

Upon successful completion of these exercises, you will be able to:

1. Identify and define key terms and concepts related to interdental care.
2. Describe the interdental embrasures.
3. Describe the characteristics, indications, and procedures for use of a variety of interdental cleaning devices.
4. Include individualized recommendations for interdental care in dental hygiene care plans.

KNOWLEDGE EXERCISES

1. Posterior teeth have _____ papillae with a col and anterior teeth have _____ papilla that forms a small col under the contact area.

2. Identify tissue and anatomic characteristics of the col, the adjacent teeth, and the surrounding papillae that contribute to the increased risk of gingivitis in the interdental area.

   _____

   _____

   _____

3. Identify the different types of floss that you and your patient can select, based on individual preference and needs.

   _____

   _____

   _____

4. Complete Infomap 26-1 to compare the benefits and limitations of waxed (or PTFE) and unwaxed floss, as noted in the textbook.

INFOMAP 26-1

FLOSS TYPE	BENEFITS	LIMITATIONS
Waxed or expanded PTFE		
Unwaxed floss		

5. Identify the location, cause of, and methods for preventing floss cuts and clefts.

_____

_____

_____

6. What is a floss aid?

_____

_____

_____

7. Describe tufted dental floss.

_____

_____

_____

8. In what situations should you recommend the use of tufted floss, knitting yarn, or gauze strips instead of regular dental floss or tape for your patient?

_____

_____

_____

9. What kind of flossing motion can be applied with tufted floss, knitting yarn, or gauze strips that is not typically applied with regular floss?

_____

_____

_____

10. Describe the shapes of interdental brushes.

_____

_____

_____

11. Describe a situation in which the interdental brush is a better choice than dental floss for complete biofilm removal or for application of chemotherapeutic agents on proximal surfaces of teeth.

_____

_____

_____

12. End-tuft brushes are usually recommended for a single area that is difficult to reach with a regular toothbrush. In what specific situations can you recommend the use of an end-tuft brush?

_____

_____

_____

13. In your own words, describe a wooden interdental cleaner, state how it is used, and identify factors you must consider when recommending it for a patient.

_____

_____

_____

14. Describe an interdental tip and a toothpick in holder and explain how they are used.

■ *Interdental tip*

_____

_____

_____

Everyday Ethics

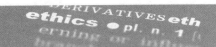

Refer to the Codes of Ethics (Appendices I, II, and III in the textbook) and Framework for Making Decisions (Table 1-2 in the textbook) as you discuss the following scenario with your classmates.

A new patient, Jane, is excited about information she has just read on the Internet about a powered flossing device. She begins to ask Glenna, the dental hygienist, detailed questions about the product, such as whether it really works, where it can be purchased, and how much it costs. Glenna is unfamiliar with the flossing aid but doesn't want to be embarrassed in front of the patient so she tells Jane

the product doesn't work and spends an extra 5 minutes at the end of the appointment going over manual flossing techniques.

Questions for Consideration

1. In ethical terms, how would Glenna's action be described?
2. From the patient's perspective, what is the role of the dental hygienist in this situation?
3. Is it unethical to mislead the patient about a product when the value is unknown or the dental hygienist prefers the benefits of another (perhaps rival) product? Why or why not?

■ *Toothpick in holder*

_____

_____

_____

15. List the patient assessment factors that provide information to help you assess your patient's individual needs before recommending a specific device for his or her interdental care.

_____

_____

_____

bridge. He has high levels of biofilm on all proximal areas and along the gingival margin of the orthodontic band. Write two dental hygiene diagnosis statements related to these issues.

Problem	**Cause (Risk Factors and Etiology)**
_____ *related to*	_____
_____ *related to*	_____

COMPETENCY EXERCISES

1. The best way to learn how to teach a patient about flossing is to practice doing it. Use all of the information you learned in the textbook chapter to teach a family member or friend (but not one of your student colleagues, because he or she has already read this chapter) about how and when to floss.

2. After careful assessment of his current oral hygiene measures, you find that your patient, Mr. Adamson, has very large hands and has a great deal of difficulty maneuvering dental floss in his posterior teeth. He also has an orthodontic band on tooth 3, which positions a temporary appliance being used to maintain an open space for the later placement of a permanent

Factors To Teach The Patient

Use the example of a patient conversation in Appendix B as a guide to develop a conversation explaining to Mr. Adamson (introduced in question 2 of the Competency Exercises) how to assemble and use the interdental devises you are recommending.
This scenario is related to the following factors:

■ By demonstration with disclosing agent, how the toothbrush doesn't clean the interdental area thoroughly
■ Dental biofilm and how it collects on the proximal tooth surfaces when left undisturbed
■ How vulnerable the interdental area is to gingival infection
■ How to use each recommended interdental aid to clean the proximal tooth surfaces

3. Write a goal for the problems you identified in the dental hygiene diagnoses in question 2. Include a time frame for meeting the goal. How will you measure whether your patient met the goal?

■ *Goal*

_____

_____

_____

■ *Time frame*

_____

_____

_____

■ *Evaluation method*

_____

_____

_____

4. You decide to recommend a floss holder and a toothpick in a holder for Mr. Adamson. Obtain samples of these interdental devices, if you can, to help you with this exercise (they will also help with the Factors to Teach the Patient section). Write a paragraph describing the method you will use to teach Mr. Adamson about these oral care devices.

_____

_____

_____

_____

_____

_____

_____

27 CHAPTER

Dentifrices, Mouth-rinses, and Irrigation

Chapter Outline

Learning Objectives

Upon successful completion of these exercises, you will be able to:

1. Identify and define key terms and concepts related to oral irrigation, dentifrices, and mouthrinses.
2. Describe the components, action, and therapeutic or cosmetic benefits of a dentifrice.

3. Describe the purpose of, procedure for, and ingredients used in oral rinses.
4. Describe the purpose, procedures, and applications for oral irrigation.
5. Define the purpose and requirements for the ADA Seal of Approval.

Key Words and Concepts Crossword Puzzle

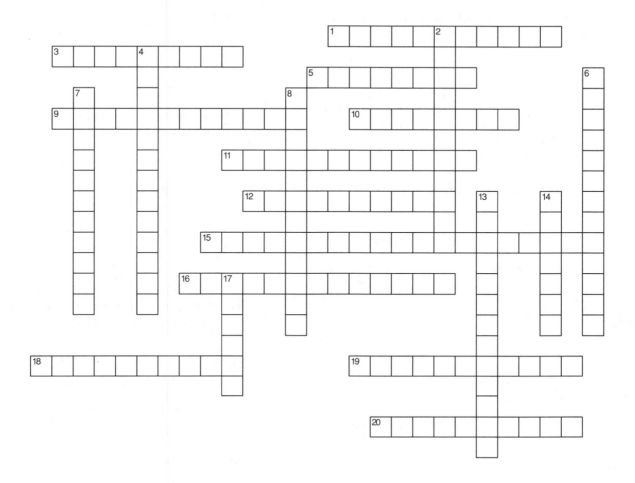

Across

1 Relating to the equilibrium of a liquid and the pressure exerted by a liquid at rest.
3 Substance in a dentifrice that retains moisture and prevents hardening upon exposure to air.
5 Substance used for flushing a specific site or area.
9 Treatment of disease by means of chemical substances or pharmaceutical agents.
10 Added to a dentifrice as a caries prevention agent.
11 Opposite of hydrostatic.
12 A substance that causes contraction or shrinkage and arrests discharges.
15 Indicates that efficacy claims of a product have been tested by research studies and are valid.
16 Ability of an agent to bind to the pellicle and tooth surface to be released and retain potency over an extended period of time.
18 A chemotherapeutic substance usually used with a toothbrush.
19 Irrigation delivered into the gingival sulcus or pocket.

20 Flushing of a specific site or area with a stream of fluid.

Down

2 An action in which one agent or drug enhances the effect of another.
4 A broad-spectrum antibacterial agent that has the ability to bind and remain in the oral cavity over a period of time.
6 A chemical with a bacteriostatic or bacteriocidal effect.
7 An agent added to a dentifrice to produce a specific preventive or treatment outcome.
8 A stream of water used for cleansing or therapeutic purposes.
13 Irrigation delivered at or coronal to the free gingival margin.
14 Placed into a cavity to introduce or drain fluid.
17 Added to a dentifrice to prevent separation of the solid and liquid ingredients during storage.

KNOWLEDGE EXERCISES

1. List three methods for self-care delivery of topical chemotherapeutic agents.

   _____

   _____

   _____

2. Identify the three components that make up the largest percentage of the ingredients found in a commercial dentifrice.

   _____

   _____

   _____

3. What is the purpose of the humectants in a dentifrice?

   _____

   _____

   _____

4. List at least three types of abrasives used as polishing agents in a dentifrice.

   _____

   _____

   _____

5. Identify two components of a dentifrice that can have sorbitol or glycerol as an ingredient.

   _____

   _____

6. What is the purpose of essential oils (e.g., peppermint) used in dentifrices?

   _____

   _____

   _____

7. The amount of therapeutic agent in a dentifrice is about _____%.

8. Which therapeutic ingredient in a dentifrice is related to prevention of dental caries?

   _____

   _____

   _____

9. Identify three therapeutic ingredients in a dentifrice that are related to reduction of supragingival calculus formation.

   _____

   _____

   _____

10. What is the most common ingredient used in dentifrices to aid in reducing sensitivity?

    _____

11. List the six basic ingredients in commercial mouthrinses.

    _____

    _____

    _____

12. List at least three general types of chemotherapeutic agents found in mouthrinses, and identify the purpose of each.

    Agent   **Purpose**

    _____

    _____

    _____

13. List at least three characteristics of an effective mouthrinse.

    _____

    _____

    _____

14. Which therapeutic agent available in mouthrinses has the greatest substantivity?

    _____

15. Which therapeutic agent available in mouthrinses acts by causing bacteriolysis?

    _____

16. Which therapeutic agent available in mouthrinses acts by inhibiting bacterial enzymes?

    _____

17. Which therapeutic agent available in mouthrinses is inactivated by a foaming agent frequently contained in commercial dentifrices?

18. Which two therapeutic agents available in mouthrinses are associated with the adverse effect of staining?

19. Describe the action and use of a mouthrinse containing peroxide.

20. Explain why rinsing with a mouthrinse that contains an effective therapeutic agent may not be effective for a patient with deep periodontal pockets.

21. In your own words, describe two types of oral irrigators.

22. For supragingival irrigation, a standard tip is usually used, and the flow of water is directed _____ to the long axis of the tooth.

23. For subgingival irrigation, a specialized tip is placed _____, and the water spray is directed _____.

24. Identify two applications for oral irrigation.

25. Identify one contraindication for recommendation of home care oral irrigation.

COMPETENCY EXERCISES

1. Using the information in the textbook, compare effectiveness, adverse effects, availability to the patient, and any other factors about therapeutic agents that might affect patient acceptance. (*Hint:* Use a separate piece of paper to make a one-page Infomap or table to aid in your comparison.) What additional information would you like to have about each of these agents that might help you inform your patients about using them?

2. Evan, a 7-year-old, has been prescribed a fluoride mouthrinse by Dr. Leiberman. Evan demonstrates a rinsing technique in which he fills his mouth with the liquid and rotates his head in all directions to distribute the rinse to all areas of his mouth.

   You plan to teach him how to rinse using the steps outlined in Box 27-4 of the textbook. Write a dental hygiene diagnosis statement that identifies a problem related to Evan's current rinsing technique.
   Problem:_____
   related to Evan's current mouthrinse techniques.

3. Write a goal for the problem identified in the dental hygiene diagnosis in question 2. How will you measure whether Evan met the goal? Include a time frame for meeting the goal.

   ■ *Goal*

   ■ *Evaluation method*

   ■ *Time frame*

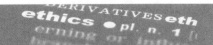

Everyday Ethics

Refer to the Codes of Ethics (Appendices I, II, and III in the textbook) and Framework for Making Decisions (Table 1-2 in the textbook) as you discuss the following scenario with your classmates.

Rachel practiced in a dental office as a dental assistant before beginning her dental hygiene education. The dentist where she worked was opposed to recommending irrigation because "it does not remove biofilm," so she is adamant that it does not work and should not be recommended. She also expressed concern that if patients use irrigation they will not floss. Rachel has made a conscious decision that she will not recommend

irrigation to any of her patients regardless of clinical findings.

Questions for Consideration

1. Using a framework for making decisions (Table 1-2, page 14), who might Rachel have to defend her decision to if she does not recommend irrigation for any of her patients? Include all individuals affected by this decision.
2. In this scenario, how does the principle of autonomy apply to the patients Rachel treats?
3. What suggestions would you offer this hygienist to make sure she continues to serve the needs of her patients as a licensed dental health professional?

---

4. You decide to recommend a self-irrigation home-care technique for your patient, Mr. Davito, because he has several areas in his mouth with 4–5-mm periodontal pocketing. Discuss the potential therapeutic benefits of daily oral irrigation for Mr. Davito.

_____

_____

_____

_____

_____

5. Using your institution's guidelines for writing in patient records, document your oral irrigation instructions to Mr. Davito.

Date	Comments	Signature
_____	_____	_____
_____	_____	_____
_____	_____	_____
_____	_____	_____
_____	_____	_____

QUESTIONS PATIENTS ASK

After you answer her questions about the ADA Seal, Ms. Leffler is very impressed with your knowledge, and she clearly believes that YOU are the expert to ask about dental products. Like many of your patients, she has questions about all kinds of oral-care products that she has heard or read about. "Does it really matter which

toothpaste I use?" "There are so many different kinds with different ingredients that claim to do different things—which one is really the best?" "Are there any negative side effects that go along with any of those extra ingredients and chemicals?" "Which mouthrinse do you recommend?" and "I read in a magazine that if I use a water irrigator at home, I don't have to floss—is that true?"

What sources of information can you identify that will help you answer your patient's questions in this scenario? What assessment information can help you determine this particular patient's needs so that you can make individualized recommendations? How will you use the evidence-based decision-making methods you learned from reading the EBDM Primer in Appendix B to help answer these questions for each specific patient?

Factors To Teach The Patient

Ms. Cerene Leffler usually prefers to use all-natural products. She has noticed that the dentifrice she likes does not display the ADA Seal of Approval on the package. She asks you during her dental hygiene appointment if that indicates that the toothpaste is not a good choice. Using patient-appropriate language, write a statement explaining to Ms. Leffler what the ADA Seal of Approval means. *This scenario is related to the following factor:*

- Significance of American Dental Association product acceptance seal (especially because it is a voluntary program, and no seal on a product does not signify that it is unsafe or not effective)

CHAPTER 28

The Patient with Orthodontic Appliances

Chapter Outline

Learning Objectives

Upon successful completion of these exercises, you will be able to:

1. Identify and define key terms and concepts related to care of patients with orthodontic appliances.
2. Identify appliances and instruments used in orthodontic treatment.
3. Describe procedures for placing and removing orthodontic appliances.
4. Provide oral hygiene instructions for a patient before, during, and following orthodontic treatment.

KNOWLEDGE EXERCISES

1. A _____ orthodontic appliance is bonded or banded to individual teeth or groups of teeth.

2. A _____ fits entirely around the tooth.

3. A _____ is bonded to the surface of a tooth to hold an arch wire.

4. _____ refers to removal of orthodontic appliances and residual adhesive.

5. A _____ is used to secure arch wires to orthodontic brackets.

6. A space _____ **prevents** closure and a space _____ **corrects** closure of a gap in the dentition that results from a prematurely lost tooth.

7. What is the purpose of an orthodontic retainer?

_____

_____

_____

8. List the advantages of bonded brackets.

_____

_____

_____

9. List the disadvantages of bonded brackets.

_____

_____

_____

10. What materials are bonded brackets commonly made from?

_____

_____

_____

11. What is a bonding pad?

_____

_____

_____

12. Elastomers hold the arch wire to the bracket. The purpose of the arch wire is to:

_____

_____

_____

13. How do you condition the enamel surface of teeth before bonding the orthodontic brackets?

_____

_____

_____

14. The procedure for applying the bonding agent is similar to the procedure for placing a dental _____.

15. After you etch a tooth before bonding the bracket, microclefts in the enamel are formed that range from _____ μm to _____ μm deep.

16. Anterior brackets may be bonded with a resin, whereas in posterior teeth, you may need to use a _____ resin to prevent detachment.

17. A patient with orthodontic appliances is at risk for a higher incidence of which two oral diseases?

_____

_____

_____

18. What two factors contribute to the demineralized areas (white spots) commonly found on a patient's teeth after removal of orthodontic brackets and bands?

_____

_____

_____

19. List two advantages of recommending a power toothbrush for your patient with orthodontic appliances.

_____

_____

_____

20. Describe how a regular toothbrush is adapted on the facial surface of teeth with orthodontic appliances.

_____

_____

_____

21. Explain how an orthodontic toothbrush, such as that pictured in Figure 28-3 in the textbook, is used.

_____

_____

_____

22. In your own words, describe the steps for removal of an orthodontic band.

_____

_____

_____

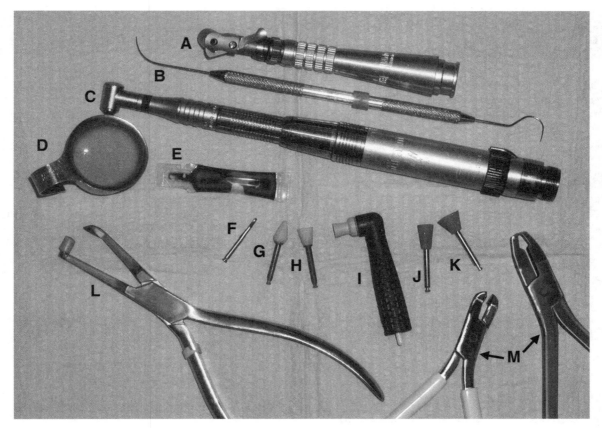

FIGURE 28-1

23. Identify one possible risk to the clinician during debonding procedures. What can you do to minimize the risk?

_____

_____

_____

_____

24. Along with careful periodontal examination, examination for demineralized areas, and removal of left-over composite resin, what other professional intervention is required after debonding orthodontic appliances?

_____

_____

_____

_____

25. **Figure 28-1** contains examples of instruments and supplies used for debanding or debonding orthodontic appliances. Name each labeled item in the spaces provided.

A. _____

B. _____

C. _____

D. _____

E. _____

F. _____

G. _____

H. _____

I. _____

J. _____

K. _____

L. _____

M. _____

COMPETENCY EXERCISES

1. Ms. Anna Moyer, a real estate agent who really relies on her smile as she interacts with the public in her job, is very excited and yet extremely nervous on the day you are to remove the brackets that have hidden

Everyday Ethics Exercise

Refer to the Codes of Ethics (Appendices I, II, and III in the textbook) and Framework for Making Decisions (Table 1-2 in the textbook) as you discuss the following scenario with your classmates.

Dorothy, a patient who had recently completed orthodontic therapy, presents for a maintenance appointment with Caroline, the dental hygienist in her general dentist's practice. The facial surfaces of tooth numbers 4–13 and 20–29 appear to harbor remnants of composite adhesive resin.

Caroline, the dental hygienist, feels an obligation to remove these adhesive remnants but does not want to make any disparaging comments about the orthodontist,

whose responsibility was to remove the adhesive. There is not enough time to remove all of the resin and complete the examination, radiographs, and dental hygiene therapy at the current appointment.

Questions for Consideration

1. Applying the principle of veracity, what obligation does Caroline have to tell Dorothy about the remaining adhesive resin on her teeth?
2. To maintain Dorothy's trust in her orthodontist, how can Caroline inform the patient of the accretions and explain the need for additional appointments?
3. Explain the treatment options that Caroline can consider, while keeping in mind the best interest of the patient.

---

her smile for so long. What important points will you make to minimize her apprehension about her personal safety and the potential for damage to her teeth when you explain the technique objectives and procedures for debonding her orthodontic brackets?

_____

_____

_____

_____

_____

_____

2. After the brackets, bands, and arch wires are removed from Ms. Moyer's teeth, it is important to remove all residual adhesive. Discuss the steps the clinician can take to ensure that all areas of each tooth are thoroughly free from adhesive.

_____

_____

_____

_____

_____

_____

3. Discuss the purpose of post-debonding preventive care that you, the dental hygienist, will provide for Ms. Moyer.

_____

_____

_____

_____

_____

_____

Factors To Teach The Patient

Do you remember Nicholas Bean from Chapter 25? He is the 12-year-old who is going right from his prophylaxis appointment to the orthodontist's office, where they will be placing full-mouth bands/brackets and arch wires on his teeth. As they are leaving, Nicholas's mother comments that they won't be seeing you again until the braces come off. You want to begin to educate Nicholas and his mother right away about the importance of the use of fluorides, thorough daily oral hygiene measures, and especially why regular maintenance appointments are necessary during orthodontic treatment.

Using the information you learned from reading this chapter and the example of a patient conversation from Appendix B as a guide, prepare an outline for a conversation that provides anticipatory guidance for Nicholas and his mother about ways to maintain good oral health status while he is undergoing orthodontic care.

This scenario is related to the following factors:

■ The significance of Biofilm around orthodontic appliances and teeth
■ How, when, and why to use fluoride rinses, toothpastes, and brush-on gels
■ The frequency for professional follow-up during and after orthodontic therapy

4. Two weeks after her fixed orthodontic appliances are removed, the orthodontist delivers a Hawley appliance to Ms. Moyer. You are responsible for educating and instructing her about the purpose and care of her retainer. What important points will you cover in your discussion?

_____

_____

_____

5. Your next patient is Missy Breckenridge. She has had her orthodontic appliances for about 2 years now, and you notice that her gingiva is not as healthy as it was when you saw her 6 months ago. When you disclose her mouth, there is a large accumulation of dental biofilm between the brackets and her gingival margins. Give examples of hints that you can give to Missy as you provide oral-hygiene instructions that address her need to ensure cleanliness on all surfaces.

_____

_____

_____

_____

29 | CHAPTER

Care of Dental Prostheses

Chapter Outline

Learning Objectives

Upon successful completion of these exercises, you will be able to:

1. Identify and define key terms and concepts related to care of dental prostheses.
2. Identify the components and characteristics of a variety of dental prostheses.
3. Describe the cleaning and care of dental prostheses.
4. Identify procedures to care for the remaining natural teeth, implants, and underlying oral tissues.

KNOWLEDGE EXERCISES

Care of Dental Prostheses Crossword Puzzle

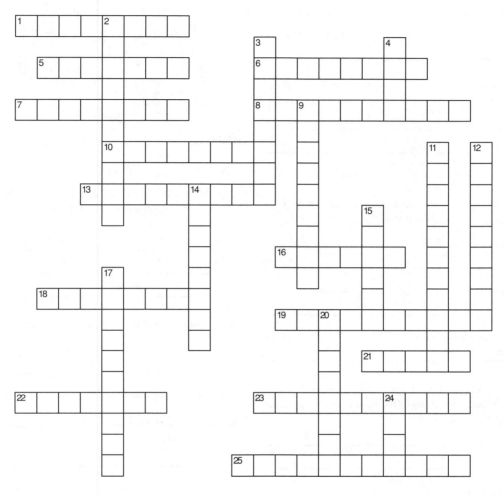

Across

1 Often placed on teeth that support an over-denture prosthesis to aid in caries prevention.

5 This term refers to massaging tissue under a removable denture with fingers and thumbs.

6 The surface of the dental prosthesis that makes contact with teeth in the opposing arch.

7 Can build up on surfaces of a denture the same way it can build up on natural dentition.

8 An artificial replacement for a body part.

10 A term that refers to cleansers used with brushes to clean removable dentures; includes denture pastes and powders, toothpastes and powders, and household agents.

13 A type of partial denture prosthesis that is cleaned and cared for outside of the oral cavity.

16 The tooth that replaces a missing natural tooth.

18 A soft material placed on the inner surface of a dental prosthesis to help hold it against oral tissues.

19 The inner surface of a dental prosthesis that rests against the mucous membrane of the alveolar ridge.

21 A type of partial denture prosthesis that is secured to natural teeth or dental implants and must be cleaned and cared for inside the oral cavity.

22 The type of dental prosthesis that replaces one or more teeth, but not all of the teeth in an arch.

23 Specially designed for difficult-to-clean areas of removable partial denture prosthesis (two words).

25 A type of removable dental prosthesis that is supported by both retained natural teeth or implants and the soft tissue of the alveolar ridge.

Down

2 The type of fluoride preparation that is contraindicated for porcelain and composite restorations.

3 A type of dental prosthesis that replaces the dentition and associated structures in an entire oral arch.

4 The part of a dental prosthesis that rests on the oral mucosa and to which teeth are attached.

9 A dental prosthesis that closes a congenital or acquired opening in oral tissues.

11 The type of dentifrice indicated for use with dental prostheses made of acrylic, or highly polished gold.

12 A type of connector that attaches a removal prosthesis to a metal receptacle included within a restoration of an abutment tooth.

14 A tooth or implant used to support a fixed or removable dental prosthesis.

15 A term that commonly refers to a fixed partial denture prosthesis.

17 Type of denture cleanser; includes ultrasonic, sonic, magnetic, and agitating mechanisms that can be combined with immersion agents.

20 The external or outer surface of a dental prosthesis is highly _____, whereas the occlusal and impression surfaces are not.

24 The rigid, stabilizing extension of a partial denture prosthesis that contacts a remaining tooth or teeth and transmits chewing force to teeth rather than mucosal tissue.

Knowledge Exercises

1. List the components of a fixed partial denture prosthesis.

   _____

   _____

   _____

2. List the criteria for an acceptable fixed partial denture prosthesis.

   _____

   _____

   _____

3. In your own words, describe the procedures for oral cleansing of a fixed dental prosthesis.

   _____

   _____

   _____

   _____

   _____

   _____

4. What characteristic of a removable partial denture prosthesis can negatively affect your patient's gingival health?

   _____

   _____

   _____

5. If your patient is unable to remove his or her own partial denture prosthesis, how do you help the patient remove it?

   _____

   _____

   _____

6. Label **Figure 29-1** with the following components.
   ◼ *Denture border*
   ◼ *Impression surface*
   ◼ *Occlusal surface*
   ◼ *Polished surface*

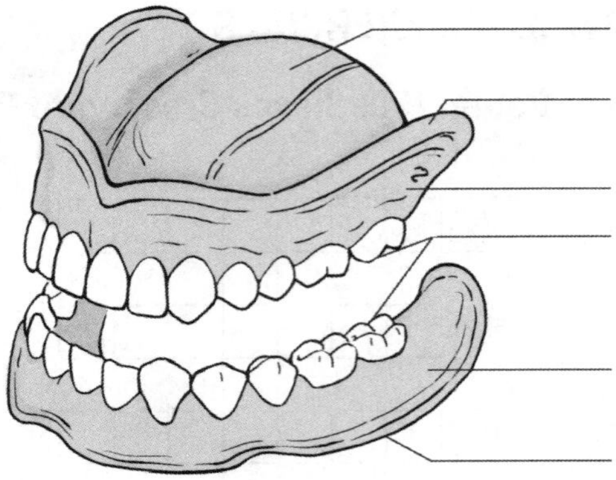

FIGURE 29-1

7. Identify two kinds of liners that may be present on the impression surface of a complete denture prosthesis.

   _____

   _____

   _____

8. Identify two kinds of complete overdenture prostheses.

   _____

   _____

   _____

9. What are the advantages of a complete overdenture prosthesis?

   _____

   _____

   _____

10. List the criteria that contribute to the success of an overdenture prosthesis.

   _____

   _____

   _____

11. What are the advantages of natural tooth and implant-retained overdentures?

   _____

   _____

   _____

12. What dental hygiene interventions can provide an added measure of protection for the oral health of a patient with a partial denture, single-arch complete

denture with natural teeth remaining in the opposite arch, or an overdenture supported by natural teeth?

_____

_____

_____

13. Describe the process you will use to remove your patient's complete denture if, for some reason, your patient is not able to remove it himself or herself.

   ▓ *Maxillary complete denture*

   _____

   _____

   _____

   _____

   _____

   ▓ *Mandibular complete denture*

   _____

   _____

   _____

   _____

   _____

   _____

14. Identify two oral conditions that can be prevented with proper cleansing and care of dental prostheses and underlying tissues.

_____

_____

15. What is the purpose of instructing your patients to remove and properly store their dental prosthesis in liquid while sleeping at night?

   _____

   _____

   _____

16. What are the requirements for the denture cleanser you will recommend to your patient?

   _____

   _____

   _____

17. Complete Infomap 29-1 below to compare the various types of cleansers that you can recommend for the care of full and partial dentures.

COMPETENCY EXERCISES

1. Imagine that you have just joined the on-site dental team at a long-term care facility or nursing home. A short time after you begin your position, you discover that many of the residents wear full or partial dentures and that that those dentures are not being cleaned regularly by the nurse's aides who are responsible for providing daily care for the residents. Most

INFOMAP 29-1			
TYPE	**ACTIVE INGREDIENT**	**CLEANSER ACTION**	**DISADVANTAGES**
Immersion Type Alkaline hypochlorite (household bleach) Alkaline peroxide (commercial powder or tablet) Dilute acids (commercial ultrasonic solutions) Enzymes (in various cleansers)			
Abrasive Type Pastes and powders (various commercial products) Household agents (salt, bicarbonate of soda, hand soap, scouring powders)			

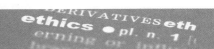

Everyday Ethics

Refer to the Codes of Ethics (Appendices I, II, and III in the textbook) and Framework for Making Decisions (Table 1-2 in the textbook) as you discuss the following scenario with your classmates.

Mr. Samuel arrived for his regular maintenance appointment with Theresa, the dental hygienist. He has a long history of treatment for periodontal disease and has generalized moderate to severe bone loss.

Mr. Samuel has an old mandibular removable partial denture. He admits it is painful to wear and difficult to chew with, but he has resisted to have it remade. He entered the treatment room with a pamphlet from the reception area that described an implant overdenture and asked if that could be a good option for him.

Theresa realizes that Mr. Samuel has questions about his treatment options. She is concerned about his periodontal disease and the problems with his prosthesis. She first discussed the need to update radiographs and for a consultation with the dentist.

Questions for Consideration

1. Given his periodontal condition, how much detail can Theresa share in reference to his request for an over-denture versus keeping his natural teeth?
2. Because Mr. Samuels seems unhappy with his current status, how can Theresa proceed to document his concerns in his record, and how will she explain to the dentist?
3. What aspects of informed consent need to be addressed with Mr. Samuel?

---

of the dentures worn by the residents are complete-arch dentures that are made of acrylic resins. Many are old and stained, and some have calculus buildup on the surfaces of the denture. The dentures are seldom removed from the patients' mouths; when they are, they are often just placed on the bedside table or in the drawer until family members come for a visit and decide that the patient looks better with the denture back in place.

You plan to provide an in-service presentation for the caregivers about the importance of denture care, and you also plan to provide hands-on training in denture-cleaning techniques for the caregiver staff.

- *List the information that you will include in your in-service presentation about denture care.*

_____
_____
_____
_____
_____
_____

- *Create a step-by-step checklist that the aides can use at the bedside to document daily cleaning of each resident's removable prosthesis as well as his or her oral tissues.*

_____
_____

Factors To Teach The Patient

Evangeline Dada has just received her brand new six-unit anterior bridge, which spans her entire smile from abutment tooth 6 to abutment tooth 11. Before placement of the fixed prosthesis, she had a removable temporary appliance made of plastic. She had no trouble cleaning her teeth when she could remove the old appliance, and she has done a good job of keeping all her oral tissues healthy. She states she is completely at a loss as to how she must take care of this beautiful new smile of hers and asks you to spend some extra time providing oral-hygiene instructions for her today.

Use the example of a patient conversation in Appendix B as a guide to develop a conversation to educate Evangeline about her new bridge, the abutment teeth that support it, and maintaining the health of the oral tissues around and underneath this new fixed prosthesis.

Use the conversation you create to role play this situation with a fellow student. If you are the patient in the role play, be sure to ask questions. If you are the dental hygienist, try to anticipate questions and answer them in your explanation.

This scenario is related to the following factors:

- How to make a self-examination of the oral tissues
- Why all prostheses need cleaning more than once a day
- The need to adapt toothbrushing, flossing, and use of other aids to the care of the abutment teeth
- How tongue cleaning contributes to complete oral health
- The significance of regular maintenance appointments to have the oral tissues checked and the prostheses professionally cleaned

_____

_____

_____

_____

2. Investigate commercially available denture cleaners so that you can make a recommendation to the long-term care center or nursing home staff. What is the active ingredient in each one? Which one (or ones) will you recommend in your in-service presentation? Provide a rationale for your choice(s).

_____

_____

_____

The Patient with Dental Implants

Chapter Outline

Learning Objectives

Upon successful completion of these exercises, you will be able to:

1. Identify and define key terms and concepts related to care of the patient with implants.

2. Discuss characteristics and factors that influence self-care or dental hygiene care of the rehabilitated mouth.
3. Discuss types, preparation and placement, and maintenance care for dental implants.

Key Words and Terms Crossword Puzzle

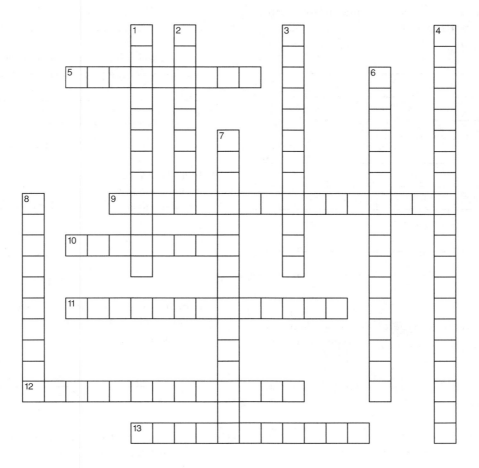

Across

5 An early form of blade- or plate-shaped endosseous implants.

9 The direct attachment of bone and alloplastic material that is required for the success of a dental implant.

10 A metal that is commonly combined with aluminum and vanadium for use in dental implants.

11 A unique characteristic of the metal titanium that makes it capable of existing in harmony with the biologic environment of the human body.

12 A dental implant in which the metal framework rests on top of the alveolar bone but under the periosteum.

13 Another name for a transosseous implant.

Down

1 Prevents microorganisms from entering the soft tissues around a dental implant (two words).

2 Refers to either the connection between the dental implant and bone or between the dental implant and soft tissue.

3 A type of dental implant that penetrates through the full thickness of the alveolar bone.

4 A layer of connective tissue between a dental implant and surrounding bone that is indicative of failed osseointegration (two words).

6 Reversible, first-stage infection of the soft tissue surrounding a dental implant.

7 Stage in which infection around a dental implant has reached the bone.

8 A dental implant that is placed within the alveolar bone.

KNOWLEDGE EXERCISES

1. In your own words, briefly describe each of the three types of dental implants.

   Subperiosteal

   _____

   _____

   Transosseous (Transosteal)

   _____

   _____

   Endosseous (Endosteal)

   _____

   _____

   _____

2. The most common type of dental implant is the _____ type that has a _____ shape.

3. Identify two biological tissues that interface with a dental implant.

   _____

   _____

   _____

4. What is the permucosal seal?

   _____

   _____

   _____

5. Identify factors that can increase a patient's risk for poor outcomes if dental implants are placed.

   _____

   _____

   _____

   _____

   _____

6. Each time the patient with dental implants is scheduled for routine dental hygiene maintenance care, you will examine the implant area carefully. List the basic criteria that indicate a healthy implant.

   _____

   _____

   _____

7. Identify two prominent contributing factors in the breakdown of the peri-implant environment.

   _____

   _____

   _____

8. Identify oral conditions that indicate that the dental implant may be ailing and should be evaluated by the oral surgeon who placed the implant.

   _____

   _____

   _____

9. Explain why it is important to instruct a patient with dental implants to select self-cleaning implements and agents carefully.

   _____

   _____

   _____

10. What type of instruments are used for removing calculus from dental implants?

   _____

   _____

   _____

COMPETENCY EXERCISES

1. Describe the dental hygienist's role in collaborative treatment planning and preparing the patient for dental implant procedures.

   _____

   _____

   _____

2. Matthew Glenn, aged 45 years, is scheduled today for a periodontal maintenance appointment. You are very excited and anxious to check the area of his dental implant–supported bridge. The prosthesis he received 3 months ago is a three-unit replacement for teeth 3, 4, and 5; each pontic supports an individual dental implant. You provided oral-hygiene

Everyday Ethics

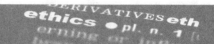

Refer to the Codes of Ethics (Appendices I, II, and III in the textbook) and Framework for Making Decisions (Table 1-2 in the textbook) as you discuss the following scenario with your classmates.

Mrs. Kent was scheduled for her appointment with Lorene, the dental hygienist. Mrs. Kent had joined this practice about 2 years ago. Every time Lorene treated Mrs. Kent, she became frustrated because it was evident that the patient was not following her prescribed guidelines for self-care. She gave Lorene the feeling that she just came to get her teeth cleaned, not for a true periodontal maintenance program. The anterior teeth had badly worn crowns and were not aesthetically pleasing. Recently a corner had chipped off no. 8.

Dr. Langly and Lorene talked about Mrs. Kent's most recent radiographs. He explained that he was going to suggest replacing tooth numbers 8 and 9 with implants.

Lorene questioned the plan based on what she had observed about Mrs. Kent's interest in caring for the appliances she already had. Lorene said in a frustrated tone of voice, "But Dr. Langly, wouldn't we be adding to her burden with more specialized home-care procedures?"

Dr. Langly smiled and responded: "Lorene, look at it this way: How about if we give her a beautiful smile? Couldn't that inspire her to really take better care of her mouth?"

Questions for Consideration

1. What value does Mrs. Kent appear to place on maintaining her oral cavity? What may have been missing in her past experiences with dental care?
2. How is it, or is it not, ethically acceptable to plan such a treatment plan for a patient who has demonstrated such poor daily oral hygiene?
3. With respect to the patient's autonomy, role play a dialogue that could ensue between Lorene and Mrs. Kent as Lorene explains the oral health and aesthetic values of the new treatment plan.

---

instructions for him both before and after his the implant procedure, but you haven't seen him since.

During your assessment today, you find out that he is not having any oral problems, and the implants have been comfortable and feel just fine. In fact, he is delighted with the implants. His daily oral care is generally fair, but you notice small areas of biofilm in the hard-to-reach areas of the prosthesis, such as the embrasure between teeth 4 and 5 and the distal surface of tooth 3. To your surprise, there is also significant calculus buildup on the facial and mesial surfaces of tooth number 2.

The gingival tissue around the implant looks healthy. Mr. Glenn also exhibits some very slight calculus buildup on the facial surfaces of the left maxillary molars and on the lingual surfaces of his lower anterior teeth. You find no other significant medical history, dental history, or dental examination findings for Mr. Glenn today.

Use a copy of the Individualized Patient Care Plan template (Appendix C) to develop a care plan for Mr. Glenn that emphasizes daily care techniques to ensure long-term success for his implants and prosthesis.

Factors To Teach The Patient

Use the Individualized Patient Care Plan you developed for Mr. Glenn (introduced in Competency Exercise question 2) and the example conversation in Appendix B as a guide to prepare a conversation to provide oral hygiene instructions for Mr. Glenn during his dental hygiene appointment today.

This scenario is related to the following factors:

- How to care for implants: special needs related to titanium surfaces
- How the health of the periodontal tissues and the duration of the implants and prostheses depend on meticulous daily self-care by the patient
- The role of biofilm in periodontitis and peri-implants; vulnerability of the implant to infection from periodontal pathogens that may be present on adjacent natural teeth
- How cleaning a mouth with complex restorations takes longer

The Patient who Uses Tobacco

Chapter Outline

Learning Objectives

Upon successful completion of these exercises, you will be able to:

1. Identify and define key terms and concepts related to the use of tobacco.
2. Explain the systemic and oral effects of tobacco use.
3. Describe the effects of nicotine addiction.
4. Describe strategies for tobacco cessation.
5. Plan dental hygiene care and tobacco cessation interventions for patients who use tobacco.
6. Identify the role of the community-based dental hygienist in tobacco-free initiatives.

KNOWLEDGE EXERCISES

1. Tobacco contains many components that are _____ to humans. Tobacco use is the single most _____ cause of disease and premature death in the world.

2. Nicotine in cigarette smoke can be absorbed into the bloodstream through which tissues?

   _____

   _____

   _____

3. List the factors that affect the amounts of nicotine and other tobacco components that are absorbed into the bloodstream.

_____

_____

_____

4. Nicotine from smokeless tobacco can be absorbed through which tissues?

_____

_____

_____

5. Nicotine spreads through the bloodstream to which tissues?

_____

_____

_____

6. Match each of the descriptive statements in the box below with the appropriate tobacco-related term. Each term may be used more than once.

7. How is nicotine eliminated from the body?

_____

_____

_____

8. List as many negative health effects of tobacco use and/or exposure to secondhand ETS as you can.

_____

_____

_____

_____

_____

_____

9. Identify as many potential oral health consequences of tobacco use as you can.

_____

_____

_____

_____

_____

_____

TOBACCO-RELATED TERMS	**DESCRIPTIVE STATEMENTS**
A. Tolerance B. Dependence C. Abuse D. Addiction E. Cotinine F. Nicotine G. Nitrosamines H. Pyrolysis I. Thiocyanate J. ETS	_____ The use of any drug in a way that causes harm to the person or other persons who are affected by the user's behavior _____ By-product of nicotine in found in body fluids _____ and _____ Substances measured to determine recent use of nicotine-containing products _____ The chief psychoactive ingredient in tobacco _____ The chief addictive agent in tobacco _____ Refers to exposure to passive, secondary, or secondhand smoke _____ Refers to a group of cancer-causing chemicals found in tobacco _____ The process of breaking down chemicals contained in tobacco by heat created at the end of a burning cigarette _____ By-product of hydrogen cyanide that is found in tobacco smoke _____ Substance found in the various aids used for smoking cessation _____ Refers to the user's need for increased tobacco use over time to create the desired feeling of well-being _____ Loss of control over the amount and frequency of use of tobacco _____ Intensifies the release of dopamine by the brain _____ One criterion is that withdrawal symptoms occur when use of tobacco is discontinued _____ Chronic, progressive, relapsing disease characterized by compulsive use of a substance _____ This chemical is not the most physically harmful substance found in tobacco _____ Released with other substances when the tobacco is ignited _____ Constitutes 1–2% of the dry weight of cigarette tobacco and 1.45–8% of smokeless tobacco

10. Peak concentration of nicotine in the blood plasma occurs _____ after the onset of smoking and _____ declines over the next _____.

11. Why are children of parents and/or caregivers who use tobacco also at high risk for disease?

    _____

    _____

    _____

12. As you are providing dental hygiene care for your patient who uses tobacco, you can identify the negative effects of tobacco use that are specific to that patient. In your own words, explain each of the following terms as they relate to your role during dental hygiene care for each patient.

    Detect

    _____

    _____

    _____

    Explain

    _____

    _____

    _____

    Relate

    _____

    _____

    _____

    Motivate

    _____

    _____

    _____

    Refer

    _____

    _____

    _____

    Ascertain

    _____

    _____

    _____

    Consult

    _____

    _____

    _____

Document

_____

_____

_____

13. Your patient, who is dependent on nicotine, may still continue to use tobacco, even though you have spent considerable time during a dental hygiene appointment educating him or her about the personal oral health effects of tobacco use. You can inform and advise your patient, but you must wait to provide support until he or she can articulate reasons for quitting and is ready to take that step. Explain two types of treatment programs that can provide support for your patient who is now ready to quit using tobacco.

    _____

    _____

    _____

    _____

    _____

    _____

14. The five *A*s provide the basis for a simple but effective tobacco dependence–intervention approach. Number the five *A*s in the appropriate order (from 1 to 5) and then *briefly* outline the basic premise of each one.

    _____ *Advise*

    _____

    _____

    _____ *Arrange*

    _____

    _____

    _____ *Ask*

    _____

    _____

    _____ *Assess*

    _____

    _____

_____ *Assist*

_____

_____

_____

15. Your patient is not yet ready to quit using tobacco. Identify the five *R*s that you will use as the basis for a continuing discussion with your patient about tobacco use.

_____ *Tailoring advice to each patient*

_____ *Potential for increased problems*

_____ *Identifying benefits of quitting*

_____ *Barriers to quitting*

_____ *Reinforcing at every visit*

16. List the methods that are available for delivering nicotine-replacement therapy if your patient is considering pharmacotherapy as a treatment for nicotine addiction.

_____

_____

_____

17. Identify nonnicotine pharmacotherapies approved by the FDA for tobacco cessation.

_____

_____

_____

18. In your own words, state the objectives and rationale for using pharmacotherapies to help your patient stop using tobacco.

_____

_____

_____

19. What factors should be considered when recommending pharmacotherapies to help your patients stop using tobacco?

_____

_____

_____

20. What are the most common oral side effects of the pharmacotherapies used for treatment of nicotine addiction?

COMPETENCY EXERCISES

1. Each of the following statements expresses a concept that some of your patients may believe. But each statement is *false*. Create a true statement and provide an explanation/rationale for each that you could use to convince your patient that the original statement is not true.

   ▓ *The use of spit tobacco is a safe alternative to smoking tobacco.*

   _____

   _____

   _____

   ▓ *It is fairly easy for smokers to stop using tobacco once they decide that they are going to do so.*

   _____

   _____

   _____

2. Use the Tobacco Use Assessment Form (Fig. 31-2 in the textbook) to assess the tobacco-using habits of a friend or relative. Use the methods outlined in the Tobacco Cessation Flow Chart to encourage your friend or relative to quit.

   _____

   _____

   _____

3. Appendix D contains a patient assessment summary for Mr. Harold Wilmot. Use the information in the summary to write at least three dental hygiene diagnosis statements for Mr. Wilmot's dental hygiene care plan that are related to his use of tobacco.

Problem	**Cause (Risk Factors and Origin)**
_____ *related to*	_____
_____ *related to*	_____
_____ *related to*	_____

4. Write a goal for each problem identified in question 3. Include a time frame for meeting the goal. How will you measure whether or not Mr. Wilmot met the goal?

Goal 1

_____

_____

_____

■ _Time frame_

_____

_____

■ _Evaluation method_

_____

_____

_____

Goal 2

_____

_____

_____

■ _Time frame_

_____

_____

■ _Evaluation method_

_____

_____

Goal 3

_____

_____

_____

■ _Time frame_

_____

_____

■ _Evaluation method_

_____

_____

_____

5. List the dental hygiene interventions you will plan to help Mr. Wilmot _arrest or control disease and regenerate, restore, or maintain_ oral health.

■ _Clinical interventions_

_____

_____

■ _Education/counseling_

_____

_____

■ _Oral hygiene instructions/home care_

_____

_____

6. Appendix D contains a Patient-Specific Dental Hygiene Care Plan for Mrs. Diane White. The care plan includes an educational intervention to explain the effects of secondhand smoke on Mrs. White's developing fetus. Make an outline of the points you will want to be sure to cover as you talk to Mrs. White during her dental hygiene and re-evaluation appointments.

_____

_____

_____

7. Using your institution's guidelines for writing in patient records, document that you have provided education and counseling related to the health effects of secondhand smoke during Mrs. White's appointment.

Date   **Comments**   **Signature**

_____

_____

8. As a dental hygienist, your role in addressing the oral and systemic health damage of tobacco use is wider than simply providing assessment, information, motivation, and guidance to individual patients in your clinical practice. Discuss your role in tobacco education and cessation from a broader community-based or advocacy perspective.

_____

_____

Everyday Ethics

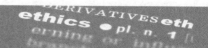

Refer to the Codes of Ethics (Appendices I, II, and III in the textbook) and Framework for Making Decisions (Table 1-2 in the textbook) as you discuss the following scenario with your classmates.

Fifteen-year-old Jason comes with his mom for a regular maintenance appointment with the dental hygienist. During the oral examination, Ellen, the hygienist notices small red and white patches in the vestibular areas of the mandible adjacent to the molar teeth. She also records moderate brownish staining on the teeth and plans to use the air-powder polisher after scaling. She questions Jason about smoking and the use of smokeless tobacco,

but he states that he has tried cigarettes only once or twice.

Questions to Consider
1. What beneficial approach can Ellen use with Jason if she suspects he is not telling the truth about his smoking habits?
2. How can Ellen maintain Jason's right to confidentiality but inform his mom of potentially serious changes in the gingival tissues?
3. Which of the ethical principles apply to this situation? Explain your response from both the dental hygienist's perspective and the patient's perspective.

 Factors To Teach The Patient

Mrs. White's husband arrives to pick up his wife following her dental hygiene appointment. He wants to discuss their insurance coverage with the office manager, but she is on the telephone, so he must wait for a few minutes to speak with her. He sits down in a chair and immediately takes out a pack of cigarettes and some matches. He asks you for an ashtray.

Use the example conversation provided in Appendix B as a guide to prepare an outline for explaining the tobacco-free policy in your office to Mr. White.

Use the conversation you create to role play this situation with a fellow student. If you are the patient in the role play, be sure to ask questions. If you are the dental hygienist, try to anticipate questions and answer them in your explanation.

This scenario is related to the following factor:

■ Nonsmokers who breath ETS can incur the same serious health problems as smokers. Children are especially suseptible.

DISCOVERY EXERCISE

Collect a variety of patient education materials—such as brochures, posters, or videotapes—that address the health and/or oral health effects of tobacco use. Encourage each of your student colleagues to collect as many materials as possible from a variety of different sources. Get together in small groups to discuss the materials.

■ *Determine the scientific accuracy of the information included in the patient-education materials.*

■ *Determine which type of patient each of the materials is best suited for.*

■ *Determine how each of the materials might best be used as part of tobacco-cessation initiatives in your clinic.*

32 CHAPTER

Diet and Dietary Analysis

Chapter Outline

Learning Objectives

Upon successful completion of these exercises, you will be able to:

1. Identify and define key terms and concepts related to providing a dietary assessment.

2. Identify vitamins and minerals relevant to oral health.

3. Plan and provide dietary assessment and patient counseling for caries control.

KNOWLEDGE EXERCISES

Crossword Puzzle

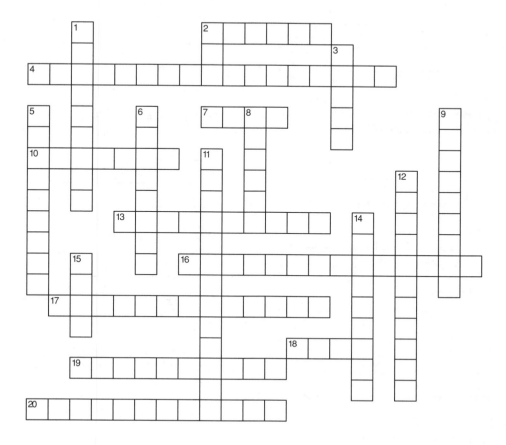

Across

2 United States Department of Health and Human Services.

4 Evaluation of diet adequacy performed by a dental hygienist to help plan appropriate interventions for a patient who may be at nutritional and oral health risk (two words).

7 Recommendations for adequate intake of essential nutrients.

10 Refers to comparing the nutrient content of a food with the amount of energy it provides.

13 Term that refers to nutritional inadequacy of specific nutrients in body tissues.

16 Foods that do not lower the pH of biofilm or that encourage remineralization.

17 Needed in small amounts in the diet; not energy yielding.

18 Agency that developed the food pyramid.

19 Foods that lower the pH of oral biofilm and increase risk for dental caries.

20 Poor nourishment.

Down

1 One factor in exposure to cariogenic food that is very significant for increasing risk for dental caries.

2 Maximum intake of a specific nutrient that is unlikely to create adverse health risks for an individual.

3 Diet consisting only of plant foods.

5 Lifestyle that includes only typical day-to-day physical activity.

6 Chemical substance in foods that is needed by the body for building and repair.

8 Lifestyle that includes an increased amount of physical activity.

9 Developed by the USDA to illustrate the five important food groups important in a balanced diet.

11 Carbohydrate, protein, and fat are examples.

12 Carbohydrates that produce acids when they are acted on by specific biofilm organisms.

14 Listing of various foods and measurements of amounts eaten during a specific time period.

15 Comprehensive term that encompasses all categories of dietary reference guidelines.

Knowledge Exercises

1. List the major food categories included in the MyPyramid.

   _____

   _____

   _____

2. Identify two other food categories listed in the MyPyramid Food Intake Patterns (Fig. 32-3 in the textbook) that contribute to an individual's caloric intake.

   _____

   _____

   _____

3. The Food Intake Patterns sheet contains a table that outlines daily amount of food that is appropriate based on 12 different _____.

4. Identify the three charicteristics used to determine the appropriate calorie intake level for an individual person's diet.

   _____

   _____

   _____

5. Look at Figure 32-2 in the textbook to find the appropriate calorie level for yourself. Then identify the daily amount of food from the vegetable group that is suggested to meet your nutritional needs.

   _____

6. What amount of food from the dark green vegetable subgroup is suggested for your diet?

   _____

7. Table 32-1 in the textbook provides a comprehensive list of nutrients with their functions, associated disease states, and food sources. Your instructor will let you know the level of detail you are expected to recall from the information in that table. It is most important for you to be able to link deficiencies in nutritional intake with oral manifestations you may observe while providing dental-hygiene care for your patients.

   The Infomap 32-1 located on the next page reorganizes information from the textbook to help you associate nutrient deficiencies with specific intraoral findings. Use information in Chapter 32 of the textbook to help you complete the infomap with (a) the oral findings you might observe if your patient is deficient in each listed nutrient and

(b) food sources for that nutrient that you can recommend to your patient.

8. Which vitamins and minerals are associated with healthy skin and mucous membrane?

   _____

   _____

   _____

9. Which nutrients are important for healthy wound healing and tissue repair?

   _____

   _____

   _____

10. Which nutrients are essential for the development of healthy tooth structure?

    _____

    _____

    _____

11. Dental caries is the result of _____ _____ and not a nutrient deficiency.

12. Identify four factors that interact to result in dental caries.

    _____

    _____

    _____

13. Any incident of sucrose intake lowers the pH in the dental biofilm. But what two major factors interact to enhance cariogenic exposure and increase your patient's risk for developing dental caries?

    _____

    _____

    _____

14. In your own words, discuss the purposes of a dietary assessment.

    _____

    _____

    _____

15. Summarize the information you will provide for patients when you are explaining the dietary

INFOMAP 32-1

NUTRIENT	ORAL MANIFESTATIONS OF DEFICIENCY	FOOD SOURCES
Vitamin A		
Thaimin (Vitamin B_1)		
Niacin (Vitamin B_3)		
Riboflavin (Vitamin B_2)		
Pyridoxine (Vitamin B_6)		
Cobalamin (Vitamin B_{12})		
Ascorbic acid (Vitamin C)		
Vitamin D		
Calcium		
Fluoride		
Foliate		
Iron		
Magnesium		
Phosphorus		
Zinc		
Protein		

assessment intervention before asking them to complete a food diary.

_____

_____

_____

16. Identify some common dietary omissions that you will want to be sure to review with your patient as you explain the food diary form.

_____

_____

_____

17. In your own words, explain how to calculate a patient's caries risk using the Sweet Score. (*Hint:* Use the information in Fig. 32-6 in the textbook to guide your answer.)

_____

_____

_____

_____

_____

_____

18. If, after calculating the Sweet Score, you determine that your patient is at moderate or high risk for dental caries, what recommendations will you be sure to provide during your oral-health education session with that patient?

_____

_____

_____

19. Identify *patient* factors that can affect your success in providing nutritional counseling for your patients.

_____

_____

_____

20. Identify *communication* factors that can affect your success in providing nutritional counseling for your patients.

_____

_____

_____

21. For a patient who is especially caries susceptible, what ingredient in chewing gum will help promote remineralization if chewed immediately after each meal?

_____

_____

_____

COMPETENCY EXERCISES

1. Use **Table 32-1**, in the next column, to create a food diary for everything you ate yesterday. (No cheating, now; no one will ever see this but you.) What nutrients are missing from your diet?

_____

_____

_____

TABLE 32-1	FOOD DIARY	
TYPES OF FOOD/ BEVERAGE	QUANTITY EATEN (IN CUPS, OZ., TSP., ETC.)	PREPARATION METHOD
Breakfast		
Snack		
Lunch		
Snack		
Dinner		
Snack		

2. Make a copy of the Scoring the Sweets form (Fig. 32-6 in the textbook). Use the information in your 24-hour food diary to calculate your personal risk for dental caries. What recommendations will you give yourself to reduce your caries risk?

_____

_____

_____

3. Ask a student colleague, friend, or member of your family to complete a 3- or 5-day food diary. Make a copy of the Dietary Analysis Recording Form (Fig. 32-7 in the textbook) to complete a dietary analysis for that person. Use the MyPyramid Web-based analysis program available at _www.mypyramid tracker.gov_ to analyze the diary. This online dietary analysis program is not difficult to learn and has a tutorial that will help you get started.

4. Identify topics you would include in a patient education program based on the dietary analysis you completed for question 3.

_____

_____

_____

5. Use the MyPyramid nutritional guidelines and copies of Figure 32-9 in the textbook to create _your_ ideal caries-control diet that contains foods you like to eat. Create menus for several days, and make sure that your diet provides adequate nutrition for a person who is just like you. Compare your menus with the menus created by your student colleagues.

Discuss how your colleagues' food preferences, cultural considerations, or personal eating practices compare with yours. What does this exercise help you realize about possible barriers when you are providing diet counseling for your diverse individual patients?

_____

_____

_____

_____

_____

6. Because individualized dental hygiene care plans are based on individualized patient needs determined by assessment data, not every dental hygiene care plan you write will include dietary assessment or dietary counseling. Discuss patient assessment findings that would indicate the need to include a 24-hour or 3- to 7-day dietary assessment as part of your patient's dental hygiene care plan.

_____

_____

_____

Everyday Ethics

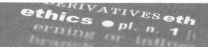

Refer to the Codes of Ethics (Appendices I, II, and III in the textbook) and Framework for Making Decisions (Table 1-2 in the textbook) as you discuss the following scenario with your classmates.

Ms. Carlson presents with type I diabetes and several significant changes in her oral cavity since her last dental-hygiene appointment, including angular cheilosis, glossitis, and several proximal carious lesions. The hygienist, Bettina, believes that Ms. Carlson has advanced dietary needs beyond the scope of practice of a dental hygienist and, therefore, avoids any chairside dietary assessment with the patient. Routine personal daily oral care instructions are given. Upon completion of the examination, Bettina mentions her concerns about Ms. Carlson's dietary status to the dentist but does not record any recommendations in the patient's permanent record.

Questions for Consideration
1. What professional protocol for referrals can be followed by the dental hygienist because she believes giving dietary advice to a patient with diabetes is beyond the scope of practice for a dental hygienist?
2. By eliminating the chairside dietary assessment, did Bettina act nonmaleficently toward the patient? Explain your response.
3. Which ethical principles would be ignored if Bettina does not educate the patient about the preventive measures for her dental caries or document this information in the patient's record?

Factors To Teach The Patient

Use the care plan you prepared for Christopher Michaels in Competency Exercise 7 and the example conversation in Appendix B as a guide to prepare an outline for a conversation with Christopher's mother explaining his risk for caries and the importance of changing the boy's daily dietary habits. One more piece of information to add to your conversation is that because of the abscess associated with the caries on his mandibular molar, Christopher has just received a prescription for a (sucrose-enhanced) antibiotic liquid preparation that he will take three times a day for the next 10 days. He absolutely refuses to take any medication in a pill form, so the antibiotic syrup is the only answer.

Use the conversation you create to role play this situation with a fellow student. If you are Christopher's mother in the role play, be sure to ask questions and try to identify a couple of real-life barriers to behavior change. If you are the dental hygienist, try to anticipate questions and answer them in your explanation. Also try to adapt for the barriers identified by Christopher's mother.

This scenario is related to the following factors:

- Reasons to avoid frequent daily use of medications with sucrose
- Reasons for rinsing with water after a medication contained in a syrupy sucrose mixture
- How dental caries on the tooth surface starts and progresses
- How the interaction of cariogenic foods, tooth surface, saliva, and microorganisms act together in the dental caries process
- How repeated, frequent acid production and the pH in the dental biofilm adversely affect the teeth

7. In Appendix D of this workbook, you will find a Patient Assessment Summary for Christopher Michaels, age 10 years, who has evidence of rampant caries and increased risk for continued caries activity. Use the Dental Hygiene Care Plan template in Appendix C to prepare a plan for Christopher that includes a dietary assessment.

_____

_____

_____

Fluorides

Chapter Outline

Learning Objectives

Upon successful completion of these exercises, you will be able to:

1. Identify and define key terms and concepts related to the use of fluorides.
2. Explain fluoride metabolism, mechanism of action, and effect/benefits of fluoride on pre-eruptive and posteruptive teeth.
3. Describe historical aspects, water supply components, and effects/benefits of water fluoridation.
4. Describe topical fluoride compounds and application methods.
5. Discuss fluoride safety.
6. Plan individualized fluoride prevention interventions.

Fluoride Word Search Puzzle

To solve the puzzle, first solve the clues; then find the answers in the grid. The answers can run across, down, or diagonally and can start at the right or left or top or bottom. When you have found all the words, the first 22 unused letters in the grid will spell out a hidden message.

Hidden message: Remember that the most effective agent for dental caries prevention and control is spelled

_____

_____

```
f l U O r i d e c a r i o s t a t i c e a n h
d n o t t o x i c i t y c f l f D O t U r s i
d W h i t e S p o t e i l f l r l i t d i Z G
l r g b d y m w l y p f l u F k t k L n S b r
r r w m c t P b n o n u o r r a k c r u A h a
f h z l h n k M r d o r e D p q g a b x c y n
t y y l d x g t v r i d w a m n v s e m i d d
x t c p c e o p a d e m y N o r u d f k d r R
T g H l o x f p e r r x l i k r y l f j u o a
r z w a i c a l i f o r t l f V t m i r l x p
p p g h l t a c u r v a H a R V K N c t a y i
j T t a i o k l d o z K c r v k g g a w t a d
f m r t p S E y c i r e v p k x V x c m e p s
l h e p M a h f l i L i m n s t g l y z d a M
B g R c T r t a f e f q d i k b n n n k P t i
p f K k o c r i s e l i s a b g v g c r h i c
t a l u Z e k i t G c o c p t d y t d k o t h
y n l l n N o h G e r t L a z i g t l t s e i
L f w i d n g t B o j m Y x t h o l g n p T g
h k m p z R B d u z f t n q C i h n t r h z a
f e t p n K r l n k m h l z z j o v r N a m n
r C Q m r z f m p O T C M p k l P n y l t d y
k l d e m i n e r a l i z a t i o n b b e y m
```

Word Search Clues

■ A fluoride compound with a pH of 3.5 that may etch porcelain (two words)

■ The researcher who associated Colorado brown stain with drinking water (four words)

■ The first research city and state in the United States to add fluoride to its municipal water supply in January 1945 (two words)

■ The result of unintentional fluoride incorporated into a food or beverage during processing (two words)

■ Over the counter (acronym)

■ A small area on the tooth that may be the first clinically detectable caries lesion or an area of demineralization (two words)

■ An area of demineralization below the enamel surface that can become remineralized with fluoride application (two words)

■ The crystalline mineral component of bones and teeth containing $Ca_{10}(PO_4)6X_2$

■ Inhibiting dental caries

■ The removal of fluoride from a water supply that has a naturally occurring higher-than-optimum fluoride level

■ Breakdown of the tooth structure with a loss of calcium and phosphorus

■ Term referring to the ability of clinically tested products to produce a significant health benefit

■ Fluoride ions have replaced some of the hydroxyl (OH) ions in this type of hydroxyapatite

■ A less-soluble apatite that is more resistant to acids

■ A systemic nutrient that enhances tooth remineralization

■ Small white spots to severe brown staining and pitting of the enamel caused by pre-eruptive ingestion of excessive amounts of fluoride

■ The form of apatite that is the principal mineral component of teeth, bones, and calculus

■ Refers to enamel with deficient calcification

■ Parts per million (abbreviation)

■ Fluoride enhances this process, which returns minerals to the tooth

■ A type of gel that becomes fluid under stress to permit flow

■ This can occur as a result of a rapid intake of high concentration fluoride over a short period of time

■ A form of professional topical fluoride application that is easily applied to root surfaces and sets up in the presence of saliva.

KNOWLEDGE EXERCISES

1. Identify two ways fluoride is made available to the tooth surface.

_____

_____

_____

2. Describe how dietary fluoride is absorbed by and distributed to body tissues.

_____

_____

_____

3. Approximately 99% of fluoride in the body is located in _____, such as _____.

4. Fluoride concentration in the saliva ranges from _____ to _____ ppm.

5. Fluoride is absorbed in the _____ and excreted mostly through the _____.

6. During the formation of enamel, fluoride is deposited starting at the _____.

7. Fluoride concentration is greatest at the _____ of the dentin.

8. Too much fluoride ingested during tooth development can result in _____.

9. Before the tooth erupts but after the crown is completely mineralized, systemic fluoride is deposited on the _____.

10. Fluoride, from drinking water or from topical fluoride treatments, continues to be deposited on the surface of the tooth after the tooth has _____.

11. Topical fluoride uptake on the tooth surface is most rapid during _____.

12. Topical fluoride concentration in the enamel is highest at the _____ of the enamel.

13. Fluoride level in cementum is high and increases _____.

14. In your own words, describe demineralization.

_____

_____

_____

15. Where does demineralization occur?

_____

_____

_____

16. In your own words, describe remineralization.

_____

_____

_____

17. What is the role of fluoride in the demineralization–remineralization process?

_____

_____

_____

18. What is the effect of fluoride on bacteria?

_____

_____

_____

19. What is dental fluorosis?

_____

_____

_____

20. Who pinpointed fluorine as the element related to the observed changes in tooth enamel and risk for dental caries?

_____

_____

_____

21. Who was Dr. H. Trendley Dean?

_____

_____

_____

22. What is the optimal level of fluoride concentration in drinking water for caries prevention?

_____

_____

_____

23. How does the climate in the area you live affect the optimal fluoride concentration that is placed in the community water system for prevention of dental caries?

_____

_____

_____

24. Adding fluoride to the school water supply in communities that do not have access to a fluoridated community water system is one way to benefit children in rural areas. Why is the concentration of fluoride increased from the optimum levels when fluoride is added to only the school water supply?

_____

_____

_____

25. When fluoride is removed from the water in a community, one of two possible effects is noted. What are the two possible effects?

_____

_____

_____

26. What compounds are used to fluoridate water supplies?

_____

_____

_____

27. List factors to investigate when you are trying to determine if your patient needs fluoride supplements.

_____

_____

_____

28. In what forms can supplementary fluoride be given?

_____

_____

_____

29. If the fluoride water concentration in the community is 0.045 ppm and there is no additional fluoride in the water supply at school, what is the dose of supplemental fluoride that is recommended for a 5-year-old child?

_____

_____

30. The ideal fluoride regime for most patients is high frequency, low concentration. That is why fluoridated water is so effective in preventing dental decay for most people. What factors indicate the need for you to include a professionally applied fluoride treatment in your patient's care plan?

_____

_____

_____

_____

_____

31. What are the objectives for a professionally applied topical fluoride?

_____

_____

_____

32. What is the concentration of fluoride ions in a 1.23% acidulated phosphate gel, which you apply to your patient's teeth using a tray?

_____

_____

33. What professionally applied solution is recommended for infants and small children who are at high risk for dental caries?

_____

_____

34. What are the advantages of the solution you identified in question 33?

_____

_____

35. Which fluoride application(s) is(are) considered effective to reduce dentinal hypersensitivity?

_____

_____

_____

36. If your patient presents with a four-unit porcelain anterior bridge, which fluoride preparation is not appropriate for you to recommend and why?

_____

_____

_____

37. How are the patient's teeth prepared before painting on a fluoride solution, applying a fluoride varnish, or placing the trays during a professional fluoride application?

_____

_____

_____

38. Briefly list the steps for applying a fluoride varnish.

_____

_____

_____

39. Briefly describe the techniques for using self-applied fluorides.

_____

_____

_____

_____

40. Match each of the following descriptions with the appropriate self-applied fluoride mouth-rinse preparation. Each type of mouth rinse is used more than once.

DESCRIPTION	MOUTH RINSE TYPE
_____ Once per week use	A. Low potency/high frequency
_____ Recommended for daily use	B. High potency/low frequency
_____ Available only as a sodium fluoride preparation	
_____ Available as a sodium fluoride, acidulated phosphate fluoride, or a stannous fluoride preparation	
_____ Can be purchased as an over-the-counter preparation	
_____ Is available in a 0.5% solution	
_____ Is available in a high-potency solution that is commonly diluted with water before use	
_____ Is sometimes used in school-based fluoride rinse programs	
_____ Has been shown to reduce the incidence of dental caries by 30–40% with reports of a 42.5% reduction in caries in primary teeth	

41. Use **Infomap 33-1** to help you compare type of fluoride ion and concentrations available in each type of preparation available for recommendation to patients who are at risk for dental caries.

INFOMAP 33-1		
PREPARATION TYPE	**TYPE OF FLUORIDE ION**	**RANGE OF FLUORIDE ION CONCENTRATION AVAILABLE**
Professional topical fluoride foam or gel preparations		
Self-applied fluoride gel preparations		
Self-applied fluoride rinse preparations		
Fluoride dentifrice preparations		
Fluoride varnish preparations		
Optimally fluoridated water		

42. In your own words, briefly list important safety measures to discuss with patients when educating them about the use of home fluorides.

_____

_____

_____

43. Briefly describe the signs and symptoms of a toxic dose of fluoride.

_____

_____

_____

44. If your patient feels nauseated and has stomach pain after receiving a professional fluoride treatment in your clinic, what is the first thing you should do?

_____

_____

_____

45. What dental-related symptom is linked to a larger-than-safe dose of systemic fluoride ingested over a long period of time?

_____

_____

_____

46. Supply the acronym or chemical formula that is used to identify each type of fluoride preparation— just one more time to help you remember!

■ *Acidulated phosphate fluoride*

_____

■ *Sodium fluoride*

_____

■ *Sodium monofluorophosphate*

_____

■ *Stannous fluoride*

_____

COMPETENCY EXERCISES

1. A dental hygienist experienced an unfortunate incident a few days ago when she was preparing a fluoride treatment for a 6-year-old child patient in her clinic.

She filled a set of trays with the maximum allowable amount of neutral sodium fluoride foam for children (*Hint:* consult Table 33-4 in the textbook) and left the trays sitting on the counter while she exited the room briefly to get permission for the fluoride treatment from the child's mother. She returned moments later to find that the child had picked up the trays and licked every bit of the fluoride foam out of both the upper and the lower tray. Calculate the dose of fluoride that the child received in this incident.

_____

_____

_____

_____

_____

2. Is the child described in question 1 in danger of an acute reaction?

_____

_____

_____

3. A 10-year-old mentally challenged child who weighs 50 lb accidentally ingested 200 mL of fluoridated toothpaste that contained 0.8% Na_2PO_3F. Is this child in danger of an acute toxic reaction?

_____

_____

_____

_____

_____

4. Give an example of a situation that could lead to chronic fluoride toxicity, and discuss what you would include in an education presentation for your patient (or patient's parent) to prevent this from happening.

_____

_____

_____

5. Appendix D contains a Patient-Specific Care Plan for Melody Crane (aged 15 months). Use the information in the care plan to determine the components of a complete fluoride-intervention program that you will recommend for Melody. Include all

Everyday Ethics

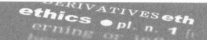

Refer to the Codes of Ethics (Appendices I, II, and III in the textbook) and Framework for Making Decisions (Table 1-2 in the textbook) as you discuss the following scenario with your classmates.

Daniel was an extremely well-behaved and cooperative 4.5-year-old boy at a moderate to severe risk for dental caries because of having one carious lesion and living in a nonfluoridated area. When it came time for the fluoride treatment, the dental hygienist, Nina, spent a few extra minutes explaining to Daniel how she will paint a coating on his teeth to make them stronger. Although Daniel's parents did not have insurance coverage, the hygienist decided it would be important for him to receive a fluoride application regardless of the fee. Daniel tolerated the procedure well. After the appointment, Nina explained to Daniel's mother the varnish postoperative instructions. Daniel's mother became upset and said, "Why did you give my son a fluoride treatment without my permission? My husband just lost his job, and I cannot afford this added cost."

Questions for Consideration

1. Do the benefits of attempting the fluoride treatment outweigh the possible negative experience with Daniel's mother? Why or why not?
2. His mom was upset when she was informed of the cost of her son having the fluoride without her permission. Explain the protocol for obtaining informed consent. Would it really be necessary in this situation? Why or why not?
3. Were there any fluoride recommendations that Nina could have made for Daniel in lieu of the professional varnish application?
4. What ethical principles support/do not support Nina's decision or course of action with Daniel?

---

types of recommended fluoride intervention, and identify any additional information that you will provide Mrs. Crane as you discuss your recommended program for the infant.

_____

_____

_____

6. Appendix D contains a Patient Assessment Summary for Mrs. Rosalee Ayers (aged 55 years). Mrs. Ayers has an increased risk for root caries owing to slight generalized recession. Determine the compo-

nents of a complete fluoride intervention plan for Mrs. Ayers.

_____

_____

_____

7. Appendix D contains a Patient Assessment Summary for Ms. Marie Tonawonda. What components would be appropriate to include in a fluoride intervention plan for this patient?

_____

_____

_____

8. If you provided a professional fluoride treatment for Ms. Tonawonda during her dental hygiene appointment, how might you consider altering the standard fluoride tray procedure to ensure complete coverage of all vulnerable tooth surfaces?

_____

_____

_____

_____

_____

_____

Factors To Teach The Patient

In Competency Exercise question 5, you developed a plan for a patient specific fluoride intervention for Melody Crane. Use the plan you developed and the example conversation in Appendix B as a guide to prepare a conversation that you might use to educate Melody's mother about the fluoride intervention you have planned.
This scenario is related to the following factors:

- Personal use of fluorides
- Need for parental supervision
- Determining need for fluoride supplements
- Fluorides being a part of the total preventive program
- Fluoridation
- Bottled drinking water

DISCOVERY EXERCISES

Your patient, Mrs. Edmons, makes a frantic telephone call to the clinic this morning. Her normal, healthy, and very curious 2-year-old son, Nick, has sucked out and eaten most of a tube of fruit-flavored children's toothpaste. She estimates that he has consumed about 3 oz. of toothpaste. The first question you ask her is to identify the kind and amount of fluoride in the toothpaste. She states that the back of the tube indicates 0.15% sodium fluoride. Discover how to convert Mrs. Edmons's estimate of the amount of toothpaste Nick has eaten into the approximate amount in milliliters. Has Nick ingested more than the safely tolerated dose of fluoride?

_____

_____

_____

_____

_____

_____

Sealants

Chapter Outline

Learning Objectives

Upon successful completion of these exercises, you will be able to:

1. Identify and define key terms and concepts related to dental sealants.
2. Identify sealant materials and classifications.
3. Describe how dental sealants work to penetrate and fill tooth pits and fissures.
4. Discuss indications for use, clinical procedures for application, and maintenance of dental sealants.

KNOWLEDGE EXERCISES

Terms and Concepts Crossword Puzzle

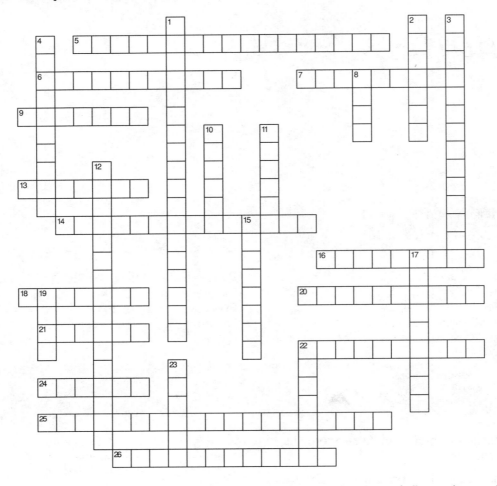

Across

5 Inked ribbon used to determine high spots in a recently placed dental sealant by marking contacts between maxillary and mandibular teeth (two words).

6 A substance added to another substance to increase its usability; refers to the acid etchant that prepares enamel for bonding with the sealant.

7 Resistance to flow as a result of molecular cohesion.

9 A compound of high molecular weight formed by a combination of a chain of simpler molecules.

13 Refers to procedures that are used to clean debris or biofilm from the surface of a tooth before etching during sealant application.

14 The physical adherence of a dental sealant to the microspaces between the enamel rods of the tooth structure (two words).

16 Caries limited to the enamel.

18 An organic polymer that flows into the pit or fissure of a tooth and bonds to the enamel surface by mechanical retention.

20 The type of acid used in a 15–50% solution to etch the tooth before placement of a dental sealant.

21 The process by which plastic becomes rigid.

22 Refers to examination of a just-placed dental sealant for voids or air bubbles in order to determine if adjustment or replacement is necessary.

24 The appearance of the surface of a tooth after it is adequately etched and thoroughly dried during sealant application.

25 Polymerization with the use of an external light.

26 Expression of the degree of adherence between the tooth surface and the sealant (two words).

Down

1 The self-curing, hardening process of pit-and-fissure sealants.

2 Under laboratory conditions (two words).

3 The reaction in which a polymer is produced.

4 Tiny openings such as those created during the acid etch step of sealant placement.

8 Term that refers to polymerizing of the sealant during application.

10 Bisphenol A-glycidyl methacrylate (abbreviation, without the hyphen).

11 Within the living body (two words).

12 The ability of things to exist together without harm.

15 Term referring to an absorbent pad placed in the cheek over the opening of the Stensen's duct to aid in maintaining a dry field when placing sealants.

17 Refers to procedures that maintain a dry field during placement of dental sealants to keep saliva from contaminating the area to be etched.

19 Refers to the process of creating irregularities or micropores in the enamel.

22 Phosphoric acid used to prepare the enamel surface of the tooth to provide mechanical retention for a dental sealant.

23 The type of sealant that contains glass, quartz, silica, and other composite materials in addition to Bis-GMA that makes the sealant more resistant to abrasion.

Sealants for Prevention

1. In your own words, describe the purpose and action of a dental sealant.

   _____

   _____

   _____

2. List the criteria for an ideal dental sealant.

   _____

   _____

   _____

3. The many types of dental sealants have, to some extent, combined or overlapping characteristics. For example, autopolymerized dental sealants can be either clear or opaque in color. Identify all of the classifications and types of dental sealants.

   _____

   _____

   _____

4. Study Table 34-1 in the textbook and review the section "Clinical Procedures" in Chapter 34 of the textbook to learn the basic procedures for application of dental sealants. List the general rules for sealant application.

   _____

   _____

   _____

5. What is the purpose of debriding and cleaning the tooth surface before etching for sealant placement?

   _____

   _____

   _____

6. What materials are necessary for isolating the area receiving a dental sealant?

   _____

   _____

   _____

7. After the tooth surface is etched, rinsed, and redried, what should you observe?

   _____

   _____

   _____

8. What will prevent the dental sealant from penetrating to the bottom of the occlusal fissure?

   _____

   _____

   _____

9. Identify the factors that affect sealant retention.

   _____

   _____

   _____

COMPETENCY EXERCISES

1. You are collecting assessment data during an initial dental hygiene appointment for Dimitri Albergo, who is 12 years old. Dr. Donovan expects you to evaluate the need for dental sealants, record your findings on an assessment form, and then discuss your specific recommendations when he comes in to examine Dimitri. Together, you will make decisions for including sealants in Dimitri's dental hygiene care plan. What oral findings indicate a potential need for the placement of dental sealants?

   _____

   _____

   _____

2. Discuss why Dimitri's second molars are the most important teeth to evaluate for sealant placement.

   _____

   _____

   _____

3. During your oral examination of Dimitri, you find a pit-and-fissure area on tooth 30 that is questionable for the placement of a dental sealant. What is the next step to follow in determining whether that specific tooth surface is appropriate for sealant placement?

   _____

   _____

   _____

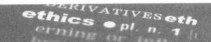

Everyday Ethics

Refer to the Codes of Ethics (Appendices I, II, and III in the textbook) and Framework for Making Decisions (Table 1-2 in the textbook) as you discuss the following scenario with your classmates.

Lillian had always enjoyed doing sealants when she was in dental hygiene school. They had been required to do quite a few, and as students they got to participate in Sealant Day, a volunteer program carried out by the local dental hygienists every spring.

Now, when she came back from the state dental hygiene meeting, she was all excited about the new interpretation of the practice act by the Dental Board and greeted her employer, Dr. Fine, with the news the first thing Monday morning. The board had voted that the dental hygienist who had been in practice for 2 years full-time (or part-time equivalent) could make the decision whether a pit or fissure needed a sealant. There was a continuing education course and an examination required.

Lillian added: "Remember Jack—that teenager that was here last week? He had some really deep fissures that I was sure would benefit from sealants. Can I go ahead and schedule him? I told him he needed them. He has an appointment with you to have a few cavities filled, but that wouldn't fit in your book until nearly the end of the month."

Dr. Fine continued quietly to tie on his gown for the first patient, and then he smiled and said, "Well, Lil, let's wait until he comes in for his appointment with me and I'll look at them."

Questions for Consideration

1. Professionally, what action(s) can Lillian take to initiate a system of calibration between her and Dr. Fine to pursue the new practice protocols?
2. What ethical issues may be involved here?
3. Which of the core values describe the friendly relationship between Lillian and Dr. Fine? And which core values describe Lillian's wishes to extend the services for Jack's (the patient's) benefit?

Factors To Teach The Patient

The dental hygiene care plan you develop for Dimitri (introduced in Competency Exercise question 1) recommends dental sealants for all four of his second permanent molars, plus teeth 14 and 3. Dimitri's mother has heard of dental sealants but does not understand why she should spend so much money to "fix" a tooth that has nothing wrong with it. In order to obtain consent from Dimitri's mother to apply the dental sealants, you must educate her.

Use the example of a patient conversation in Appendix B as a guide to develop a conversation to explain dental sealants to Mrs. Albergo.

This scenario is related to the following factors:

- Sealants as part of a preventive program but not as a substitute for other preventive measures (e.g., limiting dietary sucrose, using fluorides, and controlling dental biofilm)
- What a sealant is and why such a meticulous application procedure is required
- What can be expected from a sealant, including how long it lasts and how it prevents dental caries
- Need for examination of the sealant at frequent, scheduled appointments and need for replacement when indicated

4. When you evaluate Dimitri's bitewing radiographs, no occlusal or proximal surface dental caries are present on tooth 14. What is the next step in deciding whether to select that tooth for placement of a dental sealant?

_____

_____

_____

Implementation: Prevention

■ Chapters 23–34

COMPETENCY EXERCISES

Maria Hernandez is a 19-year-old single mother who has just received health insurance, including dental insurance. This is only her second visit ever to a dentist. The first was when she had a tooth extracted, because of dental caries, at age 14. She presents with swollen gingiva, multiple areas of severe dental caries, and extensive biofilm along the gingival margins of all her teeth. She is 5 months pregnant with her second child and has no other health issues.

Maria is nearly fluent in English, although Spanish is her first language; she lives with her mother and younger siblings. Maria's first child, who is 4 years old, has been receiving care in the clinic and has, within the last 6 months, had extensive dental work, including crowns and extractions because of dental caries.

1. Outline the points you will cover as you educate this young mother about the influences of maternal and family oral health on the health of infants and toddlers.

   _____

   _____

   _____

   _____

   _____

   _____

2. What aspects of prevention will you focus on during a series of perhaps four dental hygiene appointments with Maria?

   _____

   _____

   _____

   _____

   _____

3. What factors are likely to affect your efforts to communicate with and educate Maria about preventing dental disease for herself and her young family?

   _____

   _____

   _____

   _____

   _____

   _____

4. You are working with other dental professionals to develop a pilot health-promotion and disease-prevention program that will provide a 1-year comprehensive, individualized dental-health education intervention for families with children who have been identified as most at risk for dental caries and periodontal disease.

   It is not in your job description to provide dental-hygiene services. Rather, you will educate the children and mothers, refer for needed dental care, and facilitate access to the dental services already available in nearby dental clinics. The identified children and mothers have agreed to meet with you for one 2-hour session each week for the next year.

   Today you examine Victor Azure, an 11-year-old child who lives on the nearby Navajo reservation with his mother; father; and two older brothers, who attend high school.

   The results of Victor's dental examination reveal multiple restorations in primary molars and dental sealants on first molars that were provided by the dental practice located on the reservation. He has no currently active caries, but you observe a few demineralized areas on the maxillary incisors. You also observe swollen gingiva and extensive biofilm along the gingival margins of all of Victor's teeth.

   Victor states that he brushes nearly every day with fluoridated toothpaste but really hates to do it because it is boring. Victor sometimes uses a home fluoride rinse but more often uses a strong-tasting mouthwash that his father likes. Victor states that his father uses the mouthwash because he has bad breath and some of his teeth wiggle. Victor knows that some of his remaining primary teeth are getting loose and hopes that the mouthwash will keep him from losing them.

The interview with Victor's mother, Skye, regarding his dental history indicates that Victor was exposed to fluoridated water for only the first 3 years of his life, before the family came back home from Chicago to live on the reservation, which does not have fluoridated water. Victor did not ever visit a dentist until last year, when all the restorative work was done, and his mother states that she plans to try to maintain the regular schedule of visits to the dentist that was recommended when Victor was there 6 months ago.

Skye states that the dentist told her that Victor's high rate of decay is linked to his diet, which is high in frequent carbohydrate intake, including large amounts of carbonated beverages, which he drinks all day long. But she also states that she isn't worried about the high rate of decay in the primary teeth because those are going to fall out soon anyway. She states proudly that she allowed the placement of the sealants to protect his adult teeth from decay.

When you go over Victor's medical history with his mother, you find that except for the fact that he is extremely overweight, there are no current health problems. There is, however, a family history of diabetes. Both Victor's mother and father have been recently diagnosed with type 2 diabetes, Victor's grandfather died because of complications of diabetes, and a number of Victor's aunts and uncles have diabetes. One of his older brothers is currently being tested for diabetes.

You are responsible for creating an individualized health-promotion, disease-prevention education plan for Victor and his mother that addresses all of the relevant components you studied in the prevention section of the textbook. Plan the sequence of health-promotion, disease-prevention topics you will discuss with Victor and his mother over the next year during your weekly meetings.

_____

_____

_____

_____

_____

Your next patients are Samantha Mitchell, who is a 6-year-old, first-grade student, and her older sister, Hayley, who is almost 12. Both girls have been seen regularly by a dentist since they were 2 years old, but this is their first visit to your clinic.

Samantha is in generally good health. There is no previous history of dental caries, minimal biofilm, and no gingival inflammation—except in the mandibular incisor area where the permanent central incisors are erupting. Her first permanent molars, which exhibit well-coalesced, rather shallow pits and fissures are not completely erupted. There is no proximal decay noted on the radiographs.

Hayley has already received sealants in her first permanent molars. You make a mental note to recommend sealants in 6 months after Samantha's first molars are fully erupted.

5. You prepare a care plan for Samantha that includes dental hygiene interventions based on individualized assessment data and patient need. As you present the care plan to Mrs. Mitchell, explain to her why dental sealants are not included in this care plan you prepared for Samantha. Concentrate on Samantha's assessment data and on your determination of need for services as you continue to explain to Ms. Mitchell why sealants are not indicated for Samantha right now, even when she states "But our insurance covers sealants" and "But you recommended sealants for Hayley."

_____

_____

_____

_____

_____

_____

6. Get together with a group of your student colleagues and gather examples/samples of a variety of adjunctive dental hygiene aids, such as flossing aids or holders, oral irrigators, and different types of interdental cleaners. Each one of you will then be responsible for learning how to use one oral hygiene aid, demonstrating it to all the others in the group and providing feedback to each individual as he or she practices the technique for using the aid.

7. From the patient records available in your school clinic, find cases for which the assessment data indicate the need for preventive interventions. A patient that you have personally collected the assessment data for is probably the best choice, but any patient record will do for this exercise. Use the assessment data to develop a patient-specific dental

hygiene care plan for that patient that addresses all the relevant aspects of oral-disease prevention and oral-health promotion discussed in this section of the textbook.

_____

_____

_____

_____

_____

DISCOVERY EXERCISES

1. Identify the chemotherapeutic agent/ingredient in at least one brand of mouth rinse or dentifrice that is commonly available to your patients. Go to the library to find scientific information about the ingredient you identify. You can also use product information from the company that produces the product. According to the list of characteristics found in Box 27-3 of the textbook, does the active ingredient appear to be an effective chemotherapeutic agent? If each of your classmates does this exercise using different brands of mouth rinse, you can share your findings and enhance your knowledge base about mouth rinses.

2. Identify teaching materials currently available in your school to use for patient education in your clinic. Investigate sources for new or additional materials, and request samples. When you receive them, analyze them for accuracy, readability, and appeal. Decide which ones are most appropriate and valuable for providing information for the patients you will see in your school clinic.

3. Create a product-comparison Infomap. This discovery exercise will help you compare chemotherapeutic agents used in dentistry and is best done by working together in small groups of three to six students.

   Step 1: Gather together a variety of mouth rinses, dentifrices, or other dental products that contain chemotherapeutic ingredients recommended by dental hygienists for prevention of dental disease. Have each group member be responsible for finding particular products. You can gather over-the-counter products as well as those that are commonly dispensed only by prescription. You will need to make sure that you have the available packaging information for each product.

   Step 2: Assemble small plastic cups, long cotton swabs, and some paper towels so that you can do a taste test.

   Step 3: Develop an Infomap that will help you compare these products. There are examples of Infomaps throughout this workbook to give you ideas as you develop this one. Your Infomap should allow you to compare similar products in such areas as active chemotherapeutic ingredients, alcohol content, ADA Seal of Approval, cost, taste, efficacy of the product based on current research findings, and any other topic areas you think are important for your comparison.

   The Infomap you create can be used to help you compare products when you are making recommendations to your patients. After your student group develops the basic framework for the Infomap, you can continue to add products as you become aware of them in order to keep a currently updated review of products for recommending to your patients.

4. Use the information in the textbook to create an Infomap that compares various kinds of manual toothbrushes that you can recommend for your patients. How about an Infomap comparing the various brands and types of dental floss? What other prevention products could you compare in an Infomap format?

5. Being able to apply evidence-based prevention protocols as we make recommendations for patients requires practice in accessing, analyzing, and applying information from the dental and oral health literature. Select a prevention topic, and perform a Medline search to obtain a list of current scientific research articles related to that topic. Obtain the full-text articles either online or at the library.

   Write a short review of the literature to summarize what you learned from reading the articles. Be sure to include recommendations for patient care that are based on your analysis of the literature.

6. Work with your student colleagues to create an annotated list of web sites that provide information on topics related to the prevention of oral disease. Each student should select a topic, and then perform an Internet search using the search engine of his or her choice. Make sure the Web sites you select provide valid, scientific, and reliable information.

   Write a brief summary of the information you learned from the web site, and be sure to include the correct Internet address (URL) at the top of the page. Provide electronic copies of your brief description of the Web site to your instructor or to a student colleague who is willing to compile the information into one document that can be shared by all students.

7. Investigate prevention in the news. Collect articles from the current popular literature—such as newspapers, magazines, and television or radio announcements—that provide information on prevention of oral diseases. Also look for dental product advertisements that appear in the popular press. This is the information that your patients see and will probably ask you about when you are providing patient education.

■ *Is the information that you find presented in the popular media valid and scientifically accurate?*

■ *How can this information affect the way in which the dental profession is perceived?*

■ *Does the media information you find agree with the recommendations you make for dental preventive care?*

FOR YOUR PORTFOLIO

1. Include a copy of the original product comparison Infomap your student group created in Discovery Exercise 3. As you update the Infomap with new product information, also include your most currently updated Infomap in your portfolio. Having both the original and the updated Infomaps will help you demonstrate your commitment to continued learning.

2. Provide written examples that describe dental hygiene education and counseling interventions you have provided for specific patients. Select examples that illustrate your ability to communicate, motivate, and educate particular patients so that positive health outcomes result. Structure your examples so that each includes a discussion of the following:

■ *Significant assessment findings*
■ *Prevention topics and methods presented*
■ *Oral-health techniques demonstrated*
■ *Method of patient practice used*
■ *Methods for evaluating success of the patient's compliance, motivation levels, and learning styles (Discuss any factors that affected your ability to communicate with the patient and factors that affected compliance with your recommendations.)*

3. Include copies of patient-specific care plans you have developed that illustrate your ability to plan individualized prevention for specific patient cases. Include some early attempts at developing care plans and also some care plans that you have developed near the end of your student career. Provide a short written analysis of how the early examples compare with the later examples of care planning to demonstrate your growth toward competency in care planning for prevention.

4. Include the literature review you wrote in the Discovery Exercise 7. Later you can update your search to see if there is new information available that might change any recommendations you made in your first review.

5. Collect as many examples of prevention in the news as you can during the time you are a student and jot down notes analyzing each example. Later on you can use your notes to write an analysis of all the examples you collected. Take time to identify trends in how preventive dentistry is presented in the popular media. How does the popular view of dentistry affect the way your patients perceive and are motivated by your prevention interventions and recommendations?

Implementation: Clinical Treatment

■ SECTION VI LEARNING OBJECTIVES

Completing the exercises in this section of the workbook will prepare you to:

1. Manage patient anxiety and pain during dental hygiene treatment.
2. Provide a variety of dental hygiene treatment interventions.

■ COMPETENCIES FOR THE DENTAL HYGIENIST

The following ADEA competencies are supported by the learning in Section VI.

Core Competencies: C3, C9, C10

Patient/Client Care Competencies: PC4, PC5

Anxiety and Pain Control

Chapter Outline

Learning Objectives

Upon successful completion of these exercises, you will be able to:

1. Identify and define key terms and concepts related to controlling pain and anxiety.
2. Identify the components of pain and describe a variety of mechanisms for control of dental pain.
3. Describe procedures for nitrous oxide sedation.
4. Describe the pharmacology and method of action of local anesthetics.
5. Describe clinical procedures for administration of anesthesia during dental hygiene treatment.
6. Identify and explain the indications and contraindications for use of anesthesia during dental hygiene treatment.

KNOWLEDGE EXERCISES

1. In your own words, describe interaction between the two components of pain.

_____

_____

_____

2. Each individual's reaction to pain is different. Individuals who react strongly or quickly to a painful stimulus are said to have a _____ pain threshold. Those who do not react strongly to the same painful stimulus are said to have a _____ pain threshold.

3. List the factors that can influence your patient's reaction to dental pain.

_____

_____

_____

4. Which of the five pain-control mechanisms alter pain reaction?

_____

_____

_____

5. Which of the pain-control mechanisms relies for success on your ability to communicate with and educate your patient?

_____

_____

_____

6. **Figure 35-1** shows a nitrous oxide delivery system. Label the following components on the figure. It might be useful to use colored pencil (use green for oxygen and blue for nitrous oxide, of course!). Note that some components may not be easy to identify or locate on the figure, but do your best; then investi-

gate or ask your instructor to find out if your idea was correct.

■ *Oxygen tank (add a notation to identify the gas pressure)*

■ *Nitrous oxide tank (add a notation to identify the gas pressure)*

■ *Cylinder valves used to open and close each tank* (Hint: *There is one on each tank.*)

■ *Hoses that carry only oxygen gas*

■ *Hoses that carry only nitrous oxide gas*

■ *Hoses that can carry both nitrous oxide gas and oxygen*

■ *Regulator or reducing valve (location not discussed in the textbook)*

■ *Flow meter (location not discussed in the textbook)* (Hint: *The clinician uses this to control the level of each gas administered to the patient.*)

■ *On-demand valve* (Hint: *Probably located near the flow meter.*)

■ *Reservoir bag*

■ *Nasal hood, nose piece, or mask*

■ *Scavenger system*

■ *Areas where there are connectors (It is important to know where these are, because you will regularly need to inspect and test them for potential leaks.)*

7. Conscious sedation, produced by administration of a combination of nitrous oxide and oxygen, is frequently used to reduce patient anxiety and perception of pain during short dental procedures that are expected to cause a low level of pain. Identify the two properties of nitrous oxide that are useful for reducing pain.

_____

_____

_____

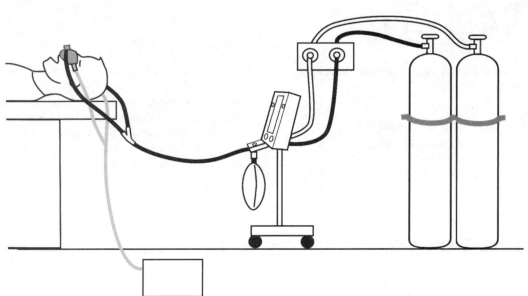

FIGURE 35-1

8. Why is nitrous oxide sedation especially useful for control of soft-tissue discomfort during dental hygiene procedures?

_____

_____

_____

9. During dental hygiene procedures, a range of _____% nitrous oxide is administered in combination with oxygen to achieve optimum pain control for most patients, with the primary saturation of blood occurring in _____ minutes.

10. What is the minimum amount of oxygen flow that is maintained by the gas delivery system for patient safety?

_____

_____

_____

11. You will administer _____% oxygen to your patient for several minutes after the completion of the dental hygiene procedure to prevent _____.

12. List contraindications for the use of nitrous oxide during dental hygiene care.

_____

_____

_____

13. Attention to the details of providing an effective scavenging system, rigorous equipment maintenance, and the initiation of other methods for preventing overexposure are imperative when nitrous oxide is used during patient care. What are the potential health hazards for clinicians who are exposed to excessive levels of nitrous oxide?

_____

_____

_____

14. Without looking in the textbook, list the steps you will use to administer nitrous oxide–oxygen analgesic during patient care. For each step, when appropriate, indicate the time frame and the amount of oxygen or nitrous flow.

_____

_____

_____

_____

_____

_____

_____

_____

_____

15. In your own words, explain how the nitrous oxide gas is titrated during administration.

_____

_____

_____

16. Identify at least three advantages and three disadvantages of using conscious sedation anesthesia (such as nitrous oxide) to reduce patient pain and anxiety during dental hygiene treatment.

◾ *Advantages*

_____

_____

_____

◾ *Disadvantages*

_____

_____

_____

17. List three important components to include in your patient's progress notes after you administer nitrous oxide during dental hygiene treatment.

_____

_____

_____

18. Which of the five basic pain control mechanisms alter pain perception?

_____

_____

_____

19. A nonopioid analgesic is effective in altering pain perception by blocking _____.

20. Pretreatment analgesics, if they are recommended, should be administered _____.

21. List the indications for applying topical anesthetic to reduce your patient's perception of intraoral pain.

    _____

    _____

    _____

22. Identify the active ingredients that are available as noninjectable or topical anesthetic preparations and the amount of time that each provides anesthesia to the tissues.

    _____

    _____

    _____

    _____

    _____

    _____

23. Match each description below with the correct amide type of local anesthesia. Each type of anesthesia is used more than once; some descriptions apply to more than one type of anesthesia.

TYPE OF AMIDE ANESTHETIC	DESCRIPTION
A. Articaine B. Bupivacaine C. Lidocaine D. Mepivacaine E. Prilocaine	_____ Long-acting amide drug _____ Short- or medium-acting amide drug _____ Citanest plain and Citanest forte _____ Carbocaine, Polocaine, Isocaine _____ Marcaine _____ Septocaine, Septanest, and Ultracaine _____ Xylocaine, Octocaine, Lignospan _____ Available in 1.8 mL of solution in cartridge _____ Most widely used amide; also available as a topical _____ Causes less vasodilation, so can be used without a vasoconstrictor _____ Diffuses best through soft and hard tissues _____ Provides extended period of analgesia to manage post-care pain _____ Metabolic by-products can temporarily reduce the oxygen-carrying capacity of blood _____ Potential drug interaction if patient is taking Cimetidine

24. Match each description below with the correct dental cartridge ingredient.

DENTAL CARTRIDGE INGREDIENT	DESCRIPTION
A. Amide anesthetic B. Antioxidant C. Sodium chloride D. Sterile water E. Vasoconstrictor	_____ Creates isotonic match with the body _____ Blocks the transfer of ions across the nerve membrane _____ Constricts blood vessels _____ Preservative for the vasoconstrictor _____ Diluent

25. Match each description below with the correct group of local anesthesia drugs. Each group is used more than once.

LOCAL ANESTHESIA DRUG GROUP	DESCRIPTION
A. Amide B. Ester	_____ Currently used only in topical anesthetics _____ Metabolized in blood plasma _____ Low incidence of allergic reactions _____ Less effective and shorter acting _____ Higher incidence of allergic reactions _____ Metabolized by the liver _____ Causes vasodilation

26. Which ingredient identified in question 22 is most likely to cause an allergic reaction in your patient?

    _____

    _____

    _____

27. Which ingredient identified in question 22 is the most likely to cause a toxic reaction in your patient?

    _____

    _____

    _____

28. In your own words, describe the techniques and armamentarium used for administering noninjectable anesthesia.

_____

_____

_____

_____

_____

_____

29. What techniques can be used to apply topical anesthesia to oral tissues?

_____

_____

_____

_____

30. Identify two vasoconstrictors that are commonly used in dental anesthesia and indicate the standard concentration of each one.

_____

_____

_____

31. A vasoconstrictor offsets the vasodilating action of the local anesthetic. List the reasons for including a vasoconstrictor in local anesthetic solution.

_____

_____

_____

32. What preservative for the vasoconstrictor can cause a potential allergic reaction?

_____

_____

_____

33. What potential drug interactions can cause an adverse reaction when dental anesthetics with vasoconstrictors are used?

_____

_____

_____

34. You will consider your patient's medical history, the type of dental hygiene procedures that are planned,

the potential for patient discomfort, and patient preference when you determine whether to include local anesthesia in your patient's plan for care. What sources of information will you use to assess your patient before providing local anesthetic?

_____

_____

_____

35. What patient risk factors will you consider when selecting which local anesthetic solution to use during dental hygiene treatment?

_____

_____

_____

36. What medical conditions indicate the need for patient-specific evaluation and very careful consideration when determining local anesthesia use during dental hygiene treatment?

_____

_____

_____

37. List the armamentarium you will assemble before providing local anesthesia.

_____

_____

_____

_____

_____

_____

38. Why do you position the patient with the head lower than the heart during a local anesthesia injection?

_____

_____

_____

39. What is prevented from happening when you aspirate before injecting local anesthesia solution?

_____

_____

_____

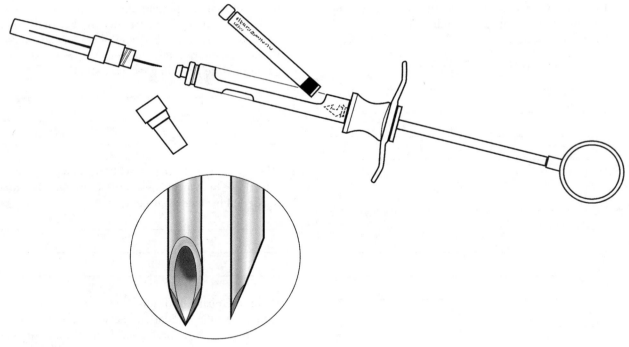

FIGURE 35-2

40. In your own words, describe the procedure for aspiration using a conventional anesthetic syringe.

_____

_____

_____

41. The steps for syringe assembly are listed below. Some of the structures are printed in boldface; label each one on **Figure 35-2**.

▪ *Step 1: Pull back on the **thumb ring.***
▪ *Step 2: Insert the **cartridge** that contains the selected type of anesthetic. Identify the **rubber stopper** and the **diaphragm end** of the cartridge. Identify the **volume** of solution in the cartridge. Identify the **window** openings in the syringe that will allow you to view the cartridge during aspiration.*
▪ *Step 3: Set the **harpoon** into the appropriate end of the cartridge, and test for lock.*
▪ *Step 4: Discard the **safety cap** from the **cartridge end** of the needle.*
▪ *Step 5: With your fingers holding the **needle hub,** screw the needle securely onto the end of the syringe. Identify the **needle** that is used for injection. Indicate the available **lengths** and **diameters** of the needles that are used for injecting dental anesthetic.*
▪ *In the detail, identify the **bevel** of the needle, and draw a line to indicate where the **bone** will be relative to the bevel when the needle is inserted for injection.*

42. Describe what you will do if you see blood in the anesthetic cartridge when you aspirate while providing local anesthetic for your patient.

_____

_____

_____

43. The local anesthetic solution is deposited slowly, _____ minutes for a full cartridge, to prevent _____ and to reduce potential for a _____.

44. What injections will ensure complete soft- and hard-tissue anesthesia for your patient when you are providing periodontal treatment for all of the teeth in the mandibular left quadrant?

_____

_____

_____

45. Which injection will be needed to anesthetize the lingual tissue so that complete patient comfort is achieved during dental hygiene procedures in this area of the mouth?

_____

_____

_____

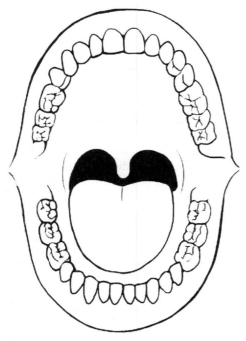

FIGURE 35-3

46. Use a colored pencil to mark **Figure 35-3** to identify the areas that are anesthetized after a middle superior alveolar (MSA) injection on the right side of the patient's mouth.

47. Use a colored pencil to mark Figure 35-3 to identify the area that is anesthetized after an ASA injection on the right side.

48. What structure in the molar teeth is not anesthetized after a posterior superior alveolar (PSA) injection?

_____

_____

_____

49. Which injections anesthetize only the terminal nerve endings for one individual tooth?

_____

_____

_____

50. It is important that you are able to identify the type and the cause of any patient reaction quickly when you are providing local anesthesia. Match each description with the correct symptom. Some symptoms are used more than once; some descriptions apply to more than one type of symptom.

SYMPTOM	DESCRIPTION
A. Adequate anesthesia B. Allergy C. Epithelial desquamation D. Hematoma E. Overdose F. Paresthesia G. Psychogenic reaction H. Trismus	_____ Anxiety reaction _____ Can be the result of too rapid absorption of a drug into bloodstream _____ Can indicate that topical anesthetic was left in contact with the tissue for too long _____ Can result from reduced ability to eliminate or metabolize the local anesthesia drug _____ Caused when a vein or artery is opened and leaks blood into the surrounding tissue _____ Experience of a profound effect for the duration of the procedure _____ Extended duration of anesthesia effect _____ Hypersensitive state that can result in exaggerated response to a subsequent exposure to local anesthesia drug _____ Onset may range from a few seconds to many hours later _____ Patients will sometimes report this reaction as an allergy to local anesthesia _____ Response can range from mild to generalized life-threatening anaphylaxis _____ Spasm of jaw muscle that restricts opening after injection _____ Syncope and hyperventilation are the most common responses _____ Tissue sloughing _____ Toxic levels of local anesthesia drug are present in the bloodstream _____ Prevention of these complications relies on the use of excellent injection technique _____ This response can be made less likely if you use excellent patient communications skills and gentle administration techniques when you are injecting local anesthesia

COMPETENCY EXERCISES

1. Today you are presenting your dental hygiene care plan for four-quadrant, initial therapy scaling and

root planing for Mr. Shizoka. You will ask the patient to sign an informed-consent form before you begin your treatment. Mr. Shizoka does not have much previous dental experience. When you were collecting assessment data for the care plan, he appeared to be very nervous. He asked lots of questions about what you were doing and stopped you frequently when you were trying to probe because he was concerned about whether he would feel pain.

Mr. Shizoka's medical history indicates that he has iron-deficiency anemia and takes a daily ferrous iron supplement. He has hypertension and takes an antihypertensive medication; but he tells you that whenever he is highly stressed, he gets a headache. Write a dental hygiene diagnosis statement related to Mr. Shizoka's anxiety about receiving dental hygiene treatment.

Problem	Cause (Risk Factors and Origin)
_____ related to	_____
_____ related to	_____

2. In the dental hygiene care plan you have developed, you plan to use nitrous oxide–oxygen for pain and anxiety control during Mr. Shizoka's four scaling and root-planing appointments. You have already explained to Mr. Shizoka what nitrous oxide–oxygen sedation is and how it works. Explain the advantages and disadvantages so that he can be completely informed about the use of this pain and anxiety control measure.

_____

_____

_____

_____

_____

_____

3. Mr. Shizoka agrees to try the nitrous oxide–oxygen sedation for at least his first dental hygiene appointment to see if he is comfortable with it. Use your institution's guidelines for writing in patient records to document that you have fully informed Mr. Shizoka and that he has agreed to the use of nitrous oxide analgesia during his dental hygiene treatment

Date	Comments	Signature

4. At his next appointment, you carefully titrate the nitrous oxide–oxygen combination for Mr. Shizoka, and he shows all the signs of ideal sedation. When you begin the injection of local anesthesia into the area where you will be providing care, Mr. Shizoka becomes agitated and starts moving his arms and legs. His rate of respiration increases significantly, he starts to sweat, and his eyes tear up. You immediately stop injecting the local anesthesia. He says he feels sick to his stomach and wants to sit up. Discuss _two_ possibilities for what is happening in this scenario.

_____

_____

_____

Everyday Ethics

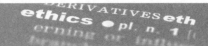

Refer to the Codes of Ethics (Appendices I, II, and III in the textbook) and Framework for Making Decisions (Table 1-2 in the textbook) as you discuss the following scenario with your classmates.

Mr. Denver, in for a dental hygiene appointment, stated that he has not been to a dental office for the past 5 years because he is fearful of oral treatment owing to past painful experiences. Oral examination revealed bleeding on probing, generalized 5- to 6-mm pockets, and heavy biofilm and calculus deposits. Proposed treatment is four appointments for periodontal débridement with patient instruction, followed by a reevaluation.

Questions for Consideration

1. What anxiety and pain management methods could be used for this patient, and which methods are legal for a dental hygienist to administer in your state or province?
2. What are the ethical issues of providing treatment that would predictably cause pain without at least offering adequate pain management?
3. Is the standard of care for pain management different if a dentist or a dental hygienist provides the deep scaling? Explain.

5. What will you do next in the situation described in question 4?

_____

_____

_____

_____

_____

_____

6. Use your institution's guidelines for writing in patient records to document what happened today at Mr. Shizoka's dental hygiene appointment.

Date	Comments	Signature

7. Explain, in patient-appropriate language, how the noninjectable local anesthesia patch is administered.

_____

_____

_____

Factors To Teach The Patient

Because a scheduled patient did not arrive and you have some time free, you are asked to spend the time speaking to Miriam's mother. Miriam Carroll is 9 years old. She has many dental problems but is always cooperative during treatment. At Miriam's appointment today, Dr. Steve will extract three primary molar root tips, and both the maxillary and mandibular arches on the left side of her mouth will be anesthetized for the extractions. This is the first time Miriam will experience the effects of local anesthesia.

Use the example of a patient conversation in Appendix B as a guide to prepare a conversation that you might use to provide postoperative follow-up information to Miriam's mother.

This scenario is related to the following factors:

■ Be careful not to bite lip, cheek, or tongue while tissues are without normal sensations. Warn and watch children to prevent injury. Do not test anesthesia by biting the lip.

■ Avoid chewing hard foods and avoid hot food and drinks until normal sensation has returned.

36 | CHAPTER

Instruments and Principles for Instrumentation

Chapter Outline

Learning Objectives

Upon successful completion of these exercises, you will be able to:

1. Identify and define key terms and concepts related to dental instruments and instrumentation.
2. Identify the components of dental instruments.
3. Describe the purpose, characteristics, and principles for use of a variety of types of dental instruments.
4. Describe methods for developing dexterity and preventing cumulative trauma injuries during dental hygiene instrumentation.
5. Identify techniques for maintaining sharp dental instruments.

Principles for Instrumentation Crossword Puzzle

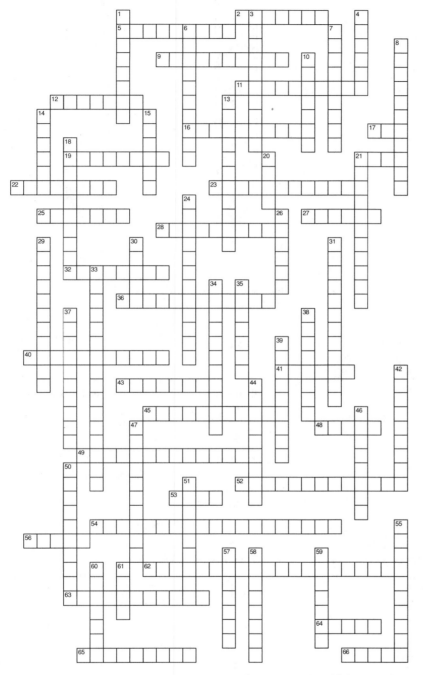

work area with the nondominant hand and the stone is applied at the appropriate angle (two words).
48 The thick, stronger, less flexible instrument shank needed for the removal of heavy calculus deposits.
49 A sharpening stone that is attached to a rotary motor (two words).
52 Refers to a fine-grained instrument sharpening stone made of natural mineral materials (two words).
53 Refers to the cutting edge of an instrument that visually presents a rounded, shiny surface that reflects light.
54 Area of the tooth where treatment is indicated and the stroke of the dental instrument is applied (two words).
56 Connects the handle and the working end of a dental instrument.
62 An artificial sharpening stone material (three words).
63 This type of instrument has paired working ends that may be either mirror image or complementary.
64 Refers to the cutting edge of an instrument that is a fine line, has no width, and does not reflect light.
65 The type of instrument shaft that is designed to help give better access to very deep pockets.
66 A scaling instrument with a rounded working end; there are two types: universal and area-specific.

Down

1 A working stroke that is parallel with the long axis of the tooth being treated.
3 Refers to sharpening stones made with materials other than natural mineral stone.
4 The position of the blade of an area-specific Gracey curet.
6 A sharpening method in which the flat stone is placed on a steady surface and the instrument is moved across the surface of the stone.
7 Refers to development of the control, coordination, and strength needed to become proficient in the efficient and effective use of dental instruments.
8 Refers to a light pressure stroke that disrupts dental biofilm from the root surface of a previously root-planed tooth surface.
10 Refers to the instrument stroke that is applied with an instrument to accomplish a task, such as removing calculus.
13 Dental hygiene instrument that is usually held by the non-dominant hand using a modified pen grasp (two words).
14 Refers to an Arkansas stone that has metal particles ground into the surface and needs to be cleaned by rubbing with emery paper.
15 Refers to any scaling instrument with two cutting edges that meet in a point; can have a curved or straight blade.
18 Refers to the acceptable state for the sharpening stone and testing stick before use for sharpening dental instruments.
20 The type of stroke that is used when activating most scaling instruments.
21 A coarser grain-sharpening stone useful for preliminary sharpening of an excessively dulled instrument.
24 The type of instrument shank that is designed to help adapt the instrument to difficult-to-reach areas, such as the distal surfaces of molars (two words).
26 Single, unbroken movement of the instrument as it is applied against the tooth surface.
29 Refers to a stroke that is dependent on the surface texture of the area being instrumented; lighter pressure is applied progressively as strokes continue and the surface becomes smooth (two words).
30 Another term for the sharpened working end of a dental instrument.
31 This type of lateral pressure when scaling contributes to burnishing of calculus.
33 The hand position that is used to hold a dental instrument (three words).
34 Refers to the fine line where the face and the lateral surfaces of a well-sharpened dental instrument meet (two words).
35 One of three types of strokes that can be applied against the tooth surface with an instrument; a diagonal stroke.
37 The finger that establishes a fulcrum when using a modified pen grasp during instrumentation (two words).
38 Refers to a scaling instrument in which the relationship of the shank, blade, and handle are in a flat plane; indicates that the instrument is primarily used in anterior teeth.
39 A name for a type of scaler; refers to a straight scaler.
42 An artificial sharpening stone that is cleaned by scrubbing with water and repaired by using a Joe Dandy disc to remove grooves (two words).
44 Relaxed and level when working in the neutral position.
46 Refers to the size of the instrument handle; usually available in four sizes.
47 A working stroke that is applied parallel with the occlusal surface of the tooth being treated.
50 Refers to the unique area of each instrument that is used to carry out the purpose and function of that instrument (two words).
51 Removal of inflamed soft tissue inside a periodontal pocket.
55 Refers to the instrument stroke that is used to magnify tactile sensitivity; uses a light pressure in order to magnify tactile sensitivity.
57 Stroke that applies definite, well-controlled pressure on the surface of a tooth; refers to instrumentation of a tooth to remove calculus.
58 The thinner type of instrument shank that may provide more tactile sensitivity and is used to remove fine calculus or for maintenance root débridement.
59 To smooth and polish the surface of calculus (usually with an instrument that is not sharp) instead of removing it completely with a well-sharpened instrument.
60 The position of wrist, forearm, elbow, and shoulder that prevents occupational pain risk for dental hygienists.
61 A type of scaling instrument that has multiple cutting edges lined up on a round, oval, or rectangular base.

Across

2 The combined push-and-pull stroke commonly used to activate a periodontal probe (two words).
5 This type of lateral pressure can result in gouging of the root surface, patient discomfort, and clinician fatigue.
9 Describes the relationship between the working end of the instrument and the tooth surface being treated.
11 The place on a tooth where the third finger of the hand is placed during instrumentation to provide stabilization and control (two words).
12 The pressure that is required of an instrument to the tooth during a scaling procedure.
16 Refers to the angle formed by the working end of the instrument and the tooth surface; usually 60–80°.
17 A type of scaling instrument that has a single straight cutting edge that is turned at a 99° angle to the shank.
19 Used to sharpen files (two words).
21 A cylindrical-shaped sharpening stone that is applied to the face of the instrument rather than angled along the side of the cutting edge.
22 Refers to the using the mirror to view or provide light to any area of the mouth.

23 When you are using the modified pen grasp, the position of the instrument against this finger is extremely important to instrument control (two words).
25 The support upon which your scaling hand finger rests so that force can be exerted during the scaling procedure in order to remove calculus.
27 A type of instrument handle that is lighter weight, enhances tactile sensitivity, and lessens clinician fatigue.
28 A type of instrument that permits exchange or replacement of the working end.
32 Refers to the hand that is usually used for holding a scaling instrument during treatment.
36 The number used to identify a specific instrument (two words).
40 This type of instrument has only one working end (two words).
41 This instrument is used to dislodge heavy calculus by pushing horizontally from facial to lingual on the proximal surface of teeth.
43 Metal particles removed during sharpening that remain attached to the edge of the instrument; sometimes referred to as the bur (two words).
45 Refers to a sharpening technique in which the dental instrument is stabilized against the edge of an immovable

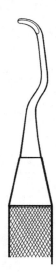

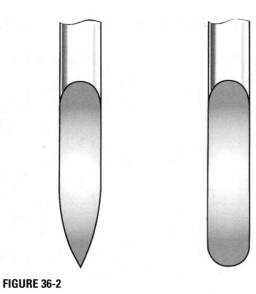

FIGURE 36-1

FIGURE 36-2

KNOWLEDGE EXERCISES

The following questions help you look at each type of instrument from several perspectives. If possible, have real instruments available to look at as you are doing these exercises so you can thoroughly understand the instruments' similarities and differences and visualize their parts.

1. Locate and label each of the following parts on the instrument shown in **Figure 36-1**.
   - Blade
   - Shank
   - Lower shank
   - Handle
   - Serrated surface of the handle

2. The instrument shown in **Figure 36-1** has a relatively _____ shank shape and is probably intended for use on anterior teeth.

3. Label the instruments shown in **Figure 36-2**.
   - Scaler
   - Curet

4. Label the following areas of both instruments shown in **Figure 36-2**.
   - Pointed tip
   - Rounded toe (tip)
   - Cutting edges
   - Area of the cutting edge that is adapted to the tooth during scaling
   - Face of the blade
   - Terminal shank

5. Match each description below to the letter that indicates the appropriate instrument shown in

Figure 36-3 by writing the correct letter in the space provided.

_____Area-specific curet

_____Scaler

6. Label the following areas on the working ends of each of the instruments shown in **Figure 36-3**.
   - Rounded toe (tip)
   - Pointed tip
   - Face of the blade
   - Cutting edges
   - Area of the cutting edge that is adapted to the tooth when scaling
   - Terminal shank
   - Lateral surface and back of the blade

7. Match each description below to the letter that indicates the appropriate instrument shown in **Figure 36-4** by writing the correct letter in the space provided.

_____Area-specific curet

_____Universal curet

_____Scaler

8. Label or mark the following areas on the working ends of each instrument shown in **Figure 36-4**.
   - Face of the blade
   - Cutting edges
   - Terminal shank
   - Lateral surface(s)
   - Back of the blade

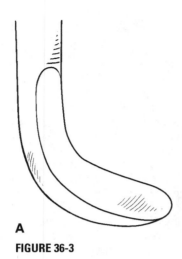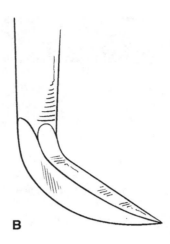

A   B

FIGURE 36-3

9. Without looking at the figure in the textbook, draw a straight line on **Figure 36-4** to indicate how the face of the sharpening stone would be placed (and angled) to sharpen *each* of the cutting edges of each instrument shown. After you draw your lines and label each angle, use a protractor to measure those angles. If your diagram is not correct, erase your lines and redraw them, using the protractor to help you place the angle of your sharpening stone correctly.

10. Imagine that you are using the moving-stone technique to sharpen the instruments shown in **Figure 36-4**. Draw an arrow to indicate the direction of the stroke in which you would apply the most pressure as you move the stone. (*Hint:* This is also the direction you would finish each area as you are sharpening.)

11. List the disadvantages of using a power-driven sharpening technique.

_____

_____

_____

12. When you are activating your instruments during dental hygiene treatment, the proper modified pen grasp is controlled and firm, but not tight and rigid. What are the effects of a grasp that is too tight and rigid?

_____

_____

_____

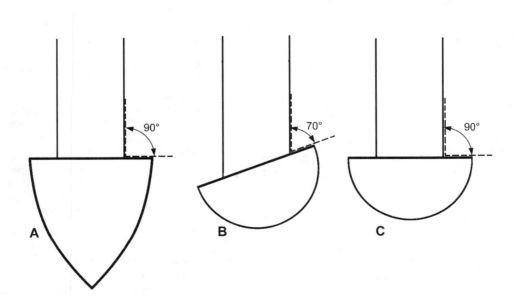

A   90°   B   70°   C   90°

FIGURE 36-4

Everyday Ethics

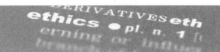

Refer to the Codes of Ethics (Appendices I, II, and III in the textbook) and Framework for Making Decisions (Table 1-2 in the textbook) as you discuss the following scenario with your classmates.

Leslie is eager to begin a new position in her first year of clinical practice as a dental hygienist. Dr. Shepherd has been in practice for 15 years, and most staff members have been with him at least the past 10, including Ann, the dental hygienist with whom she will be practicing. Leslie is glad to have someone with experience take her under her wing.

A dental assistant takes care of instrument sterilization and tray setups for the dental hygienists. As she sat down to her first patient, she noticed the instruments on her tray were all sickle scalers, and she wanted curets. On closer inspection, however, she discovered that all but one instrument were indeed curets; they had just been missharpened, leaving them with no contour (curvature) at the toe.

She excused herself to go into the instrument supply room only to find that all of the curets had sharp, pointed toes. Going back to the clinical area, she peeked in to ask Ann if the assistant did the sharpening for her, noting the curets on Ann's tray were equally sharpened to a distinct point. Ann answered, "No, I do all the sharpening myself because I am very picky."

Leslie pondered what she would do to address this situation—especially how to approach it without alienating her new coworkers.

Questions for Consideration

1. Given Leslie's neophyte status as a clinician, how could she approach her new colleague—an experienced practitioner—with her concerns? Which core values of dental hygiene are involved?
2. What harm, if any, is there to Dr. Shepherd's patients? Discuss why or why not the dentist needs to be notified about the condition of the instruments.
3. Using an ethical decision framework (Table 1-2, page ___), describe realistic alternatives for Leslie's course of action in this situation.

---

13. What factors can influence your risk for cumulative trauma injury and pain from incorrect use of instruments during dental hygiene procedures?

_____

_____

_____

DISCOVERY EXERCISES

The only real way to become competent in the skills described in this chapter of the textbook is to practice. It is, of course, difficult to help you do that in a workbook format. But here are some exercises you can do on your own to help you become competent in identifying instruments and practicing the principles of instrumentation. If you'd like, work in small groups with two or three of your student colleagues. Using the information and descriptions in Chapter 36 in the textbook, group members can provide feedback about each person's instrument technique.

1. Gather together a variety of instruments and lay them out on a table in front of you. Examine them carefully and thoroughly, identifying the instrument parts, the types, and the adaptation characteristics (such as the angle of the shank) of each instrument you have available. Then practice picking up the

Factors To Teach The Patient

Today is your first scaling and root-planing appointment with Mrs. Lorna Patel. (You spent a lot of time with her in the assessment chapters of this workbook; see her Patient-Specific Care Plan in Appendix D.) When you open your sterilized instruments and line them up on the tray, Mrs. Patel expresses amazement at the number of them and comments on their different shapes. When you begin to check each instrument for sharpness before using them, she wants to know what you are looking for.

Use the example of a patient conversation in Appendix B as a guide to write a statement explaining to Mrs. Patel why you have so many instruments on your tray and why you need to make sure they are well sharpened before you begin her treatment. Use the conversation you create to educate a patient or friend who is not a student colleague. *This scenario is related to the following factors:*

- Why it is necessary to use a variety of instruments for scaling
- Benefits of using a finely sharpened instrument for calculus removal
- Harmful effects of using dull instruments

instrument in the modified pen grasp, placing a fulcrum on the tip of the thumb of your nondominant hand, and adapting the blade of the instrument on your fingernail in the correct position for activation.

2. Examine each instrument to determine its characteristics—such as balance, shank length, fabrication materials, and shape and rigidity of the shank. Discuss the purpose and uses of each instrument. Think about area of the mouth the instrument is appropriate for, the technique the instrument is intended for (heavy calculus or root planing, for example), and any other indications/contraindications for use that pertain to the instrument's design.

3. Examine each instrument to determine whether the cutting edge is sharp. Practice the correct placement of a sharpening stone to sharpen each instrument.

4. To develop your dexterity, practice each of the strength, stretching, writing, and instrument exercises described in the "Dexterity Development" section of Chapter 36 in the textbook.

5. Sit comfortably in a chair that has no arms. Practice placing shoulders, arms, elbows, and wrists in a neutral position. While you are sitting there, practice each of the exercises in Figures 36-20 and 36-21 in the textbook.

Nonsurgical Periodontal Instrumentation

Chapter Outline

Learning Objectives

Upon successful completion of these exercises, you will be able to:

1. Ildentify and define key terms and concepts related to nonsurgical periodontal treatment.
2. Define the scope, purpose, and effect of nonsurgical periodontal therapy.
3. Describe appointment preparation and follow-up procedures for nonsurgical periodontal treatment.
4. Identify and describe techniques used for nonsurgical periodontal instrumentation.
5. Identify the types and components of power-driven scalers.
6. Describe techniques for using and maintaining power-driven scalers and manual instruments.

Key Words and Concepts Crossword Puzzle

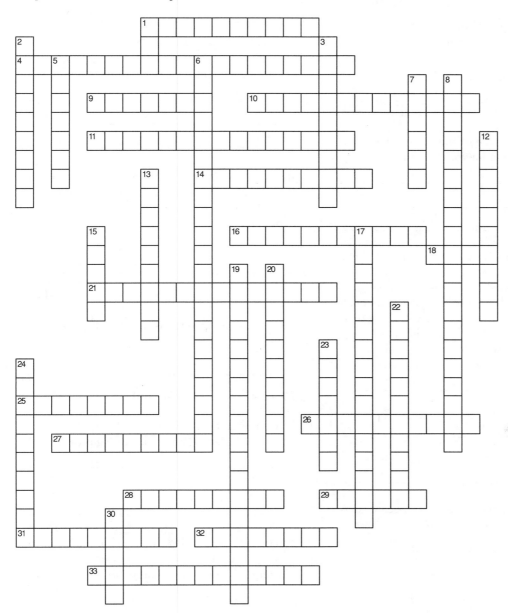

Across

1 A device that converts energy or power from one form to another.
4 Area of the tooth where scaling and root planing are performed (two words).
9 Refers to an area of calculus on a tooth.
10 Metal rod used in magnetostrictive ultrasonic unit inserts.
11 Refers to the procedure of using manual instruments or power-driven instruments for débriding the surfaces of teeth during nonsurgical periodontal therapy.
14 Formation and collapsing of bubbles in the water surrounding an ultrasonic tip.
16 Refers to the removal of endotoxins and microorganisms from the crowns and roots of teeth; scaling and root planing.
18 Can be produced if a power-driven scaler is not used appropriately; can cause damage to the pulp tissue of a patient's tooth.
21 Refers to the overlapping strokes used to ensure complete removal of calculus from a tooth or root surface (two words).
25 Calcified dental biofilm.
26 Another term for lavage.
27 Refers to the area between the roots of a multirooted tooth.
28 The distance of the tip movement of a power-driven scaler; determines the power output of the instrument.
29 Therapeutic washing.
31 One characteristic of the predominant microflora present in infected periodontal pockets.
32 Varies during instrumentation depending on the nature of the calculus deposit and the type of therapy being performed.
33 The type of power-driven scaler that produces tip vibrations by dimensional changes in crystals housed in the handpiece.

Down

1 Refers to the outermost third of the instrument cutting edge that is kept in contact with the tooth surface during instrumentation.
2 kHz; 1000 cycles per second.
3 Lipopolysaccharide (LPS) complex found in the cell wall of many gram-negative microorganisms; toxic to human tissue.
5 A term that refers to instrumentation of the crown or root surfaces of a tooth.
6 Can be used for coolant and lavage in some ultrasonic units to help reduce levels of pathogens in aerosols when using a power-driven scaler; can also be used as a preprocedural rinse to reduce microorganisms.
7 Resolving inflammation, shrinking spongy tissue, and converting a pocket to a sulcus brings your patient's gingival tissue to _____.
8 Reduces aspiration of contaminated materials by both the patient and the clinician during the use of a power-driven scaler (three words).
12 The last step of calculus removal in which the clinician uses an explorer to determine the end point of the treatment.
13 The speed of movement of the tip of a power-driven scaler; expressed as cycles per second.
15 Another name for magnetostrictive inserts in the handpiece of a power-driven scaler.
17 The type of power-driven scaler that produces tip vibrations by expansion and contraction of a metal stack or rod.
19 Agitation in the fluids surrounding a rapidly vibrating ultrasonic tip; has a disruptive effect on surface bacteria (two words).
20 Operates in a frequency range between 25,000 and 50,000 cycles.
22 Definitive periodontal treatment that removes altered cementum or contaminated surface dentin from the root surface of a tooth (two words).
23 Refers to the direction of the pressure of the cutting edge of a scaling instrument against the surface of the tooth; if the force is not sufficient, calculus may not be totally removed.
24 The presence of bacteria in the blood.
30 The type of power-driven scaler that is driven by compressed air.

KNOWLEDGE EXERCISES

1. What is the aim of periodontal debridement interventions you provide for your patients?

   _____

   _____

   _____

2. List procedures that can be included when you plan periodontal debridement for your patient.

   _____

   _____

   _____

3. Nonsurgical interventions for periodontal disease can provide the definitive treatment for many of your patients with periodontal infections. Some patients with more advanced disease will require additional treatment after the initial debridement therapy that you provide for them. Describe the aims and expected outcomes of providing complete and carefully performed nonsurgical periodontal therapy.

   _____

   _____

   _____

   _____

   _____

4. What are the clinical end points that indicate successful nonsurgical instrumentation?

   _____

   _____

   _____

5. What changes occur in the subgingival microflora after instrumentation procedures during periodontal debridement?

   _____

   _____

   _____

   _____

   _____

6. List situations that indicate the need to plan multiple appointments for completion of periodontal debridement procedures.

   _____

   _____

   _____

7. In your own words, describe tissue conditioning.

   _____

   _____

   _____

8. If multiple dental hygiene appointments are planned for nonsurgical periodontal therapy, when should you evaluate the success of your initial periodontal debridement?

   _____

   _____

   _____

9. Identify the components of an immediate evaluation.

   _____

   _____

   _____

10. What postcare instructions will you provide your patient after scaling and root planing procedures?

    _____

    _____

    _____

11. What factors are taken into account when determining a maintenance interval after completion of nonsurgical periodontal treatment?

    _____

    _____

    _____

12. In your own words, explain full-mouth disinfection.

    _____

    _____

    _____

13. A recommended plan for dental hygiene care includes complete and thorough scaling of each segment of the mouth. List the problems associated with providing an incomplete or preliminary, partial scaling at the first appointment and then planning to have your patient schedule

additional appointments for more definitive treatment.

_____

_____

_____

_____

_____

14. What assessment strategies will you use to assess your patient to formulate a plan for instrumentation?

_____

_____

_____

15. What will you look for during a visual examination of your patient's gingival tissues that will help you formulate your strategy for instrumentation?

_____

_____

_____

16. Why will you perform a tactile subgingival examination, using a periodontal probe and explorer, before beginning periodontal instrumentation to remove calculus?

_____

_____

_____

17. Why is it important to have your patient's radiographs available for review during scaling and root-planing procedures?

_____

_____

_____

18. List the factors that affect which instruments you will select for calculus removal during an individual patient's nonsurgical care.

_____

_____

_____

19. Removal of subgingival calculus is more difficult than removal of supragingival calculus and is complicated by several significant factors. List the fac-

tors and variables that make instrumentation of subgingival surfaces more complex.

_____

_____

_____

_____

_____

20. The steps for providing manual scaling are listed below. Put the list in the correct order (1 = first step; 10 = last step).

_____ *Select the correct cutting edge of the instrument.*

_____ *Stabilize your hand in your patient's mouth, using a finger rest.*

_____ *Adapt the toe of the cutting edge of the instrument against the tooth surface.*

_____ *Use smooth, overlapping, light-pressured finishing strokes that provide maximum sensitivity to minute irregularities of the tooth surface.*

_____ *Apply sufficient (moderate to heavy) lateral pressure for calculus removal.*

_____ *Angle the instrument blade for insertion to the base of the periodontal pocket.*

_____ *Apply light lateral pressure for instrument insertion and confirmation of soft-tissue attachment.*

_____ *Activate the instrument, maintaining the angulation and adaptation of the cutting edge evenly during the stroke.*

_____ *Pick up the instrument using a light modified pen grasp.*

_____ *Repeat in overlapping, channeled strokes to remove all calculus.*

21. Explain how a well-sharpened instrument reduces the amount of lateral pressure necessary for complete calculus removal.

_____

_____

_____

22. Describe the clinician's hand motion that helps maintain adaptation of the toe of the cutting edge of the instrument to the tooth surface during scaling procedures.

_____

_____

_____

INFOMAP 37-1

TYPE	FREQUENCY	MODE OF ACTION	TIP TYPE AND MOVEMENT	WATER USE	CONTRAINDI-CATIONS, PRECAUTIONS, AND RISK FACTORS FOR USE	PRINCIPLES OF INSTRUMEN-TATION AND TECHNIQUE FOR USE
Sonic scaler						
Ultrasonic magnetostrictive						
Ultrasonic piezoelectric						

23. Your dental hygiene care plan for a patient may include a blended approach that uses both manual and power-driven dental hygiene instrumentation techniques. List general clinical preparation measures that you will follow before using a power-driven scaler during patient care.

_____

_____

_____

24. List the steps used to prepare an ultrasonic unit.

_____

_____

_____

25. List the steps for preparing your patient before you use a power-driven scaler.

_____

_____

_____

26. Complete **Infomap 37-1** with information from the textbook to help you compare the different types of power-driven scaling devices.

27. **Figure 37-1** shows four ultrasonic tips. Identify the following components for each one. One way to do this is to use a different colored pencil to fill in or identify each area on the drawing.

   ■ *The point of the tip*
   ■ *The tip*
   ■ *The grip*
   ■ *The area in which you would likely find the O-ring on a magnetostrictive insert*

   ■ *The area in which the metal stack would be located on a magnetostrictive insert*

28. Match each description to the appropriate tip shown in **Figure 37-1** by writing the correct letter in the space provided next to each statement. Each letter is used more than once; some descriptions apply to more than one tip.

   _____ Designed for removal of heavy supragingival calculus

   _____ Thinner tip designed for subgingival instrumentation

   _____ Universal tip generally used for removal of moderate to heavy deposits from supragingival or relatively shallow pockets

(continued on p 245)

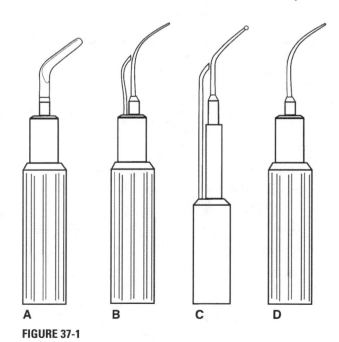

A   B   C   D

FIGURE 37-1

Everyday Ethics

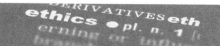

Refer to the Codes of Ethics (Appendices I, II, and III in the textbook) and Framework for Making Decisions (Table 1-2 in the textbook) as you discuss the following scenario with your classmates.

Lorna and Christine both practice as hygienists in the same office approximately 2.5 days per week. Lorna graduated from dental hygiene school about 15 years ago, and Christine was licensed just 3 years ago. They generally had their own patients that were routinely scheduled with the same hygienist. One day Mrs. Border, a patient routinely scheduled with Christine, showed up in Lorna's appointment book because she wanted to fit in her regular maintenance appointment before going to stay with her daughter.

Because she was going to be gone all winter, the receptionist scheduled her with the first available hygienist. Lorna reviewed the patient's medical history and made a mental note that she suffered seasonal asthma attacks. Following the oral examination, Lorna began to explore, finding rough areas that she assumed was the tooth surface. Upon further instrumentation, the areas turned out to be deep calculus. Lorna worked diligently but needed to reappoint Mrs. Border for a second visit. The patient was outraged and complained that Lorna should have used the "sprayer-machine" like Christine usually does.

Questions for Consideration

1. While respecting both the patient's autonomy and Christine's role as a professional, how can Lorna proceed to address this dilemma?
2. What action needs to be taken to ensure that the patient's rights and that Lorna's duties are being fulfilled?
3. Realizing the deep calculus could not all have formed since the previous appointment, how can Lorna best handle the situation? She knows Mrs. Border will make her next appointment with Christine and possibly complain to the dentist.

_____ Tip designed for use in furcation areas

_____ Tip that is intended for use on only low or medium power if it is attached to a magnetostrictive insert

_____ Tip intended for use in removing orthodontic cement

_____ Tip designed with an external water-flow system

_____ Tip designed with an internal water-flow system

COMPETENCY EXERCISES

1. In your own words, explain why the interrelationship among dental biofilm, endotoxins, cementum, and calculus is important to consider when you plan dental hygiene treatment to eliminate the cause of periodontal infection.

   _____

   _____

   _____

2. You are watching your student colleague, Mary Neely, while she is scaling. You have been designated as her mentor colleague, and your task for today is to give her verbal feedback about all areas of her clinical performance while she is providing patient care. Tomorrow she will observe you providing patient care and will have feedback for you.

   While you are observing Mary, you notice that as she is scaling in the maxillary posterior areas she is having some trouble placing a comfortable fulcrum during her activation stroke. You also observe that as she activates the instrument, her wrist motion seems to move the instrument handle from side to side, and her hand pivots back and forth on her finger rest.

   Explain what this type of hand motion might indicate about the angle of the blade of the instrument against the surface of the tooth down inside the periodontal pocket. Explain what Mary is doing incorrectly and how she might change the motion of her hand to increase her ability to remove calculus. (*Hint:* You can practice moving your instrument on a typodont or model to help you visualize what you are trying to describe.)

   _____

   _____

   _____

Factors To Teach The Patient

When you present your dental hygiene care plan to Mr. Diamond (introduced in Competency Exercise question 3) before asking him to sign the consent form for treatment, he questions the need for so many appointments to just clean his teeth.

Use the example of a patient conversation in Appendix B as a guide to prepare a conversation that you will use to explain your appointment plan to Mr. Diamond. Use the conversation you create to educate a patient or friend. Then modify your conversation based on what you learned.

This scenario is related to the following factors:

- The importance of and necessity for complete removal of calculus to the health of the oral tissues in the prevention of periodontal infections
- Basic reasons for needs of, and the advantages of, multiple appointments to complete the scaling and root planing

3. A patient assessment summary for Nicholas Diamond is in Appendix D of this workbook. Use the information in his case summary, the "Appointment Plan" section of the Dental Hygiene Care Plan template in Appendix B, and the information in Chapter 37 of the textbook to write a plan for a series of initial-therapy dental hygiene appointments for Mr. Diamond. Plan to scale each quadrant at a separate appointment. As part of your written plan, indicate whether you will use manual or power instruments, how you will prepare your patient for the procedures you plan, and the postoperative instructions you will provide. Make sure to include an evaluation appointment in your plan for Mr. Diamond's treatment.

_____

_____

_____

CHAPTER 38

Nonsurgical Periodontal Therapy: Supplemental Care Procedures

Chapter Outline

Learning Objectives

Upon successful completion of these exercises, you will be able to:

1. Identify and define key terms and concepts related to nonsurgical, supplemental periodontal therapy.

2. Describe and compare delivery methods and types of supplemental antimicrobial therapies for periodontal disease.

Supplemental Care Procedures Word Search Puzzle

To solve the puzzle, first solve the clues; then find the answers in the grid. The answers can run across, down, or diagonally and can start at the right or left or top or bottom. When you have found all the words, the first 45 unused letters in the grid will spell out a hidden message.

Hidden message: The success of all periodontal therapy, including supplemental care procedures, depends on __ __ __ __ __   __ __ __ __ __ __ __ __ __   __ __ __ __ __ __   __ __ __ __ __

__ __   __ __ __ __ __ __ __   __ __   __ __ __   __ __ __ __ __ __ __ .

```
D  A  I  L  Y  P  E  R  P  S  O  N  A  L  B  R  L  D
E  N  T  A  L  B  I  I  I  O  F  I  L  I  M  E  I  C
O  E  N  P  T  R  H  R  O  L  C  B  O  Y  T  A  Q  M
H  N  E  O  P  C  S  A  R  I  T  D  I  E  N  T  U  I
T  D  M  R  M  Z  R  L  M  I  E  F  E  K  C  T  I  N
G  O  Y  T  L  L  F  E  O  G  G  X  P  I  F  A  D  I
H  G  T  B  T  T  A  R  W  O  A  T  Y  N  C  P  -
D  E  Y  M  P  S  A  A  T  G  R  O  T  W  V  H  O  B
L  N  Q  C  Y  L  D  F  E  T  I  E  V  I  C  M  L  L
P  O  Y  S  U  A  I  N  X  B  A  K  L  C  O  E  Y  A
Z  U  H  N  B  B  O  H  I  T  T  C  P  E  Y  N  M  D
X  S  N  L  E  U  T  T  Z  R  R  R  H  M  A  T  E  E
C  A  E  R  S  D  N  B  L  R  L  Z  Y  M  Z  S  R  D
C  J  G  G  L  A  C  C  T  C  T  K  N  B  E  T  E  L
G  C  H  E  M  O  T  H  E  R  A  P  Y  Y  B  N  X  P
C  T  L  O  C  A  L  D  E  L  I  V  E  R  Y  J  T  N
M  F  C  Q  W  A  N  T  I  M  I  C  R  O  B  I  A  L
L  B  N  R  Z  O  P  P  O  R  T  U  N  I  S  T  I  C
```

Word Search Clues

- An agent produced by or obtained from microorganisms that can kill other microorganisms or inhibit their growth
- Refers to controlled-release substances inserted directly at the site of infection (two words)
- Can be broken down by a biological process, such as by bacterial or enzymatic reaction
- Method of delivering antibiotics to the infected area through blood circulation
- Method of delivering any liquid substance directly into subgingival spaces
- Method of delivering chlorhexidine directly into subgingival spaces
- Method of delivering doxycycline directly into subgingival spaces (two words)
- Method of delivering metronidazole directly into subgingival spaces
- Method of delivering tetracycline directly into subgingival spaces
- Refers to therapy that uses chemical or pharmaceutical agents for the control or destruction of microorganisms

- Refers to the placement of antimicrobials directly into the subgingival pocket, directly at the site where they are needed (two words)
- Refers to the position of the periodontal tissue at the base of a sulcus or pocket as measured from a fixed point
- Reunion of epithelium and connective tissues with the root surface and bone; a goal of periodontal therapy
- The opening at the end of the cannula
- Treatment by means of a chemical or pharmaceutical agent
- Tubular end of an instrument placed in a cavity that is used to introduce or withdraw fluid
- Type of infection caused by normal flora from the skin, nose, mouth, intestinal, or urogenital tracts
- Type of infection that is caused by acquired organisms that are not normal flora
- Type of infection that can occur from organisms that are not usually harmful if an individual's immune system is impaired or altered
- A type of area-specific instrument or Gracey curet that is useful for fitting into confined areas of furcations during root planing

KNOWLEDGE EXERCISES

1. Antimicrobial therapy is only one supplemental care procedure that you will plan for your patients. List additional supplemental procedures carried out by dental hygienists.

   _____

   _____

   _____

2. What is the objective of antimicrobial therapy?

   _____

   _____

   _____

3. Identify two situations in which professional subgingival irrigation can be helpful to reduce microorganisms.

   _____

   _____

   _____

4. What conditions may indicate a recommendation of antimicrobial therapy for your patient who is in the maintenance phase of periodontal treatment?

   _____

   _____

   _____

5. What factors increase the likelihood of success of local delivery methods for antimicrobial therapy?

   _____

   _____

   _____

6. What is the dose of systemic tetracycline? What is the dose of tetracycline in a local delivery fiber?

   _____

   _____

   _____

7. How long must the tetracycline fiber remain in the pocket to be effective? When will you schedule the patient's reappointment to remove the fiber?

   _____

   _____

   _____

8. List the contraindications for placing a tetracycline fiber.

   _____

   _____

   _____

9. A biodegradable doxycycline polymer is delivered in a syringe containing liquid _____% _____ and using a _____-gauge, narrow-diameter cannula.

10. Describe the method for preparing the cannula to make it easier to insert into the periodontal pocket.

    _____

    _____

    _____

11. What steps follow the irrigation of a pocket with doxycycline polymer liquid?

    _____

    _____

    _____

12. How is minocycline hydrochloride delivered?

    _____

    _____

    _____

13. What is the dose in a chlorhexidine gluconate chip?

    _____

    _____

14. How large is the chlorhexidine chip? Use a periodontal probe to measure it, and make a full-size drawing of a chip.

    _____

    _____

    _____

15. What factors do you consider when placing chlorhexidine chips if more than one pocket is to be treated?

    _____

    _____

    _____

16. Why doesn't the chlorhexidine chip have to be removed after it is placed?

_____

_____

_____

COMPETENCY EXERCISES

1. Describe how advanced instrumentation strategies described in Chapter 38 can enhance outcomes of treatment for patients with advanced periodontal disease.

_____

_____

_____

_____

_____

2. Explain why it is important to be extremely careful to control the pressure with which you express the liquid when using a cannula to provide irrigation into a periodontal pocket.

_____

_____

_____

3. Develop an Infomap to help you compare information about the type and amount of active ingredient or agent that is delivered to the sulcus, delivery methods, placement procedures, and care and storage of each of the different types of local delivery antimicrobials.

   ◾ To make this a Discovery Exercise, gather samples of each of the products that are described in the book, and use the packaging information to complete the Infomap.

   ◾ To enhance your ability to make evidence-based decisions for planning patient care, consult the Primer on Evidence-Based Decision Making in the front of this workbook to help you complete a review of the current literature about one or more of the local delivery systems described in this chapter.

_____

_____

_____

_____

Everyday Ethics

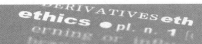

Refer to the Codes of Ethics (Appendices I, II, and III in the textbook) and Framework for Making Decisions (Table 1-2 in the textbook) as you discuss the following scenario with your classmates.

At the first 3-month maintenance appointment for Mrs. Orban, who had had a series of six sextant appointments of deep scaling and root planing with anesthesia, the tissue still showed many areas of inflammation, with probing depths greater than 4 mm and bleeding on probing. She had received repeated personal instruction with each of the appointments, and she had never achieved a truly favorable score on her biofilm disclosing tests.

　Gretchen, the dental hygienist, showed her maintenance charting and oral tissue review to Dr. Finley, and they both examined the original radiographs. Gretchen had made two vertical bitewings for the molars at this current appointment.

　Gretchen told Dr. Finley that she thought the best procedure was for Mrs. Orban to see the periodontist.

"I think she will take her condition more seriously. She never acts as though she believes what I tell her," Gretchen said. "She still talks as though she just came to have her teeth 'cleaned.'" Dr. Finley agreed to recommend the periodontist, and he personally explained the choice of treatment to Mrs. Orban. Mrs. Orban definitely told them she was not going to a periodontist under any circumstance and asked for further treatment from Dr. Finley.

Questions for Consideration
1. What ethical issues may be involved when a patient asks for the general practitioner to take over treatment that is customarily carried out by the dental hygienist?
2. Is this an ethical issue or dilemma for Dr. Finley? Explain the rationale.
3. Select terms from the core values to help in the discussion of this problem.

Factors To Teach The Patient

Your care plan for Ms. Johnetta Sullivan outlines a series of four quadrant scaling and root planing appointments plus a variety of educational and counseling interventions, with the goal of arresting her significant periodontal disease, which is characterized by generalized deep probing depths and attachment loss. When you are explaining the care plan to Johnetta in order to obtain informed consent, she asks many, many questions. She has heard about the concept of putting antibiotics "right into the gums" from her friend, who has recently received this treatment in one area of her mouth. Johnetta wants to know why she cannot receive this procedure instead of having to undergo all the "scraping and hurting" that is outlined in your care plan. You know that it is important for the interventions you have planned to come first.

Use the example of a patient conversation in Appendix B as a guide to prepare a conversation that you might use to educate Johnetta about why and how local delivery supplemental care procedures are used in the treatment of periodontal disease and about why they are not appropriate for her at this time.

Use the conversation you create to role play this situation with a fellow student. If you are the patient in the role play, be sure to ask questions. If you are the dental hygienist, try to anticipate questions and answer them in your explanation.

This scenario is related to the following factors:

- What a periodontal pocket is and why it needs to be treated
- How the treatment using minocycline hydrochloride, chlorhexidine chip, or doxycycline polymer affects the infection in the pocket
- The success of all periodontal therapy depends on the daily personal dental biofilm control by the patient

4. You are filling out the patient record for Bruce McDonald after his appointment. Today you placed the minocycline hydrochloride your dentist prescribed in a 6-mm pocket on the mesiolingual surface of tooth 3 and in a 7-mm pocket on the mesial surface of tooth 5. You educated Mr. McDonald about the home care regimens he will follow for the next few days, and you scheduled an appointment for follow-up procedures. Using your institution's guidelines for writing in patient records, document Mr. McDonald's appointment procedures.

Date	Comments	Signature

Acute Periodontal Conditions

Learning Objectives

Upon successful completion of these exercises, you will be able to:

1. Identify and define key terms and concepts related to acute periodontal conditions.

2. Identify the causes, clinical signs and symptoms, and risk factors for acute periodontal infections.

3. Plan dental hygiene care for a patient with an acute periodontal infection.

KNOWLEDGE EXERCISES

1. In your own words, explain the difference between an acute and a chronic condition.

   _____

   _____

   _____

2. Describe what you would observe during the examination of a patient diagnosed with necrotizing ulcerative gingivitis.

   _____

   _____

   _____

   _____

   _____

3. What is a pseudomembrane?

   _____

   _____

   _____

4. Identify and describe the four microscopic layers of the gingival tissue that contain spirochetes in necrotizing lesions.

   _____

   _____

   _____

5. What types of microorganisms are found in greater numbers in necrotizing lesions?

_____

_____

_____

6. What health-related factors can predispose your patient to necrotizing oral conditions?

_____

_____

_____

7. What personal factors predispose an individual to necrotizing oral conditions?

_____

_____

_____

8. What is NUP?

_____

_____

_____

9. Briefly describe necrotizing stomatitis.

_____

_____

_____

10. What is malaise, and what additional health-related symptoms may accompany a diagnosis of necrotizing oral conditions?

_____

_____

_____

11. When you are taking the medical history of a patient who presents with signs of necrotizing ulcerative oral lesions, what additional questions will you ask to aid in the diagnosis?

_____

_____

_____

12. In your own words, describe an abscess.

_____

_____

_____

13. What is a fistula?

_____

_____

_____

14. In your own words, define the term _gum boil_.

_____

_____

_____

Everyday Ethics

Refer to the Codes of Ethics (Appendices I, II, and III in the textbook) and Framework for Making Decisions (Table 1-2 in the textbook) as you discuss the following scenario with your classmates.

Sue has not seen Mr. Rufus for more than a year. He called requesting an appointment because he is overdue and is suddenly having mouth pain and a "horrible metallic taste." When he arrives, Mr. Rufus says "Hello," and Sue is overtaken by a strong mouth odor.

    Upon review of his medical history, Mr. Rufus appears to be quite healthy, but he describes the heartbreaking details of his divorce proceedings. His dental problems started about the same time. He confides in Sue that he has hardly eaten or brushed his teeth for the past 2 days.

    Sue begins an extraoral and intraoral examination, but Mr. Rufus says it is too painful for her to retract his cheeks

and lips. During the brief examination, she noticed punched-out papillae and pseudomembrane formation over much of his gingiva. She immediately suspects necrotizing ulcerative gingivitis (NUG) or perhaps necrotizing ulcerative periodontitis (NUP).

Questions for Consideration

1. At what point should Sue consult with the dentist to confirm diagnosis of NUG or NUP before discussing the details with the patient?
2. Sue has empathy for all that Mr. Rufus has gone through personally, but she feels it is her duty to mention the offensive mouth odor. How can she do this without offending or embarrassing him?
3. Is it ethical for Sue to ask questions about the patient's personal life with particular reference to his divorce? Why or why not?

15. Identify the factors that can cause the formation of a gingival or periodontal abscess.

_____

_____

_____

16. List the classic signs of a periodontal abscess.

_____

_____

_____

17. What are the objectives for immediate treatment if your patient presents with a periodontal abscess?

_____

_____

_____

18. What two methods are used to establish drainage of a periodontal abscess?

_____

_____

_____

19. What posttreatment instructions will you give your patient after you have provided dental hygiene care for a periodontal abscess?

_____

_____

_____

20. What is pericoronitis?

_____

_____

_____

Factors To Teach The Patient

After you complete the care plan for Mr. Rufus in Competency Exercise question 1, use it and the example of a patient conversation in Appendix B as guides to prepare a conversation educating Mr. Rufus about the condition in his mouth. Explain the dental hygiene interventions you have planned so that Mr. Rufus can give his informed consent for treatment.

This scenario is related to the following factors:

- Premature discontinuation of treatment for NUG because acute signs have subsided and can lead to recurrence of the infection
- The role of diet, rest, and dental biofilm control in the prevention of NUG
- The avoidance of an oral irrigating device in the presence of acute inflammatory conditions (Microorganisms may be forced into the tissues beneath a pocket, and bacteremia can be produced.)

COMPETENCY EXERCISES

1. Mr. Rufus is introduced in the Everyday Ethics scenario in this chapter. Read about the details of his health history and oral inspection. Then use the Patient-Specific Dental Hygiene Care Plan Template (Appendix C) to develop a complete care plan for the dental hygiene treatment of Mr. Rufus's condition. Include a plan for follow-up procedures.

_____

_____

_____

_____

_____

Sutures and Dressings

Chapter Outline

Learning Objectives

Upon successful completion of these exercises, you will be able to:

1. Identify and define key terms and concepts related to sutures and periodontal dressings.
2. Identify components/materials used for sutures and periodontal dressings.
3. Explain procedures for placement and removal of sutures and periodontal dressings.
4. Discuss rationale for and provide posttreatment instructions to patients with periodontal dressings.

Dressed for Success Word Search Puzzle

To solve the puzzle, first use the clues to determine the words; then find the words in the grid. Words in the grid can run across, down, or diagonally and can start at the right or left or top or bottom. When you have found all the words, the first 82 unused letters in the grid will spell out a hidden message.

Hidden message: __ __ __ __   __ __ __ __ __   __ __ __ __ __ __ __   __ __ __ __ __ __ __ __   __ __

__ __ __ __ __ __ __ __ __ __   __ __ __ __ __ __ __   __ __ __ __ __ __ __   __   __ __ __

__ __ __ __   __ __ __   __ __ __ __ __ __ __ __ __   __ __ __   __ __ __ __   __ __   __ __ __

__ __ __ __ __!

```
M S A N Y P E R I P R O T E C T I V E O
D P U O N T M O N O F I L A M E N T A L
S E U T R G I C A L P R O C E D U R E S
E R R E U Q U I B O R D E R M O L D R P
U I E S U R T U R S A G E A S S T H A R
G O T H A V E E U H N B P I O U R P S E
E C A T I E N O E I T P S C S A L L W S
N A T I E D U M S S O Y U O O P I N A S
O R K N O N O S B S L E T S R A ! P G U
L E G L I S E L I O L I K L R B P M E R
Z B J T T R A T R I F L N L N Y A T D E
K L N A D N I D R R K M N G B W R B M L
T O S T K O Y E L I G A T I O N K L L L
C I K E N H T B Z H G K V C G K V W F E
S X T K Z S R K K I N T E R D E N T A L
```

Word Search Clues

- Suture that is broken down by body enzymes or by water
- Suture that holds the margins of an incision together
- Suturing procedure that forms loops on one side of an incision and a series of stitches directly over the incision; also called a continuous lock
- Shaping of the peripheries of a dressing by manual manipulation to prevent displacement (two words)
- Approximate the edges of a wound with no overlap
- Suture that is an uninterrupted series of stitches tied at one or both ends
- Material used to cover or protect a wound; also called a pack
- A constituent of clove oil used in early periodontal dressings for its alleged antiseptic properties
- Termination of bleeding by mechanical or chemical means
- Process in which water penetrates and causes breakdown of a suture
- Suture that joins flaps on both the lingual and the facial sides of the dental arch
- Application of a suture to hold or constrict tissue
- Single-strand suture
- Paste–gel type of chemical-cured dressing; a brand name
- Type of dressing used to control bleeding
- Type of dressing that shields an area from injury or trauma
- Suture used when the flap is only one side; also called a suspension suture
- Important characteristic of a suture or needle for preventing infection
- Stitch or series of stitches made to secure apposition of the edges of a surgical or traumatic wound
- Eyeless end of a needle that allows suture material and needle to act as one unit
- Sounds like the name of a superhero but is really a well-known brand name of a zinc oxide with eugenol dressing (two words)

KNOWLEDGE EXERCISES

1. List three functions of postsurgical suture placement.

   _____

   _____

   _____

2. Which type of suture is capable of causing adverse tissue reaction?

   _____

   _____

   _____

3. What type of intraoral sutures must be removed by a dentist or dental hygienist within a specific period of time?

   _____

   _____

   _____

4. Many types of suturing needles are available. What three factors influence selection of a specific type?

   _____

   _____

   _____

5. Which part of the needle is grasped by a needle holder during the suturing procedure?

   _____

   _____

   _____

6. List at least three requirements of an acceptable surgical suture needle.

   _____

   _____

   _____

7. Suture knots tied on the _____ surface of the alveolar ridge and tied with a _____-mm suture tail left in place are easy to remove later.

8. Removable sutures should not be left in place longer than _____ days.

9. When removing a suture, it is necessary to raise the knot and hold it with a slight tension, slightly depress the tissue with the back of the scissors blade, and cut the suture in the part that was previously buried in the tissue. In your own words, describe why this procedure is followed.

   _____

   _____

   _____

10. Describe the characteristics of an acceptable dressing material.

    _____

    _____

    _____

11. List three disadvantages of zinc oxide with eugenol dressing material.

    _____

    _____

    _____

12. List three advantages of chemical-cured dressings.

    _____

    _____

    _____

13. An absorbable dressing that can be placed directly on clean moist or bleeding wounds to promote wound healing is a _____ dressing.

14. A surgical dressing is typically left in place for _____ days.

COMPETENCY EXERCISES

1. Mrs. Belinda Hawkins had periodontal surgery about 10 days ago. She is scheduled with you this afternoon for suture removal. List and explain the purpose of all the items and instruments you will need to set up in your treatment room to prepare for her postsurgical dressing and suture-removal appointment.

   _____

   _____

   _____

   _____

   _____

   _____

2. When you read Mrs. Hawkins's patient record, you note that three polyester sutures were placed in the left maxillary molar area, and six were placed in the left mandibular molar area. An interdental suturing pattern was used for all areas. Visible-light-cured dressings were placed to cover the surgical areas in both the mandibular and maxillary arches. You also look closely at Mrs. Hawkins's medical history questionnaire. What is the purpose for carefully checking the medical history when the only procedure being performed today is the suture removal?

_____

_____

_____

3. After you seat Mrs. Hawkins and update her medical history, you examine the surgical areas and find out that the dressing is completely intact on the maxillary arch but that the dressing on the mandibular arch has partly broken off and the sutures are uncovered. One suture appears as though it may be partially embedded in the dressing material. You note that all areas are fairly free of debris, and the surrounding mucosal tissue looks healthy. Describe the procedure you will use for removing the periodontal dressings.

_____

_____

_____

4. Next, you gently rinse Mrs. Hawkins's mouth with an antiseptic solution and examine the sutures. You can count all nine that were placed, and the tissue around them looks healthy—with the exception of the area where the suture was embedded in the dressing. That area is bleeding slightly but stops when you gently press gauze on the surface. After cutting each suture with the scissors, you pull gently on the _____ end with cotton pliers.

5. Explain why you need to place each suture on a gauze sponge for postprocedural counting.

_____

_____

_____

6. You gently rinse and examine Mrs. Hawkins's mouth. All areas appear to be healing well, with only slight redness in the area of tooth 30, where the suture had been embedded in the dressing. Explain follow-up bacterial biofilm control procedures to Mrs. Hawkins.

_____

_____

_____

7. Use the information provided in Chapter 40 to document Mrs. Hawkins's suture-removal procedure.

Everyday Ethics

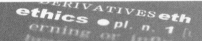

Refer to the Codes of Ethics (Appendices I, II, and III in the textbook) and Framework for Making Decisions (Table 1-2 in the textbook) as you discuss the following scenario with your classmates.

Miss Osgood arrives for a suture removal appointment with Agnes, the dental hygienist, and immediately explains the discomfort she is feeling. When asked why she didn't come in sooner to have the area observed, she said it was so close to the removal appointment she might as well wait. Agnes notes from the record that no dressing was placed. The area appears inflamed, with a slight cyanotic appearance circumscribing the suture area. The patient prerinsed with a 0.12% chlorhexidine, and Agnes began removing the sutures. Moderate bleeding and discomfort were present.

Upon removal, Agnes noted that only three sutures could be found, but four had been placed. When she conferred with the dentist, Agnes was told to dismiss the patient and to prepare a prescription for penicillin V to "take care of the infection. Eventually the suture will be absorbed by body tissues."

Questions for Consideration
1. Given the sequence of events, what issues of professionalism are exhibited in the working relationship between the dentist and the dental hygienist?
2. Was the treatment provided within an acceptable standard of care for this patient? Why or why not?
3. What information needs to be documented in the progress notes concerning the services rendered and dialogue that occurred with the patient?

Factors To Teach The Patient

Because you provided initial therapy care for Mr. Bruce Barrimundi, you are very interested in observing when he is scheduled for periodontal surgery. After the surgical procedure is complete and the sutures and dressings are placed, you are asked to give him the printed instructions for posttreatment care you created based on Table 40-1 in the textbook.

You know that compliance with recommendations is always better if you provide verbal instructions as well as written. Besides, there are several factors that you think are important to emphasize. You know that Mr. Barramundi is still smoking (although you have told him how bad it is for his periodontal health). You also know that he has a very vigorous toothbrushing style and is always working very hard to make sure every tiny area of dental biofilm is completely removed.

Use the patient instructions for posttreatment care (Table 40-1 in the textbook) and the example of a patient conversation in Appendix B as a guide to prepare an outline for a verbal reinforcement of posttreatment instructions for Mr. Barramundi.

Use the conversation you create to role play this situation with a fellow student. If you are the patient in the role play, be sure to ask questions. If you are the dental hygienist, try to anticipate questions and answer them in your explanation.

This scenario is related to the following factors:

■ Explanations for the items in Table 40-1 in the textbook
■ Care of the mouth during the period after treatment while wearing a periodontal dressing
■ That tobacco use is detrimental and delays healing

Follow your institution's guidelines for writing in patient records.

Date	Comments	Signature

QUESTIONS PATIENTS ASK

When you greet Mrs. Hawkins in the reception room and walk with her back to your treatment room for her suture removal appointment, she is clearly nervous about the impending procedure. She asks, "Will it hurt? Will there be any bleeding?"

What sources of information can you identify that will help you answer your patient's questions in this scenario?

Dentin Hypersensitivity

Chapter Outline

Learning Objectives

Upon successful completion of these exercises, you will be able to:

1. Identify and define key terms and concepts related to dentin hypersensitivity.
2. Discuss the etiology of hypersensitivity and the hydrodynamic theory of pain transmission.
3. Identify factors that influence desensitization.
4. Interview a patient to characterize pain and identify potential differential diagnoses.
5. Plan dental hygiene interventions to manage dentin hypersensitivity.

KNOWLEDGE EXERCISES

1. In your own words, define *hypersensitivity*.

   _____

   _____

   _____

2. List at least three *patient* behaviors that can trigger a hypersensitivity pain response.

   _____

   _____

   _____

3. What condition precedes the development of dentinal hypersensitivity?

   _____

   _____

   _____

4. Describe the role of dentinal tubules in the development of hypersensitivity.

   _____

   _____

   _____

5. How are odontoblasts related to the transmission of pain as explained by the hydrodynamic theory?

   _____

   _____

   _____

6. There are many, many factors that contribute to gingival recession, subsequent root exposure, and potential dentin hypersensitivity. Name as many as you can before looking in the textbook to check your answer.

   _____

   _____

   _____

7. In about _____% of teeth, the enamel and the cementum do not meet, leaving an area of exposed dentin.

8. What two factors can contribute to erosion on an exposed root surface?

   _____

   _____

   _____

9. In your own words, describe how *abfraction* occurs.

   _____

   _____

   _____

10. Which natural desensitization mechanism is related to narrowing of the inside wall of the dentin tubules?

    _____

    _____

    _____

11. A smear layer can reduce dentin sensitivity by blocking the dentin tubules. What causes a smear layer?

    _____

    _____

    _____

12. What is the *negative* effect of a smear layer?

    _____

    _____

    _____

13. Two different patients can experience pain from hypersensitivity in different ways; in other words, pain perception is subjective. What does that mean?

    _____

    _____

    _____

14. List the components to include in your patient's dental history of hypersensitivity.

    _____

    _____

    _____

    _____

    _____

15. Identify two patient response–related diagnostic tests that can be used to determine location and severity of tooth pain.

    _____

    _____

    _____

16. Without looking at the textbook (you won't always have it with you when you are interviewing a patient), identify at least three trigger questions you can ask your patient about tooth pain.

    _____

    _____

    _____

    _____

    _____

    _____

17. You can use a VRS to rate the level of pain your patient is feeling. If your patient describes her tooth-related pain as a level 3, what does she mean?

    _____

    _____

    _____

18. Identify at least five clinical techniques used to differentiate among the variety of potential causes for dental pain.

    _____

    _____

    _____

_____

_____

19. No one best method has been identified for the treatment of hypersensitivity. Treatment options offered to the patient should begin with the most _____ and least _____ _____ measures.

20. List five factors that you can take into consideration when selecting a desensitizing agent.

_____

_____

_____

_____

_____

_____

21. What patient action, if used as part of a daily oral hygiene regimen, can contribute to the formation of a smear layer or reparative dentin and thereby reduce hypersensitivity?

_____

_____

_____

22. Identify the ingredients in over-the-counter (OTC) desensitizing dentifrices.

_____

_____

_____

23. Identify therapeutic ingredients that block the pain response by occluding the dentinal tubules.

_____

_____

_____

24. List three means of covering exposed dentinal tubules at the CEJ.

_____

_____

_____

25. The highest prevalence of hypersensitivity is found in _____. Prevalence and severity _____ in older folks due to the

occurrence of natural mechanisms of desensitization.

COMPETENCY EXERCISES

1. Explain how abfraction differs from abrasion.

_____

_____

_____

_____

_____

_____

2. Using patient-appropriate language, describe the hydrodynamic theory.

_____

_____

_____

_____

_____

_____

3. Compare and contrast the two different subjective pain assessment scales (the VAS and the VRS) identified in Box 42-3 in the textbook. Why would you use them together for patient assessment?

_____

_____

_____

_____

_____

_____

4. Mr. Mustafa's chief symptom is a frequently occurring, sharply painful sensation on the right side of his mouth. The pain often occurs when he grinds his teeth together during stressful moments at work. He says that area of his mouth sometimes causes pain when he drinks very cold water or chews on cold foods or hard, crunchy foods.

   Your intraoral examination notes many areas of deep recession along the facial cervical margins, toothbrush abrasion along the facial surfaces of all his molar teeth, and numerous large MOD restorations that were placed a very long time ago. Several of the restorations are beginning to break down, but you do not find any current large, carious lesions.

Everyday Ethics

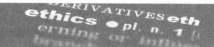

Marcy practices in a dental practice where the dentist, Dr. Goldman, sees the patient at every other dental hygiene visit unless requested for special needs.

Mrs. Stuart arrives for her dental hygiene appointment but is not scheduled to see Dr. Goldman until her next visit. She is reporting discomfort "on the lower back teeth" when she chews and when she eats or drinks something cold. The pain may last up to an hour.

At the completion of the scaling and débridement, Marcy gives Mrs. Stuart a sample of desensitizing toothpaste and suggests they will see how it is at the next appointment. Marcy then advises Mrs. Stuart to call the office if the discomfort gives her more trouble. The patient is not classified as having a periodontal condition, nor is she particularly dental caries prone, so her next visit will be in 6 months.

Questions for Consideration

1. What obligation, if any, do Marcy and Dr. Goldman have to this patient to conduct an oral/dental examination during this appointment to establish a differential diagnosis?
2. Discuss several aspects of informed consent that apply to this patient's right to know about dental sensitivity.
3. How should the maintenance recall interval be structured to meet the needs of this patient? Explain the rationale.

You know that you will need to do a very thorough clinical examination and question your patient carefully before you can begin to make statements regarding what is happening with Mr. Mustafa. But using the information you have here, what conditions may potentially be causing Mr. Mustafa's tooth pain? Which differential diagnoses can you eliminate? Support your selections using the information in Table 41-1 in the textbook.

_____

_____

_____

_____

_____

_____

QUESTIONS PATIENTS ASK

Some patients express concerns related to a friend's experiences. "My friend bleached her teeth and said that it caused sensitivity. Should I avoid bleaching my teeth?"

A patient may express concern over the diagnosis of hypersensitivity for a specific area. "How do you know that I have sensitivity and not a cavity?"

Many patients will want to understand more completely how the desensitizing agents will work to help their problem. "How soon after I start using sensitivity toothpaste will I notice an improvement in my hypersensitivity? Will I need to use a desensitizing product forever? Will I ever be able to have ice in my summer drinks again? Should I drink my morning orange juice before or after I brush my teeth?"

What sources of information can you identify that will help you answer your patients' questions? How will you use the evidence-based decision-making methods you learned from reading the EBDM Primer in the front of this workbook to help answer these questions for each patient?

Factors To Teach The Patient

You are at your desk writing out a dental hygiene care plan for Mrs. Jernigan. Her chief symptom of tooth pain has been diagnosed by Dr. Hockwater as dentin hypersensitivity. Mrs. Jernigan is scheduled with you later this week for education and counseling. This is the first patient you have counseled regarding the management of dentin hypersensitivity, and you want to be thorough.

Use the example of a patient conversation in Appendix B of this workbook as a guide to create a conversation and to role play this situation with a fellow student. *This scenario is related to the following factors:*

- Activities and habits that may contribute to dentin hypersensitivity
- Importance of appropriate oral hygiene self-care techniques, such as using a soft toothbrush and avoiding vigorous brushing, which may contribute to gingival recession and subsequent abrasion of root surface
- That toothbrushing should not immediately follow consumption of acidic foods or beverages or use of acidic mouthwashes

Extrinsic Stain Removal

Chapter Outline

Learning Objectives

Upon successful completion of these exercises, you will be able to:

1. Identify and define key terms and concepts related to removal of extrinsic dental stain.

2. Identify the effects, indications, contraindications, precautions, and procedures for selective dental polishing.

3. Describe polishing agents, instruments, and techniques used for removal of extrinsic stains.

KNOWLEDGE EXERCISES

1. Coronal polishing can remove _____ and _____, but does not remove _____.

2. The use of polishing agents for stain removal is a selective procedure that not every patient needs, especially on a routine basis. List the potential negative effects of polishing.

    _____

    _____

    _____

3. Identify actions you can take and polishing techniques you can use to minimize the negative effects of polishing.

    _____

    _____

    _____

4. Which abrasives commonly used in dental cleaning and polishing agents have a Mohs hardness value

that indicates that they are less likely to scratch your patient's exposed tooth surfaces?

_____

_____

_____

5. What characteristics and application principles affect the abrasive action of polishing agents?

 ▪ _Characteristics of abrasive particles_

 _____

 _____

 _____

 ▪ _Application principles_

 _____

 _____

 _____

6. In your own words, explain the difference between cleaning and polishing agents.

_____

_____

_____

7. Ultra- or high-speed handpieces rotate between _____ and _____ revolutions per minute. Low-speed handpieces, typically used for polishing extrinsic stains, rotate between _____ and _____ revolutions per minute.

8. Describe the kinds of prophylaxis angle attachments (polishing cups) that are available for you to use when polishing stain in different areas of the tooth.

_____

_____

_____

9. In your own words, describe the procedure used for applying the polishing agent to an area of stained enamel.

_____

_____

_____

_____

10. How is a bristle brush used?

_____

_____

_____

11. How can stain be removed from proximal surfaces of teeth?

_____

_____

_____

12. What special care is required when using finishing strips to remove stain from proximal surfaces of anterior teeth?

_____

_____

_____

13. How does an air-powder polisher work, and when is it used?

_____

_____

_____

14. In your own words, describe the techniques you will use for reducing your exposure to aerosolized spray and for protecting both your patient and yourself when polishing, especially when using an air-powder polisher.

_____

_____

_____

_____

_____

_____

15. What are the indications for polishing?

_____

_____

_____

16. List the clinical findings that indicate when you should NOT polish your patient's teeth during the dental hygiene appointment.

_____

_____

_____

_____

_____

_____

COMPETENCY EXERCISES

1. What is the difference between polishing and abrasion? In what ways can you produce one but not the other when you remove stain from your patient's teeth?

_____

_____

_____

_____

_____

2. Winston Nottingham always brings you a small packet of tea from England when he comes in for his regular periodontal maintenance appointment. He drinks tea every day, and you usually notice staining on the lingual surfaces of his maxillary and mandibular anterior teeth and on a few lingual interproximal surfaces of the lower premolars. He has significant recession, especially on the facial surfaces on his lower molars and the facial and lingual surfaces of his maxillary molars owing to previous history of periodontal infection.

   Write a dental hygiene diagnosis statement identifying Mr. Nottingham's condition in relation to the stain and the recession.

Problem	Cause (risk factors and origin)

_____ _related to_ _____

3. What dental hygiene intervention is appropriate for addressing Mr. Nottingham's problem?

_____

_____

_____

4. Using your institution's guidelines for writing in patient records, document the procedure you used to remove the tea stain from Mr. Nottingham's teeth.

Date	Comments	Signature

_____

_____

_____

5. Mr. Nottingham's son, Will, who is 12 years old, is also your patient. He is in the office for a regularly scheduled 6-month prophylaxis appointment. You are glad he has returned as scheduled, because there are several areas of demineralization that you are monitoring. Will also has significant areas of dental stain because he drinks tea every morning with his parents. You point out the areas of stain to

---

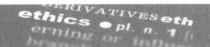

Everyday Ethics

Refer to the Codes of Ethics (Appendices I, II, and III in the textbook) and Framework for Making Decisions (Table 1-2 in the textbook) as you discuss the following scenario with your classmates.

Miss Dean, a new patient, 57 years old, was in for her second appointment. Her first one included her complete examination and treatment plan with the dentist. Her record shows generalized recession and a variety of tooth-color restorations, which Polly, the dental hygienist, now notes to guide her dental hygiene procedures. Because there were few calculus deposits and it was apparent that Miss Dean was conscientious about her daily personal oral hygiene, Polly completed the scaling and proceeded to prepare the

gel-tray for a fluoride application. This was a routine procedure for patients with recession.

Miss Dean watched for a minute and then said, "Aren't you going to polish my teeth? My other hygienist always finished with a good polishing." Polly started to explain. Miss Dean seemed perturbed.

Questions for Consideration

1. How is it an ethical issue when a patient wants a service that the hygienist deems not needed or even detrimental?
2. What choices of procedure does Polly have? Which of the alternatives would be best for her to select?
3. Describe how this episode is correctly documented in the patient's record.

him and you mention that you must polish quite a few areas in his mouth.

While you are preparing to polish his teeth, Will picks up the container of polishing paste and notices that it contains fluoride. He points that out to you and wants to know why he must also undergo the "icky" fluoride treatment after you finish polishing. He wants to know why you can't just polish all of the areas of his teeth and then skip the regular fluoride treatment completely. Discuss why the use of a fluoride-containing polishing paste is not a replacement for a conventional topical application of fluoride.

_____

_____

_____

_____

_____

_____

Factors To Teach The Patient

As noted in the Everyday Ethics case study, Polly started to explain selective polishing to Miss Dean but was apparently not successful in helping the patient understand the concept.

Use the example of a patient conversation in Appendix B as a guide to prepare an outline for a conversation for discussing the concept of selective polishing with Miss Dean. Use the outline you create as the starting point to educate a patient or friend (not a student colleague) about selective polishing.

This scenario is related to the following factors:

- The meaning of selective polishing and why it is not necessary to polish all teeth at every appointment when daily care is effective
- That stains and biofilm removed by polishing can return promptly if biofilm is not removed faithfully on a schedule of two or three times each day

43 CHAPTER

Tooth Whitening

Chapter Outline

Learning Objectives

Upon successful completion of these exercises, you will be able to:

1. Identify and define key terms and concepts related to tooth whitening.

2. Compare types of procedures, and discuss the processes of tooth whitening.
3. Discuss the risks and potential side effects of whitening.

KNOWLEDGE EXERCISES

1. Identify three types of dental stains.

   _____

   _____

   _____

2. What are the two causes of intrinsic stains?

   _____

   _____

   _____

3. Identify the most common treatment for extrinsic stain.

   _____

   _____

   _____

4. Identify the two main types of tooth whitening.

   _____

   _____

5. List the three types of vital tooth whitening.

_____

_____

_____

6. What is the active ingredient in most whitening systems for vital teeth?

_____

_____

_____

7. Explain how carbamide peroxide can be used to enhance the bleaching effect.

_____

_____

_____

8. List and describe the purpose of additional ingredients used in whitening systems.

INGREDIENT(S)	PURPOSE

9. Which type of vital tooth whitening can potentially cause adverse effects, such as necrosis of the pulp of the tooth?

_____

_____

_____

10. Which type of vital tooth whitening requires making an impression that is used to fabricate a custom-formed tray?

_____

_____

_____

11. What can happen if the tray is not correctly fitted to the patient's mouth?

_____

_____

_____

12. List and briefly describe each of the ways that over-the-counter whitening products can be delivered.

_____

_____

_____

_____

_____

_____

13. How is nonvital tooth whitening different from the procedures used to whiten vital teeth?

_____

_____

_____

14. What ingredients are used for bleaching nonvital teeth?

_____

_____

_____

15. What factors can influence the final outcome of tooth whitening treatment?

_____

_____

_____

16. What are the potential side effects of whitening treatment?

_____

_____

_____

17. Identify the potential consequences if a patient should swallow some of the tooth whitening product.

_____

_____

_____

COMPETENCY EXERCISES

1. Although many of your patients will desire to have their teeth whitened, each one must be assessed carefully to determine the safety and appropriateness of this dental procedure. Identify contraindications for tooth whitening. As you answer this question, take into consideration all of the factors you will assess in relation to each of the various types of tooth whitening systems that are available.

   _____

   _____

   _____

   _____

   _____

   _____

2. Maria Kennedy is a new patient. Right after you seat her in the dental chair, she points to a darkened front tooth and tells you that the tooth had a root canal about 5 years ago. She wants to know why the over-the-counter tooth whitening product she has applied almost made it look worse. How will you answer her question?

   _____

   _____

   _____

   _____

   _____

   _____

3. As you continue to talk with Maria, you mention that there is procedure to whiten a nonvital tooth. She gets excited about that possibility and wants to know how the procedure is done. Even though you would like to get started with her complete history assessment and oral exam first, you know that it is important to at least provide a brief answer to her question. How will you explain the procedure to her?

   _____

   _____

   _____

   _____

   _____

4. During your assessment, you determine that there are numerous demineralized areas on the surfaces of Maria's teeth, and you suspect that these are probably due to overuse of the whitening products. What interventions will you include in her care plan to address the issue?

   _____

   _____

   _____

   _____

   _____

Everyday Ethics

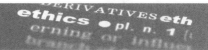

Refer to the Codes of Ethics (Appendices I, II, and III in the textbook) and Framework for Making Decisions (Table 1-2 in the textbook) as you discuss the following scenario with your classmates.

Julia is a 12-year-old dental hygiene patient who is quite verbal about the appearance of her "dark front tooth." As part of the oral care instructions, Theresa, the dental hygienist, begins to discuss possible options of nonvital bleaching to lighten the tooth. Julia becomes visibly excited and wants to whiten the tooth right away. Following Dr. Leonard's examination, Theresa brings Julia's mother in to discuss the possibility of whitening. The mother quickly tells Julia, "You don't want to do that, it's probably too expensive."

Questions for Consideration
1. Is it an ethical issue or ethical dilemma to discuss treatment options with a child patient before the parent or guardian who will make the decision for treatment? Explain.
2. Role play several possible appropriate responses Theresa could make if Julia's mother refuses to acknowledge her daughter's desire to treat her tooth and possibly improve her self-esteem.
3. In retrospect, what alternate ways could the dental hygiene appointment have been conducted with this patient to gain a more positive outcome?

QUESTIONS PATIENTS ASK

"Which whitening method is best?" "How white will my teeth actually get?" "Should I whiten my teeth before or after you place those new fillings in my front teeth?" Can I have my teeth bleached in the office now and then use an over-the-counter product to keep them white?"

What sources of information can you identify that will help you answer your patient's questions? How will you use the evidence-based decision-making methods you learned from reading the EBDM Primer in Appendix A to help answer these questions for each specific patient?

Factors To Teach The Patient

Using the example of a patient conversation in Appendix B as a guide, write a conversation you could use to obtain informed consent for a light-activated tooth whitening procedure. Use your conversation to educate a patient or a friend, and then modify it based on what you learned from the interaction.
This scenario is related to the following factors:

■ In-office whitening may produce more sensitivity than over-the-counter and at-home products.
■ In most cases, whitening must be periodically repeated to maintain desired tooth color.
■ Existing tooth-colored restorations will not change color, therefore may not match and may need to be replaced after whitening.

Implementation: Clinical Treatment

■ Chapters 35–43

COMPETENCY EXERCISES

1. In the summary exercises for Sections IV and V, you started developing a patient-specific care plan for a patient you selected from the patient assessment summary examples in Appendix D. After reading Chapters 35 to 43 in the textbook, you will be able to complete your care plan by including clinical interventions that will arrest or control disease and regenerate, restore, or maintain health for the particular patient you selected.

   Just as you did with the education and counseling interventions you planned for this patient, identify the expected outcomes of the clinical interventions you select for your patient and set goals for treatment success. Be sure to identify the methods you will use to evaluate success, and specify a time frame in which to evaluate your patient's health.

   At this point in the planning process, you can continue working on the appointment plan section of the care plan, prioritizing and sequencing the planned clinical, education, and personal daily care instructions into a schedule of appointments for your patient. Remember to establish an appropriate maintenance interval based on this particular patient's needs.

2. Describe the dental hygiene instruments and procedures you will select and use when you are providing dental hygiene care for each of the following patients. Discuss the rationale for your selections.

   ■ Mrs. Louise Gaiter presents with heavy, tenacious ledges of subgingival calculus in all areas of her mouth. In most areas of her mouth, you have recorded 3- to 5-mm pocket probing depths, but in several molar areas, there is calculus to the base of 7- to 9-mm pocket probing depths. Her gingival tissues are keratinized from long-term tobacco use.

   ■ Mr. Randall Forbes presents with spiny or nodular areas of calculus on surfaces just beneath the proximal contact areas of almost all of his teeth. His gingival tissues were bleeding heavily as you recorded probing depths during your assessment.

   ■ Mrs. Amelia Pritchert, who has had previous periodontal surgery, presents for her maintenance appointment with some areas of slight calculus and no probing depths deeper than 3 mm. But you have recorded 3 to 4 mm of gingival recession in most of the areas of her mouth.

   ■ Ms. Claudia Exeter drinks tea. She has very slight supragingival calculus in a few areas of her mouth but has a generalized moderate extrinsic stain on most of her tooth surfaces.

   ■ Amal, who is 8 years old, presents with slight lower anterior calculus, generalized dental biofilm, and moderate gingivitis with bleeding on probing in all areas of his mouth.

   ■ Mr. Robert Galen presents with slight generalized supragingival and subgingival calculus. He has a dental implant to replace tooth 38.

DISCOVERY EXERCISES

1. Spend time searching the Internet to find manufacturer and/or product Web sites that provide information about instruments and local anesthesia–related products, such as syringes, cartridges, and needle-safety devices. Create a "Webliography" (similar to an annotated bibliography) that contains a list of Web addresses (URLs) for sites providing information about specific dental hygiene–related products; include a brief description of the information that each Web site contains.

2. Use the product information you find to compare current dental hygiene instruments in terms of availability, handle size, design, and price.

3. Reread the Primer for Evidence-based Decision Making at the front of this workbook. Use the information there to help you search the literature to locate the most current evidence to support the use of a specific dental hygiene therapy, such as root planing, selective polishing, ultrasonic scaling, tooth whitening, or placement of local-delivery antibiotics during the treatment of periodontal disease. Write a brief report on your findings.

4. Search the American Dental Hygienists' Association Web site (www.adha.org) to find information about which states in the United States allow provision of local anesthesia within the scope of dental hygiene practice. Describe how the ability to provide pain control during dental hygiene procedures can affect the success of the patient's treatment.

FOR YOUR PORTFOLIO

1. Include a Webliography you create about any topic related to dental hygiene care (see Discovery Exercise 1).

2. A brief written report (make sure to cite your references accurately) about the information you gathered during your literature search for Discovery Exercise 3 would provide excellent documentation of your ability to use outside sources to find current information about dental hygiene care.

3. Include a variety of patient care plans you have developed to highlight your expertise at planning patient-specific clinical interventions for your patients.

Evaluation

■ SECTION VII LEARNING OBJECTIVES

Completing the exercises in this section of the workbook will prepare you to:

1. Identify key concepts in evaluating the outcomes of dental hygiene interventions.
2. Apply outcomes assessment findings to plan maintenance care.

■ COMPETENCIES FOR THE DENTAL HYGIENIST (Appendix A)

The following ADEA Competencies are supported by the learning in Section VII.

Core Competencies: C3, C4, C6, C10

Health Promotion and Disease Prevention Competencies: HP2, HP4, HP5, HP6,

Patient Care Competencies: PC1, PC5

Evaluation and Maintenance

Learning Objectives

Upon successful completion of these exercises, you will be able to:

1. Identify and define key terms and concepts related to evaluation of dental hygiene interventions.

2. Identify the purposes, procedures, and methods for planning dental hygiene maintenance care.
3. Discuss factors that contribute to recurrence of periodontal infection.

KNOWLEDGE EXERCISES

1. What steps will you take to evaluate the dental hygiene care you provide for each patient?

   _____

   _____

   _____

   _____

   _____

   _____

2. In your own words, identify the purpose of formative evaluation conducted during each dental hygiene appointment.

   _____

   _____

   _____

3. What is the purpose of recollecting assessment data at the end of a dental hygiene treatment cycle (summative evaluation)?

   _____

   _____

   _____

4. If a disease does not respond to routine therapy, the disease is considered to be resistant, or

_____

_____.

5. The term _____
_____ refers to the abatement of the symptoms of a disease.

6. The concept of continuing dental hygiene care is introduced to the patient in the initial dental hygiene care plan. Identify the purposes of a maintenance program for patients who successfully complete initial therapy.

_____

_____

_____

7. List the factors you will consider when deciding on a maintenance appointment interval that meets your patient's needs.

_____

_____

_____

8. After evaluating the success of your dental hygiene interventions, you will establish your patient's periodontal maintenance interval in consultation with your patient, the attending dentist, and sometimes even the patient's physician. What does the term _consultation_ mean?

_____

_____

_____

9. In your own words, define the types or categories of periodontal maintenance therapy.

_____

_____

_____

_____

_____

_____

10. Identify assessment procedures and dental hygiene interventions that are commonly provided during a dental hygiene maintenance appointment.

■ _Assessment procedures_

_____

_____

_____

■ _Dental hygiene interventions_

_____

_____

_____

11. What factors contribute to the recurrence of periodontal disease?

_____

_____

_____

12. You and the attending general dentist will decide together if there is a need to refer your patient to a periodontist for specialized periodontal therapy.

■ Under what conditions might you refer a new patient directly to a periodontist?

_____

_____

_____

■ What criteria are used to determine referral when you evaluate treatment outcomes during a maintenance appointment after you have provided the initial therapy?

_____

_____

_____

13. A dental clinic maintenance plan can be set up using a card-file system or a computer-assisted approach. Identify two administrative methods for implementing the maintenance plan and scheduling patient appointments.

_____

_____

_____

COMPETENCY EXERCISES

1. Ms. Olivia Qaba has just moved into your town and is scheduled today as a new patient in your clinic. Dr. Kish briefly examines her, then you spend the rest of

the appointment collecting thorough assessment data and providing the dental hygiene clinical interventions and education that are required to meet her needs.

When dental hygiene care is complete, you evaluate treatment outcomes. When you are planning maintenance care for Ms. Qaba (or for any patient), Dr. Kish requires that you consult with him to decide the appropriate maintenance interval for each case. Because Dr. Kish has only briefly examined Ms. Qaba before your treatment, he is unlikely to know as much about her as you do after your interaction with her during the series of dental hygiene appointments. What important knowledge do you bring to recommending a maintenance interval for your patient that Dr. Kish may not know after his brief examination? (*Hint:* Think about this question in terms of the indicators you will use to measure the success of your dental hygiene interventions.)

_____

_____

_____

_____

_____

2. What is your role in providing feedback to the dentist?

_____

_____

_____

_____

_____

_____

3. Many factors contribute to the success of periodontal therapy and the remission or recurrence of periodontal disease.

■ *For which factors are the dental hygienist's actions particularly important in arresting disease?*

_____

_____

■ *How does patient compliance affect the recurrence of periodontal disease?*

_____

_____

_____

Everyday Ethics

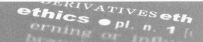

Refer to the Codes of Ethics (Appendices I, II, and III in the textbook) and Framework for Making Decisions (Table 1-2 in the textbook) as you discuss the following scenario with your classmates.

There were two full-time dental hygienists in the practice. Jeanette had been there more than 15 years, and Wilma less than a year. Wilma had previously practiced with a periodontist in another city for 6 years, and she joined this practice shortly after she moved here. Everything went well. Each hygienist had instruments of her own preference and cared for them relative to sharpening and preparation for the autoclave. Patients usually had appointments with the same dental hygienist. Jeanette scheduled a maintenance for 45 minutes, whereas Wilma never felt she had time enough even with an hour.

Occasionally, certain long-standing patients who had been with Jeanette for many years would be scheduled with Wilma when Jeanette could not be in the office.

As Wilma saw more of Jeanette's regular patients, she began to see a pattern of subgingival calculus that could

not have formed since the previous 3 or 4 months' maintenance appointment. She had decided to ask the secretary to have Jeanette's patients wait for her return for their appointments.

Mrs. Doubleday had already been scheduled and came for her appointment the next day. After the usual history review, periodontal charting, and treatment started, Wilma had to tell the patient that she needed two appointments and wanted to complete her scaling with local anesthesia. The patient was confused after having only short appointments faithfully and wanted to know whether to reschedule with Jeanette to finish because Jeanette would be back from her vacation soon.

Questions for Consideration
1. Is this an ethical issue or a dilemma? Explain.
2. Using the step procedure of Table I-2 (page 14), suggest various possible actions for Wilma.
3. Prepare possible answers Wilma could use for her reply to Mrs. Doubleday's immediate question.

■ *What risk factors for recurrence of periodontal disease are not easily modifiable by dental hygiene interventions?*

_____

_____

_____

■ *How do all these factors interplay when making decisions regarding the frequency of individualized patient maintenance appointments?*

_____

_____

_____

4. Investigate and describe the recall system that is used in your school clinic. What is your role as a student in making the system work and for making sure that complete oral health maintenance care is scheduled and delivered as needed?

_____

_____

_____

_____

_____

DISCOVERY EXERCISES

1. Before you do this exercise, take a moment to read the Primer for Evidence-based Decision Making located at the front of this workbook. Then read a bit more about your patient, Ms. Qaba, in the Factors to Teach the Patient exercise below. Develop a PICO question related to determining an appropriate

Factors To Teach The Patient

Together, you and Dr. Kish decide that a 3-month maintenance interval is appropriate for Ms. Qaba (introduced in Competency Exercise question 1). One reason for this decision is that even though her tissues are healthy right now, she is HIV positive and has a history of significant bone loss from past periodontal infection. You know from her dental history that she has previously been scheduled for 3-month periodontal maintenance, but Ms. Qaba states that she is not sure there is much point to having her teeth cleaned so often. She says that she was really hoping to stretch the interval to 6 months because she no longer has dental insurance.

Use the example of a patient conversation in Appendix B as a guide to write a statement explaining your maintenance-interval recommendation to Ms Qaba. Make sure to include a discussion of the literature articles you located when you did the discovery exercise above. *This scenario is related to the following factors:*

■ Purposes of follow-up and maintenance appointments
■ Importance of keeping all maintenance appointments

periodontal maintenance interval for Ms. Quaba. Use the PICO question you develop to find evidence in the dental literature to support your maintenance-interval recommendations.

FOR YOUR PORTFOLIO

1. Include the PICO question you develop for Ms. Qaba's case (or any other PICO question you develop for a patient case) as well as a reference list for the journal articles you find from the literature search.

Patients with Special Needs

■ SECTION VII LEARNING OBJECTIVES

Completing the exercises in this section of the workbook will prepare you to:

1. Identify treatment and education modifications necessary to meet the needs of individuals with physical, mental, and medical conditions or limitations.
2. Plan and provide dental hygiene care for individuals with special needs in both traditional and nontraditional practice settings.

■ COMPETENCIES FOR THE DENTAL HYGIENIST

The following ADEA competencies are supported by the learning in Section VII.

Core Competencies: C1, C2, C3, C4, C5, C6, C7, C8, C9, C10, C11

Health Promotion and Disease Prevention Competencies: HP1, HP2, HP3, HP4, HP5, HP6

Community Involvement: CM1, CM2, CM3, CM4, CM5, CM6

Patient/Client Care: PC1, PC2, PC3, PC4, PC5

Professional Growth and Development: PGD1, PGD2, PGD3

The Pregnant Patient

Learning Objectives

Upon successful completion of these exercises, you will be able to:

1. Identify and define key terms and concepts related to the pregnant patient.
2. Identify the oral/facial development timetable in relationship to overall fetal development.
3. Describe oral findings common in pregnancy.
4. Plan dental hygiene care that addresses the unique physical, oral, and emotional considerations of the pregnant patient.

KNOWLEDGE EXERCISES

1. The term applied to teaching ahead of time so that untoward conditions can be prevented.

   _____

2. One third of a pregnancy; a 3-month period.

   _____

3. A factor that can cause disease or malformation during fetal development.

   _____

4. An antibiotic that has the well-known effect of staining the infant's teeth if taken by the pregnant mother after 4 months of gestation.

   _____

5. A class of drug that, if taken by the mother, can cause low muscle tone and poor sucking reflex in the infant.

   _____

6. List three oral findings that are common during pregnancy.

   _____

   _____

   _____

7. In your own words, describe the clinical appearance and symptoms of a "pregnancy tumor."

_____

_____

_____

8. List three signs you might observe in your pregnant patient that would make you suspect depression.

_____

_____

_____

9. Is the following statement true or false? To ensure that the developing teeth of their unborn children will be protected, all pregnant women should receive prenatal vitamins containing fluoride. Provide a rationale for your answer.

_____

_____

_____

10. Visualizing a timeline can often help put information into perspective. Use the timeline in **Figure 45-1** to identify the oral/facial feature that is developing in the fetus during the approximate time indicated by each of the lettered segments.

■ A. _____

■ B. _____

■ C. _____

■ D. _____

■ E. *By this time (8th week), a* _____
  _____ *is apparent in the developing fetus.*

■ F. *By this time (12th week), a* _____
  is apparent in the developing fetus.

11. What are the possible adverse effects on the fetus when a woman smokes during pregnancy?

_____

_____

_____

12. Identify reasons why some women have more problems with gingivitis during pregnancy.

_____

_____

_____

COMPETENCY EXERCISES

1. Mrs. Jill Mason, who is late in the second trimester of a healthy pregnancy, presents with a toothache and a swelling on the right side of her mandible. The dentist orders a single periapical radiograph of the area. Mrs. Mason is concerned about the effect of the radiation on her developing baby. Using all the information available to you in Chapter 45, describe the educational approach, protective measures, and radiographic techniques you will use to relieve her fears and maximize safety for her and the baby.

_____

_____

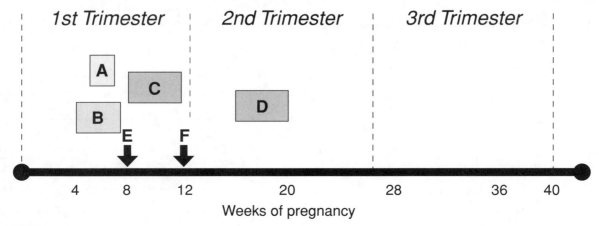

Facial Development Gestation Timeline

1st Trimester   *2nd Trimester*   *3rd Trimester*

A   B   C   E   F   D

4   8   12   20   28   36   40

Weeks of pregnancy

FIGURE 45-1

_____

_____

_____

_____

2. Describe an appropriate dental chair position for Mrs. Mason during her treatment. Also, explain the reason the modification is made.

_____

_____

_____

_____

_____

3. Mrs. White (Care Plan in Appendix D) mentions that she frequently experiences nausea, gagging, and vomiting followed by an unpleasant taste. You realize that she is at risk for several additional oral problems. Identify the possible oral problems, and provide three self-care measures that will minimize their oral effects.

_____

_____

_____

_____

4. Using the dental hygiene diagnosis format, identify a cause or factor that could result in increased risk for dental caries during the course of Mrs. White's pregnancy.

Increased risk for dental caries related to: _____

_____

5. Write a goal for the problem identified in the dental hygiene diagnosis in question 4. Include a time frame for meeting the goal. How will you measure whether your patient met the goal?

◼ *Goal*

_____

◼ *Evaluation method*

_____

◼ *Time frame*

_____

QUESTIONS PATIENTS ASK

"Because of my nausea, I have to eat frequent small snacks. I usually nibble on granola bars—those are healthy snacks, aren't they?" "I heard that pregnancy takes calcium away from my teeth, so is that why I seem to be getting more cavities?" "Should I just wait until

Everyday Ethics

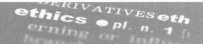

Refer to the Codes of Ethics (Appendices I, II, and III in the textbook) and Framework for Making Decisions (Table 1-2 in the textbook) as you discuss the following scenario with your classmates.

Anna, the dental hygienist, welcomed her patient, Julie, a 20-year-old single woman. She is in the first trimester of pregnancy and was referred by a nurse from the Maternal and Child Health Clinic. Anna notices the way Julie holds a hand over her mouth when she talks. Julie's history appears negative except for smoking about a half pack of cigarettes daily. Examination reveals multiple carious lesions, heavy calculus, and 4- to 5-mm proximal probing depths in several molar areas.

After making the radiographic survey and presenting initial patient instruction, there was time for one quadrant of scaling. Follow-up appointments were scheduled for dental hygiene and with the dentist. Julie does not show up for any of the appointments.

Questions for Consideration
1. How does the ethical principle of beneficence apply to this situation?
2. What is the role of the dental hygienist, if any, to make further contact with this patient, and why?
3. Describe two courses of action and the possible outcomes of the situation through a dental hygiene care plan.

Factors To Teach The Patient

Using the example Patient-Specific Dental Hygiene Care Plan for Mrs. White (Appendix D) and the example conversation provided in Appendix B as a guide, prepare an outline for a conversation that you might use to educate Mrs. White regarding one of the problems identified in the dental hygiene diagnosis. Use the conversation to educate a patient or friend, and then modify it based on what you learned by using the outline.

This scenario is related to the following factors:

■ Why control measures are learned before and in conjunction with scaling
■ Facts of oral disease prevention and oral health promotion relevant to the patient's current level of health care knowledge and individual risk factors

after the baby is born to have my fillings done?" "Is it safe to use a mouthwash while I am pregnant?"

What sources of information can you identify that will help you answer your patient's questions in this scenario? How will you use the evidence-based decision-making methods you learned from reading the EBDM Primer in the front of this workbook to help answer these questions for each specific patient?

CHAPTER 46

Pediatric Oral Health Care: Infancy through Age 5

Learning Objectives

Upon successful completion of these exercises, you will be able to:

1. Identify and define key terms and concepts related to pediatric oral health care.
2. Identify risk factors for oral disease in children.
3. Discuss the role of the dental hygienist in providing early oral care intervention.
4. Discuss anticipatory guidance for parents of infants and toddlers.
5. Explain tooth development and eruption patterns.
6. Use knowledge of specific oral health issues, child management techniques, and clinical procedures to plan dental hygiene care and oral health education for infants/toddlers and their parents.

KNOWLEDGE EXERCISES

1. Match the following term or concept with the most appropriate age-related phrase.

TERM/CONCEPT	AGE
_____ Weaning to a sippy cup	A. At 2 years of age
_____ Preschool child	B. Before 12 months of age
_____ First dental visit	C. At approximately 6 months of age
_____ Tiny touch of toothpaste	D. Tiny infant
_____ Toddler	E. 3–5 years of age
_____ Neonate	F. 1–3 years of age

2. List three indications for making a radiograph of a 3-year-old child's dentition.

_____

_____

_____

3. List at least three risk factors for oral disease in early childhood.

_____

_____

_____

4. List at least three important factors to address when interviewing parents or guardians regarding their child's risk factors for oral disease.

   _____

   _____

   _____

5. When the oral healthcare provider performs a knee-to-knee examination, who stabilizes the infant's legs and hands? For what purpose would this position be reversed?

   _____

   _____

   _____

6. How much toothpaste is appropriate for parents to place on the toothbrush of a 4-year-old?

   _____

   _____

   _____

7. List two common causes of halitosis (bad breath) in children.

   _____

   _____

   _____

8. List three indications that suggest need for orthodontic evaluation of a child patient.

   _____

   _____

   _____

9. Identify at least three areas that are appropriate to address when you are providing anticipatory guidance for the parents of a 4-year-old.

   _____

   _____

   _____

10. Provide anticipatory guidance age-related guidelines for parents regarding the following oral health care milestones.
    - Begin using fluoride toothpaste _____

      _____
    - Find a dental home _____

      _____

- Eliminate thumb and finger sucking _____

  _____
- Wean from the bottle _____

  _____
- Clean the oral cavity _____

  _____
- Avoid feeding/grazing at will _____

  _____
- Examine the mouth for oral health problems

  _____

11. List the advantages of weaning a baby from the bottle to a regular cup.

    _____

    _____

    _____

12. Identify ways a mother could provide comfort to a child who is in pain from teething.

    _____

    _____

    _____

COMPETENCY EXERCISES

1. In your own words, define *nursing bottle caries* as if you were explaining the concept to a parent.

   _____

   _____

   _____

2. Explain why knowledge of expected developmental milestones and the child's actual developmental level are necessary when providing dental care for that child.

   _____

   _____

   _____

   _____

   _____

3. Make up three terms/names for dental equipment or instruments (different from those mentioned in the textbook) that you might use to explain what is happening during a dental visit to an anxious

preschooler. For extra fun, share your names with those of your student colleagues.

_____

_____

_____

4. Angela Flores, 3 years old, sits quietly in the dental chair for several minutes while you speak with her mother. She allows you to tilt the chair into a supine position but begins to cry as soon as you approach her mouth with your mirror and explorer. She continues to cry and reach for her mother even after you explain all the fun games you will play together while you examine her teeth. Outline an appropriate response to this situation.

_____

_____

_____

_____

_____

_____

5. You are conducting an oral health education class for a mother's group at the community center near your house as part of a community service project. The mother of a darling 3-month-old girl asks you when she can expect her baby's teeth to start coming in. Explain the development and eruption patterns of primary teeth.

_____

_____

_____

_____

_____

_____

6. Explain to this young mother why healthy primary teeth are important for the growth and development of a healthy permanent dentition.

_____

_____

_____

_____

_____

_____

7. Explain how a parent can transfer _S. mutans_ from her mouth to the infant's mouth.

_____

_____

_____

_____

_____

_____

Everyday Ethics

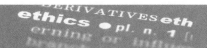

Refer to the Codes of Ethics (Appendices I, II, and III in the textbook) and Framework for Making Decisions (Table 1-2 in the textbook) as you discuss the following scenario with your classmates.

Four-year-old Charlie is accompanied by his mother to the dental office for his first dental visit. As they enter, the mother is overheard saying to her son, "Don't worry, the dentist won't hurt you." Lucy, the dental hygienist, introduces herself to the mother and child, escorts them to the treatment room, and seats Charlie in the dental chair. The mother immediately tells Charlie, "Everything will be all right, so don't be afraid." Lucy talks to Charlie and asks him

questions about his family, friends, and favorite games. He does not use eye contact, holds on tightly to the chair arms, and fidgets with his legs. He hesitates to answer, and his mother answers the questions for him.

Questions for Consideration
1. How do the ethical principles of autonomy and non-maleficence apply in this case?
2. What responsibilities does the dental hygienist have to Charlie and to his mother?
3. Describe two choices the dental hygienist can make to manage the situation and how these choices might affect Charlie, his mother, and the dentist.

Factors To Teach The Patient

Mr. and Mrs. Jacobson are in your treatment room with their son, Eric, who is 2.5 years old. The dentist has diagnosed incipient early childhood caries based on observations made during her examination. You have been asked to educate these very concerned parents about how and why this is happening to their son and what can be done to arrest the decay process and prevent further problems.

Use the example of a patient conversation in Appendix B as a guide to outline a conversation you might have with the Jacobsons. Compare your conversation with a student colleague's to identify any missing information.
This scenario is related to the following factors:

■ How the bacteria that cause dental caries can be transferred to a baby's mouth
■ How fluoride makes enamel stronger and more resistant to the bacteria that cause dental caries
■ Methods to prevent dental caries from developing in a young child's mouth
■ How feeding methods and snacking patterns can contribute to dental caries
■ How the parent can examine the infant/child's mouth and what to look for during the examination

DISCOVERY EXERCISES

Go to your local pharmacy, grocery store, or department store and find different brands and types of pacifiers available for parents to select for their baby. Use the criteria listed in Chapter 46 of the textbook to determine which brand and type of pacifier you will recommend for your patients.

CHAPTER 47

The Patient with a Cleft Lip and/or Palate

Chapter Outline

Learning Objectives

Upon successful completion of these exercises, you will be able to:

1. Identify and define key terms and concepts related to oral/facial clefts.
2. Identify prenatal risk factors and developmental time frame for oral/facial clefts.
3. Describe treatment for oral/facial clefts.
4. Use knowledge of the oral, physical, and personal characteristics of the patient to plan dental hygiene care and oral hygiene instructions.

Cleft Lip/Cleft Palate Terminology Crossword Puzzle

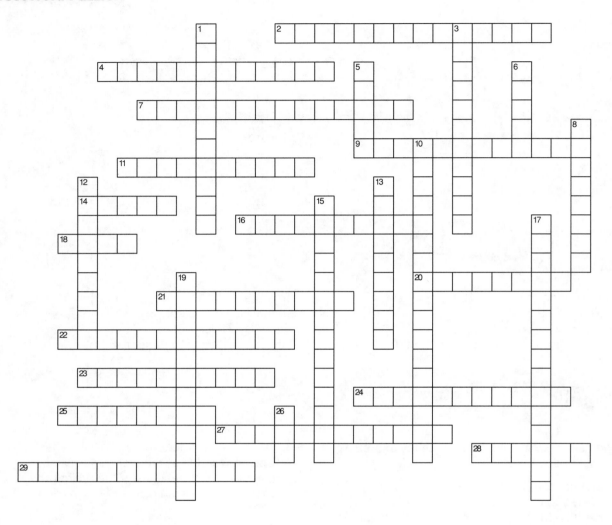

Across

2 Pertaining to or arising through the action of many factors.
4 The process of acquiring fitness for the first time; associated with persons who have acquired disabilities.
7 This insufficiency affects closure of the opening between the mouth and nose in speech, resulting in a nasal-sounding voice.
9 Insertion of an indwelling tube to facilitate passage of air or evacuation of secretions.
11 Bilateral cleft lip separates this from its normal fusion with the entire maxilla.
14 A term describing a cleft of the uvula.
16 Present at and existing from the time of birth.
18 One name for a prosthesis that closes a palatopharyngeal opening to assist with intelligible speech; can be made in either a temporary pediatric version or an adult type.
20 Genetic transmission of traits from parents to offspring.

21 Replaces or improves function of any absent part of the human body.
22 Type of surgical procedure that repositions parts of the maxilla or mandible.
23 Hereditary material contained within the ovum and the sperm.
24 An agent, such as drugs of abuse during the first trimester of a pregnancy, that can increase risk for cleft lip and palate.
25 A type of graft placed before the eruption of maxillary teeth at a cleft site to create a normal architecture through which the teeth can erupt.
27 A surgical repair of a lip defect.
28 When this normal process does not happen during development, a facial cleft can result.
29 Plastic reconstruction of the palate.

Down

1 Plastic surgery of the nose.
3 Pertaining to the function of the skeletal system and its associated functions.

5 A unilateral or bilateral congenital facial fissure.
6 Tissue transplanted and expected to become a part of the host tissue.
7 Combination of symptoms commonly occurring together.
10 Plastic surgery of nose and lip.
12 A prosthesis designed to cover the cleft of a hard palate.
13 A graft transferred from one part of the patient's body to another part.
15 The process of restoring a person's abilities to the maximum possible fitness.
17 One important member of the interdisciplinary team who will treat the patient with a cleft lip and/or palate (two words).
19 Pertaining to the part of the skull that encloses the brain and the face.
26 One source of the bone used for an autogenous bone graft.

KNOWLEDGE EXERCISES

1. Describe the direction of the formation/fusion of the lip and palatal structures during development.

   _____

   _____

   _____

2. During which embryonic weeks does the palate develop?

   _____

   _____

   _____

3. How is a class 3 craniofacial cleft defined?

   _____

   _____

   _____

4. Which classes of facial cleft involve lack of fusion in the premaxilla?

   _____

   _____

   _____

5. Which class of cleft is identified as a submucous, imperfect muscle union cleft across the soft palate, producing an incomplete closure of the pharynx?

   _____

   _____

   _____

6. List three environmental risk factors for craniofacial clefts.

   _____

   _____

   _____

7. List three common characteristics that can affect the *teeth* of a patient with a craniofacial cleft.

   _____

   _____

   _____

8. List the three categories of professionals who contribute members to an interdisciplinary team for treatment of an individual with cleft lip and/or palate.

   _____

   _____

   _____

9. Identify one of the dental specialties in which clinicians may provide care for a patient with a cleft and describe that practitioner's role in the treatment of the patient.

   _____

   _____

   _____

10. Ideally, treatment of a craniofacial cleft is begun before the infant is 6 months old. What is the purpose for such early intervention?

    _____

    _____

    _____

11. What are the goals of surgical treatment for cleft lip and palate?

    _____

    _____

    _____

12. In your own words, describe the benefits a dental prosthesis can provide for a patient with a cleft lip and palate.

    _____

    _____

    _____

COMPETENCY EXERCISES

1. Discuss why lack of prenatal care is considered a risk factor for cleft lip and/or palate.

   _____

   _____

   _____

2. Describe characteristics that may make it difficult to communicate with an individual who has an incomplete palatal closure.

   _____

   _____

   _____

Everyday Ethics

Refer to the Codes of Ethics (Appendices I, II, and III in the textbook) and Framework for Making Decisions (Table 1-2 in the textbook) as you discuss the following scenario with your classmates.

Brian is 8 years old and recently had another surgical procedure completed on his upper lip. He was born with a bilateral clefting of the lip with partial involvement of the palate. There is a university-based dental school and medical center in the city where Brian's family lives, so all treatment has been done locally.

As his dental hygienist, Leona has been delivering dental hygiene care to Brian since he was 3 years old. The status of his oral hygiene continues to decline even though Brian is at a point where he can care for his own teeth. His parents are supportive but want Brian to assume responsibility. Communication is sometimes difficult because of Brian's speech and hearing impairments.

Questions for Consideration

1. What professional role can Leona play as contributor in part of Brian's ongoing treatment plan, which includes surgical procedures related to the clefting?
2. Is Brian competent to act "autonomously" when performing home care procedures? Why or why not?
3. What issues of beneficence, veracity, and justice apply to the medical and dental care Brian receives?

---

3. Adam Horconcitos, a 12-year-old, has recently come to America from Honduras to live with Mr. and Mrs. Mehlisch, his American adoptive parents. Adam has a class 5 unilateral (left side) facial cleft that was not treated when he was an infant. He is scheduled for his first surgical procedure in about 3 weeks. You are a member of Adam's care team, and you are seeing him today for the first time to evaluate his oral status.

The only dental visits Adam has had previously were about 2 years ago with a prosthodontist in Honduras. The doctor fabricated an appliance to provide for some closure of the palatal opening to enhance Adam's ability to swallow and speak.

When you talk with Adam and the Mehlisches before the boy's examination, you find that Adam speaks fairly good English, because he went to an American school in his own country. He is a handsome, personable, and likable young man; but he is really very shy and frequently hides his mouth and nose behind his hand as he speaks to you. His voice has a kind of nasal sound, but his hearing is normal; and with a bit of concentration, you can understand him fairly well. Adam does not have any major health problems, except for a susceptibility to frequent sore throats and ear infections.

Adam did not enjoy a good dental experience during the fabrication of his prosthesis or during his recent visits with the oral surgeon to plan his surgical care. He is extremely fearful of anyone or anything that comes near his mouth. In spite of that, he is wearing the prosthetic appliance every day, and it seems to be working well for him.

You are successful in using all of your most comforting patient management techniques, and you convince Adam to allow his mouth to be examined. During your examination, you discover that he has a mixed dentition with five primary molars still being retained, significant malocclusions, and two missing anterior teeth in the area of the cleft. His level of dental caries is fortunately quite low—only one small cavity in a deciduous molar that is already loose. You conclude, from a discussion with Mrs. Mehlisch, that Adam's snacking habits are not highly cariogenic.

(continued on next page)

Factors To Teach The Patient

Today your patient is Mrs. Diane White. You first met her (see Chapter 45) when she was in her first trimester of pregnancy. About 3 months ago, her little girl was born with a class 3 cleft palate. Although the child is well cared for by an interdisciplinary team of health-care workers at the local hospital, Mrs. White notes that there is no dental hygienist on the team. She asks you for advice in providing oral care for her child as she grows.

Use information about cleft palate (Chapter 47 in the textbook) and what you learned about parental anticipatory guidance (Chapter 46 in the textbook) to role play this situation with a fellow student. If you are Mrs. White in the role play, be sure to ask questions. If you are the dental hygienist, try to anticipate questions and answer them in your explanation.

This scenario is related to the following factor:

■ Parental anticipatory guidance (Tables 46-2 and 46-3 in the textbook)

His gingival health, however, is another matter. He won't usually let anyone touch his mouth, and he doesn't like to have a toothbrush near his mouth even when he does it himself. You find extensive biofilm accumulation on his teeth, gums, and tongue as well as on the prosthodontic appliance he wears. His mother reports that his breath is often very bad. His gums bleed extremely easily when they are touched.

Using the information in the case study and a copy of the Dental Hygiene Care Plan template in Appendix C of the workbook, write an individualized dental hygiene care plan for Adam.

_____

_____

Preadolescent to Postmenopausal Patients

Chapter Outline

Learning Objectives

Upon successful completion of these exercises, you will be able to:

1. Identify and define key terms and concepts related to hormonal function.
2. Identify and describe physical, mental, emotional, and oral health factors commonly associated with adolescence and puberty.
3. Identify and describe physical, mental, emotional, and oral health factors commonly associated with menses and menopause.

KNOWLEDGE EXERCISES

1. Hormones that, together with the nervous system, maintain body homeostasis are excreted by _____ and transported to body cells or other glands by _____.

2. List the major endocrine glands.

   _____

   _____

   _____

3. Both _____ and _____ of a hormone can affect a patient's physical and mental status.

4. Identify the term defined or described by each of the following statements relating to hormones and the menstrual cycle.

   ■ *A chemical produced by the human body that has a specific regulatory function on other body cells or organs*

   _____

   ■ *A collective name for the hormones produced by the ovaries; responsible for development of female characteristics*

   _____

   ■ *A hormone that, along with estrogen, is present at various levels during the menstrual cycle*

   _____

■ A collective name for the hormones produced by the testes; responsible for development of male characteristics

_____

■ A synthetic hormone contained, either as a combination with estrogen or as a single preparation, in oral contraceptives

_____

■ The period of time from the beginning of one menstrual flow to the beginning of the next menstrual flow

_____

■ A term referring to menstruation

_____

■ Menstrual intervals >45 days

_____

■ Absence of spontaneous menstrual cycles during the reproductive years

_____

■ Difficult and painful menstruation

_____

■ A condition of the endometrium that causes pelvic pain

_____

■ The lining of the uterus

_____

■ A cluster of behavioral, somatic, affective, and cognitive disorders that appear in the luteal phase of the menstrual cycle and resolve rapidly with the onset of menses

_____

■ A feeling of fullness, soreness, or pain in the breast

_____

■ Feeling unwell, unhappy, or depressed

_____

5. Cyclic menstruation is regulated by fluctuations in estrogen and progesterone and, with some variations and irregularities, is usually about 28 days in length. In your own words, explain how the levels of each of these two hormones vary relative to menstruation and ovulation during the menstrual cycle. (_Hint:_ Describe Figure 48-1 in the textbook.)

_____

_____

_____

_____

6. Some women experience discomfort for several days preceding the beginning of their menstrual flow. If your patient mentions that she is feeling pre-menstrual, what symptoms is she likely to be experiencing?

_____

_____

_____

7. Define the two types of dysmenorrhea.

_____

_____

_____

8. If your patient is experiencing irregularity or other problems with her menstrual cycle, a careful assessment and review of her health history is imperative, because she can also be experiencing other _____ problems.

9. List the side effects of oral contraceptives that will be of concern when you are providing dental hygiene care for your patient.

_____

_____

_____

10. Identify the term defined or described by each of following statements relating to adolescents.

■ Chronic skin disorder associated with hormone fluctuation in adolescents

_____

■ Early is 10–13 years of age, middle is 14–17 years and late is 18–21 years of age

_____

■ The period during which the gonads mature and begin to function

_____

■ Referring to someone around the age of puberty

_____

■ Coming to the age of sexual maturity

_____

■ Identifies the onset of menstruation

_____

■ The process of male sperm production

_____

11. Summarize the effects of puberty-linked hormone increases on the physical development of both boys and girls.

_____

_____

_____

12. List the three health basics that teens need for general well-being.

_____

_____

_____

13. What dental disease related to eating habits has a higher incidence during adolescence than any other age group?

_____

_____

_____

14. A healthy diet is important at any age. Identify two eating disorders that are especially associated with teens who have a distorted body image.

_____

_____

_____

15. What nutritional deficiency is related to the onset of menstruation in teenage girls?

_____

_____

_____

16. Hormonal changes during puberty can cause an _____ response to bacterial biofilm and increase your adolescent patient's risk for _____.

17. List factors that increase your adolescent patient's risk for periodontitis.

_____

_____

_____

18. Between 5% and 47% of adolescents around the world demonstrate evidence of periodontal loss of attachment. Which two periodontal diseases are most likely implicated?

_____

_____

_____

19. List examples of oral problems you may observe when you perform an oral assessment of a teenage patient.

_____

_____

_____

20. The dental hygienist who understands the psychosocial development that adolescents are undergoing as they mature can communicate more successfully while teaching them about their oral health. List common emotional and behavioral changes that can affect teaching/learning of oral health measures during *early* adolescence.

_____

_____

_____

_____

_____

21. List educational approaches you can take that will have the most impact on motivation and compliance of your teenage patients and thus the most significant influence on their oral health status.

_____

_____

_____

22. Identify the term defined or described by each of the following statements relating to menopause.

■ *A normal condition of aging in which there is complete and permanent cessation of menstrual flow*

_____

■ *Physiologic reaction that causes the hot flashes and night sweats characteristic of menopause*

_____

■ *A prescription of purified or synthetic hormone to correct or prevent undesirable symptoms of menopause*

_____

23. Most adverse oral changes related to menopause can be prevented or diminished with adequate nutrition and thorough daily oral hygiene care. List the oral changes that can be associated with menopause.

_____

_____

_____

COMPETENCY EXERCISES

Charin Woodmacher, 15 years of age, and her mother both arrive for Charin's scheduled dental hygiene appointment. You haven't seen Charin in almost 2 years, because, as her mother told you on the telephone, Charin has simply refused to come for dental appointments. Mrs. Woodmacher also told you that Charin's braces were finally removed about 6 months ago, and the treatment was never completed because of Charin's attitude.

You greet Charin in the reception room, and she just rolls her eyes. She continues to slouch in the comfortable chair and keeps her book open. Mrs. Woodmacher sighs and pulls Charin upright; they both follow you down to the treatment room.

When you update the teen's medical history, her mother informs you that Charin has recently been diagnosed with bulimia and is currently under medical and psychological treatment for the disorder. Charin has iron-deficiency anemia and is taking a daily supplement; she also takes a combination estrogen/progestin oral contraceptive.

Mrs. Woodmacher finally goes back to the waiting room, and you direct your next few questions to Charin. She states, "That tooth on the lower left side has been bothering me and my mother says that I need my teeth cleaned." Your intraoral assessment findings include deep occlusal decay on tooth 30, with evidence of an abscess on the periapical radiograph of that area.

You document evidence of enamel erosion on the maxillary anterior teeth, generalized biofilm accumulation and heavy calculus in all areas, and generalized erythematous and bleeding tissues. Probing depths in the anterior teeth are generally 4 mm, and there are numerous areas of 6 to 7 mm in depth in the posterior teeth.

1. What are Charin's oral and general health risks based on the significant findings from her assessment data?

_____

_____

_____

_____

_____

_____

2. Dr. Hillcrest, the dentist where you practice, prescribes antibiotics for the abscess on Charin's lower right molar. What specific counseling/patient-education topic will you need to address with Charin because of this prescription?

_____

_____

_____

_____

3. Write at least two dental hygiene diagnosis statements for Charin's dental hygiene care plan.

Problem	Cause (Risk Factors and Origin)
_____ *related to*	_____
_____ *related to*	_____

Everyday Ethics

Refer to the Codes of Ethics (Appendices I, II, and III in the textbook) and Framework for Making Decisions (Table 1-2 in the textbook) as you discuss the following scenario with your classmates.

Amy, an 18-year-old, returns home from her first semester of college and presents with swollen gingiva, weight gain, and stories about considerable amounts of alcoholic beverages being consumed at parties. She also tells Sally, the dental hygienist, that she has just started taking birth control pills. Sally acknowledges Amy's desire to exercise her independence while away at school but also notes the term "risky behaviors" in the patient's chart

Questions for Consideration
1. Ethically, what is Sally's role as a primary dental health provider in referring this patient to other professionals for counseling and/or a physical examination?
2. Role play a discussion that might occur between Sally and Amy's parents, who are still financially responsible for the services rendered. Consider what has been entered into the patient's chart—"risky behaviors."
3. Using a decision framework, prioritize the content of the home care information needed to educate Amy about her oral conditions.

4. What dental hygiene interventions will you plan to address in each of the dental hygiene diagnosis statements written in question 3?

Oral Hygiene Clinical	Education/ Counseling	Instructions

5. Write one goal for each problem identified in the dental hygiene diagnoses in question 3. Include a time frame for meeting the goals. How will you measure whether your patient met the goals?

Goal 1

_____

_____

_____

◼ *Evaluation method*

_____

_____

_____

◼ *Time frame*

_____

_____

_____

Goal 2

_____

_____

_____

◼ *Evaluation method*

_____

_____

_____

◼ *Time frame*

_____

_____

_____

6. Chapter 48 in the textbook describes the unique challenges of trying to communicate with and motivate an adolescent. Given what you have observed about Charin's attitude and what you have learned about communicating with adolescents, what spe-

cific communication measures will increase your success in helping Charin attain and maintain oral health?

_____

_____

_____

Factors To Teach The Patient

Today is the first time you are providing dental hygiene care for Rosalee Ayers, age 55 years. She arrives late and mentions that because she is under high stress these days and hasn't been eating or sleeping very well, she overslept this morning. Rosalee is a high-powered businesswoman who takes great pride in her youthful appearance and her healthy lifestyle. As you update her health history, you note that she has received regular dental hygiene care for the last 15 years. Her general health status is very good, and she takes no medications. A notation in her record states that she is in menopause; her menses ceased 1 year ago.

When you begin your oral examination, Rosalee mentions that because of the oral hygiene instruction she has received at this clinic, she has always brushed and flossed every day. Lately, however, she has noticed that her mouth frequently feels really dry, and sometimes she feels a burning sensation on her tongue, palate, and inside her lips.

Your assessment findings indicate that her biofilm levels are very low, there are very few dental restorations, and there are no current carious lesions.

Her oral tissues are generally very healthy looking. Periodontal pocket depths are all <3 mm. Past periodontal charts have recorded generalized 2- to 3-mm recession in all premolar and molar areas, but there are no changes in the level of recession when you do your periodontal charting today.

After your assessment is complete, you write a brief care plan and, because of your patient's increased risk for root caries, you include a recommendation for fluoride treatment.

When you discuss your care plan with Rosalee, she chuckles and says, "Look, I'm not a kid any more. What on earth do I need a fluoride treatment for?"

Use the example of a patient conversation in Appendix B as a guide to write a conversation explaining your recommendations to Rosalee.

This scenario is related to the following factors:

◼ The benefits of fluoride throughout life
◼ The importance of nutrition, exercise, and sleep for good health

The Elderly Patient

Chapter Outline

Learning Objectives

Upon successful completion of these exercises, you will be able to:

1. Identify and define key terms and concepts related to aging.
2. Identify physical, general health, and oral health changes that are characteristic of aging.
3. Describe the effects of osteoporosis and Alzheimer disease on oral health status.
4. Describe dental hygiene interventions and health education approaches that enhance the oral health of the elderly patient.

KNOWLEDGE EXERCISES

1. In your own words, define the following terms related to aging.

   ▓ *Aging*

   _____

   _____

   _____

   ▓ *Senescence*

   _____

   _____

   _____

   ▓ *Gerontology*

   _____

   _____

   _____

■ *Geriatrics*

_____

_____

_____

■ *Biologic age*

_____

_____

_____

■ *Chronologic age*

_____

_____

_____

■ *Psychologic age*

_____

_____

_____

■ *Life expectancy*

_____

_____

_____

2. There are two common classifications used to define individuals from elderly populations: age related and function related. These two systems used together can help provide an accurate description of your aging patients. List the categories for each of these classifications.

■ *Age-related classifications*

_____

_____

■ *Function-related classifications*

_____

_____

_____

3. Differentiate between the terms *primary aging* and *secondary aging*.

_____

_____

_____

4. For each of the following body systems, describe at least two changes that occur as a result of primary aging.

■ *Musculoskeletal*

_____

_____

■ *Skin*

_____

_____

■ *Cardiovascular*

_____

_____

■ *Respiratory*

_____

_____

■ *Gastrointestinal*

_____

_____

■ *Central and peripheral nervous*

_____

_____

■ *Senses*

_____

_____

■ *Endocrine*

_____

_____

■ *Immune*

_____

_____

5. The elderly may react differently to disease from your younger patients. Identify the differences mentioned in the textbook.

_____

_____

_____

6. List four of the most common chronic health conditions of the elderly.

_____

_____

_____

7. Why are the elderly more at risk from alcohol consumption?

_____

_____

_____

8. List the causes of osteoporosis.

_____

_____

_____

9. Your older patient with osteoporosis is considered to be at greater risk for periodontal bone loss. List the factors that relate osteoporosis to periodontal disease.

_____

_____

_____

10. What medications used in treatment for osteoporosis increase bone formation?

_____

_____

_____

11. List and briefly describe the four progressive stages of Alzheimer disease.

_____

_____

_____

_____

_____

12. Identify the age-associated oral conditions described by each of the following statements.

   ▨ _Difficulty swallowing_

   _____

   ▨ _Oral lesion that appears as skinfolds with fissuring at the corner of the mouth; not specifically an age-related lesion but frequently seen among elderly persons_

   _____

   ▨ _Burning, smooth, shiny, bald tongue with atrophied papillae; related to nutritional deficiencies_

   _____

   ▨ _Deep red or bluish nodular masses commonly found during an intraoral examination of older individuals on either side of the midline on the ventral surface of the tongue_

   _____

   ▨ _Oral condition often noted in the elderly that is related to pathologic states, drug-induced changes, or radiation-induced degeneration of salivary glands_

   _____

   ▨ _Dental disease occurring in older folks that is related to cementum exposed by periodontal infections and often to xerostomia_

   _____

13. A dry, purse-string opening of your elderly patient's lips may make wide opening difficult during dental hygiene treatment. What causes this condition?

   _____

   _____

   _____

14. In your own words, describe common age-related degenerative changes to oral mucosa.

   _____

   _____

   _____

   _____

15. Identify the risk factors for oral candidiasis that may be present in your elderly patient.

   _____

   _____

   _____

16. Identify risk factors that may contribute to root caries in the elderly.

_____

_____

_____

_____

_____

17. Periodontal findings reflect the patterns of health and disease over the years of your older patient's life. Describe the range of tissue changes that may be noted when examining an older patient.

_____

_____

_____

_____

_____

_____

18. Identify the barriers that can negatively affect access to dental hygiene care for an elderly individual.

_____

_____

_____

19. Older patients often use more prescription drugs and more over-the-counter medications than other age groups. List the ways you can be sure that you know what drugs your patient is taking and that you make appropriate decisions when you plan dental hygiene care.

_____

_____

_____

20. List factors likely to occur in your elderly patient that can contribute to accumulation and retention of dental biofilm and increased difficulty in removal.

_____

_____

_____

21. Describe specific biofilm removal methods and techniques that you can recommend for an elderly patient.

_____

_____

22. Caloric intake must decrease to control weight as elderly individuals become less physically active. However, nutritional needs of older individuals are not different from those of younger adults. What factors can contribute to dietary and nutritional deficiencies in your older patients?

_____

_____

_____

_____

COMPETENCY EXERCISES

1. Explain why an older patient's slowness to learn new oral hygiene techniques does not necessarily mean an inability to learn.

_____

_____

2. Alzheimer disease typically progresses in stages. Define the dental hygienist's role in caring for a patient and providing oral hygiene instructions as a patient advances through these stages.

_____

_____

3. Discuss why it is important to develop an aggressive preventive care plan for a patient in the early stages of Alzheimer disease.

_____

_____

_____

_____

4. Today your patient is Marie Tonawonda, age 89 years. Refer to her Patient Assessment Summary

TABLE 49-1	OSCAR ASSESSMENT TABLE

A SYSTEMATIC APPROACH TO IDENTIFYING FACTORS THAT NEED TO BE EVALUATED WHEN PLANNING DENTAL HYGIENE CARE FOR: MARIE TONAWONDA

Issue	Factors of Concern
Oral	
Systemic	
Capability	
Autonomy	
Reality	

(Appendix D) as you complete the following exercises.

Ms. Tonawonda has been a patient in your clinic for many, many years, and she comes in every 4 months, like clockwork, for her periodontal maintenance appointments. Her father was a dentist, and she was his dental assistant when she was a young girl, so she loves to talk about the changes she has observed in dentistry.

As her nephew, Stan, escorts her slowly into your treatment room, you notice that although she greets you cheerfully as usual, she is becoming increasingly frail. As Stan helps with a health history update, he mentions that his aunt has recently been placed on an antidepressant by her physician. Stan visits his aunt in her home nearly daily and recently noticed that she hasn't been eating regular meals. There has been other evidence that Ms. Tonawonda has been decreasingly able to provide her own daily self-care, and Stan says that even when he reminds her, she does not always remember to brush her teeth or comb her hair every day.

Next week Ms. Tonawonda is moving to a nearby extended-care facility, where she will have her daily needs met by the staff. Stan states that he will continue to bring her in for her regular dental care and that Ms. Tonawonda's insurance will continue to cover the cost of any dental needs she has.

While your dental assistant is taking radiographs of Ms. Tonawonda's teeth, you begin to jot down notes for her dental hygiene care plan. You suddenly remember the OSCAR assessment approach to identifying the needs of older individuals (see Table 21-2 in the textbook). Complete the OSCAR Assessment Table (**Table 49-1**) on this page to describe the OSCAR factors of concern for Ms. Tonawonda.

Everyday Ethics

Refer to the Codes of Ethics (Appendices I, II, and III in the textbook) and Framework for Making Decisions (Table 1-2 in the textbook) as you discuss the following scenario with your classmates.

Mr. and Mrs. Bracken were among Doc Roberts's first patients when he began his practice almost 30 years ago. They keep a strict 4-month maintenance plan with the dental hygienist. Rosemary, the new hygienist, is looking forward to meeting and treating the Brackens for the first time as she has heard many wonderful things about this lovely elderly couple.

Upon completion of the oral examination with Mrs. Bracken, Rosemary recorded significant dental biofilm retention and evidence of xerostomia. She immediately begins to give the patient detailed home care instructions and asks for a complete listing of medications that Mrs. Bracken is taking for her arthritis, angina, and diabetes. Mrs. Bracken left the appointment confused and upset.

Questions for Consideration
1. Considering that Mrs. Bracken seemed overwhelmed at the end of her appointment, how may Rosemary have erred in her judgment of the patient and the instruction she gave? Suggest alternative approaches.
2. To ensure the autonomy of Mr. and Mrs. Bracken while acknowledging their longevity in the practice, how can the medical status of these patients be clarified?
3. With an intent to act beneficently toward Mrs. Bracken and improve her oral health, explain several factors that Rosemary needs to assess in the self-care plan she uses.

5. Using Ms. Tonawonda's Patient Assessment Summary (Appendix D), your OSCAR assessment notes, and the information in Chapter 49 of the textbook, write three dental hygiene diagnosis statements for Ms. Tonawonda's care plan.

Problem	Cause (Risk Factors and Origin)
_____ *related to* _____	
_____ *related to* _____	
_____ *related to* _____	

6. Because Ms. Tonawonda's cognitive abilities are declining, her need for education and oral hygiene instruction are very different from that of most of your other patients. Ms. Tonawonda will need ways to receive reminders for daily oral care. It is likely that staff at the extended-care facility will be ultimately responsible for Ms. Tonawonda's oral care (as well as the oral care of others who live there). What dental hygiene interventions will you plan to control disease and maintain her current state of oral health?

◾ *Clinical interventions*

_____

_____

_____

◾ *Education counseling interventions*

_____

_____

_____

◾ *Oral hygiene instruction/home-care interventions*

_____

_____

_____

Factors To Teach The Patient

After Marie Tonawonda (introduced in Competency Exercise question 3) moves to the extended-care facility, her nephew, Stan, comes in for his regular appointment. Stan thanks you again for all the information you provided when Ms. Tonawonda was in for her appointment, and he reaffirms his commitment to maintaining his aunt's oral health.

He mentions his concern about your direction to limit Ms. Tonawonda's exposure to high-sucrose foods. In order to increase nutritional intake, the residents at Sunshine seem to have access to food at any time they desire and, unfortunately, that includes availability of cookies all the time. Stan has encouraged the staff to provide support for his aunt's efforts at limiting sweets and conducting daily brushing and flossing, but he isn't sure his wishes are being met.

You decide that you will investigate the possibility of volunteering to provide staff in-service presentations about oral health to the caregivers at the extended-care facility. Develop an outline of the topics you would cover in these presentations.
This scenario is related to the following factors:

- That dentition can last a lifetime
- The value of a well-balanced diet
- Importance of drinking fluoridated water

QUESTIONS PATIENTS ASK

A healthy, functionally independent 70-year-old patient asks you if, at her age, she should consider dental implants for the molar teeth that were recently extracted. How will you respond?

What sources of information can you identify that will help you answer your patient's question in this scenario? How can you use the evidence-based decision-making methods you learned from reading the EBDM Primer at the front of the workbook to help answer this question?

The Edentulous Patient

Chapter Outline

Learning Objectives

Upon successful completion of these exercises, you will be able to:

1. Identify and define key terms and concepts related to an edentulous patient.
2. Identify potential adverse effects of dental prostheses on oral tissues.
3. Plan dental hygiene interventions that address patient needs before and after insertion of a denture.
4. Identify criteria and procedures for marking dentures.

Terminology Word Search Puzzle

To solve the puzzle, first use the clues to determine the words; then find the words in the grid. Words in the grid can run across, down, or diagonally and can start at the right or left or top or bottom.

```
W E R M T S P E C I A L I Z E D H V N L Z L K
M M X A F V G C O M P L E T E N T T P G L T E
Y A F O N V D F W P Z V N X T V K A A X C I P
M S D Q S O M M D H D X G R T M S M P T H M U
Z T M H J T D A Y P Z V W W D O V D I J A P L
K I B B B T O O N A Z H G N C M M P L T R L I
K C L F M Q H S N D D N P U K A F K L D A A S
L A Y F B R B P I T I H M H N N G V A E C N F
W T J V Z R V T N S I B E G N H T L R N T T I
X O M P N C L O H W U A U S C R T Z Y T E P S
L R P L Z P I T F S G L O L I K B C H A R R S
C Y G K F T R M R N A V P H A V K J Y L I O U
Z G D X C L Y N I R E C R P F R E L P P Z S R
P Q R E Q N Y L C R C N T P M Z I L E R A T A
Y G S X K K E H D J V C V K N Z I S R O T H T
L E L N C D E E T T K F Y P R N C Y P S I E U
R V J Y O I N Z G F R V N K I G R E L T O S M
N X L M L T K P L C K P F N J D R B A H N I J
M D E I U L F J T G X T G H J U G K S E X S T
N R T R B M R T R P V C M H T V G P I S T Z Z
C I E K P A L A T I N U S N X T R L A I B G N
S T O M A T I T I S L K E T B B K Q T S T R R
K V I M M E D I A T E D E N T U R E M T D J R
```

Word Search Clues

- Term for an artificial replacement of one or more teeth and associated oral structures (two words)
- Term for an artificial substitute for missing natural teeth
- Type of denture that replaces the entire dentition and associated structures of the maxilla or mandible
- Complete denture fabricated for placement directly after the removal of natural teeth or surgical preparation of dental arches (two words)
- Any prosthesis that uses dental implants for retention, support, and stability (two words)
- Removable prosthesis that covers remaining teeth, roots, or implants
- Modification of the form and color of the denture base and teeth to produce a more lifelike appearance
- The mucosa that covers the floor of the mouth, vestibules, and cheeks
- Type of mucosa that covers the edentulous ridge and hard palate
- The cushion of connective tissue, vessels, nerves, adipose tissue, and glands between mucosa and bone on the edentulous ridge
- Excision of a segment of any part (for example, of the jawbone) or removal of bones forming a joint
- The tori usually removed from the lingual premolar area before fabrication of a denture

- Bony enlargement (torus) that is surgically removed before fabrication of a maxillary denture
- Bony changes in the alveolar ridge over time that can lead to loss of denture support, changes in facial structure, and changes in oral functioning
- Material used to adhere a denture to the oral mucosa; should not be used long term to compensate for poorly designed, constructed, or ill-fitting dentures
- Fissuring at the corners of the mouth of a patient who wears dentures (two words)
- A generalized redness on the tissues that support a denture; your patient may experience a burning sensation
- Red, pebble-shaped, edematous lesions on the palate that are related to ill-fitting dentures, poor oral hygiene, and possible *Candida albicans* infection (two words)
- Chronic inflammatory oral lesion that appears in elongated folds related to the border of an ill-fitting denture (two words)
- Congenital absence of teeth that may require construction of dentures for a child patient
- Bony protuberance located on the buccal aspect of the alveolar ridge
- Mucosa that covers the dorsal surface of the tongue and contains filiform papillae

KNOWLEDGE EXERCISES

1. Identify reasons for wearing a denture to replace the missing teeth in an edentulous arch.

   _____

   _____

   _____

2. List three reasons why a denture may be constructed to replace primary dentition for a child patient.

   _____

   _____

   _____

3. What is the purpose of a provisional or interim dental prosthesis?

   _____

   _____

   _____

4. Why is it often necessary to reline or remake an immediate denture approximately 6 months after initial placement?

   _____

   _____

   _____

5. As a dental hygienist, you may provide counseling and education for your patient both before and after he or she receives a new denture. Explain the purpose of predelivery patient counseling.

   _____

   _____

   _____

6. When a denture is placed immediately after extractions, you instruct your patient to leave the denture in place for _____ without removing it to aid in control of bleeding and swelling.

7. Because adjustments can be expected when a new denture is placed over healed ridges, you instruct your patient to return within _____; you then make reappointments as needed.

8. What is the purpose of a postinsertion appointment with the dental hygienist after a new denture is placed? (*Note:* The dentist will adjust the new denture, if needed, not the dental hygienist.)

   _____

   _____

   _____

   _____

9. List the potential effects of alveolar ridge remodeling after placement of a complete denture.

   _____

   _____

   _____

10. Your patient may resort to _____ remedies to counter the effects of alveolar remodeling or poor denture fit, but you will counsel him or her to seek dental care if there are any problems, because these remedies are _____ if used improperly or over time.

11. List factors that contribute to the varying tissue reactions experienced by patients who wear dentures.

    _____

    _____

    _____

12. Xerostomia can adversely affect denture _____ and tissue _____.

13. List two negative oral effects related to the sensory changes that may be experienced by your patient who wears complete dentures.

    _____

    _____

    _____

14. For most of your patients who wear complete dentures, a _____ maintenance appointment frequency is adequate, unless they are experiencing problems.

15. At dental-hygiene appointments, it is important to thoroughly examine the oral tissues of a patient who wears complete dentures. In your own words, describe the tension test for examining the mouth of your edentulous patient.

    _____

    _____

    _____

16. List the three *most common* causes of oral lesions under a dental prosthesis.

   _____

   _____

   _____

   _____

17. What is the effect of xerostomia for your patient who wears dentures?

   _____

   _____

   _____

18. Trauma from an ill-fitting denture or rough spot on a denture surface can result in _____.

19. Name the common fungal infection that can result in denture stomatitis.

   _____

   _____

   _____

20. List three factors that can contribute to angular cheilitis in your patient who wears dentures.

   _____

   _____

   _____

21. If you observe a localized ulcer-shaped lesion related to an overextended denture border that persists longer than normal healing times, you should bring the situation to the attention of the dentist so that the lesion can be _____
   _____.

22. List the topics to include when you are educating your patient about ways to prevent damage to oral tissues related to wearing dentures.

   _____

   _____

   _____

23. List three reasons to mark your patient's denture with identifying information.

   _____

   _____

   _____

24. In your own words, briefly summarize the criteria for an adequate denture-marking system relative to the following issues.
   ■ *The denture*

   _____

   _____

   _____

   ■ *The material used*

   _____

   _____

   _____

   ■ *The procedure used*

   _____

   _____

   _____

25. List two areas in which identification information can be incorporated as a denture is fabricated.

   _____

   _____

   _____

26. Where should an inclusion identification marker be placed on an existing denture that was not previously labeled?
   ■ *Maxillary denture*

   _____

   _____

   _____

   ■ *Mandibular denture*

   _____

   _____

   _____

27. Identify two methods for marking identification information on the surface of a denture.

   _____

   _____

   _____

28. What information is included when marking the denture of a patient who is in a long-term-care nursing home?

   _____

   _____

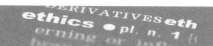

Everyday Ethics

Refer to the Codes of Ethics (Appendices I, II, and III in the textbook) and Framework for Making Decisions (Table 1-2 in the textbook) as you discuss the following scenario with your classmates.

Mr. Ryan presents for his yearly denture examination and oral cancer screening. He faithfully keeps his appointment every year because the cigarette stains build up on his full upper and lower dentures, and he likes the way his dental hygienist, Kaitlin, gets them very clean.

    During this visit, Kaitlin notices a small area on the alveolar ridge under the denture near the area of tooth no. 29. Mr. Ryan is aware of the lesion and sometimes doesn't wear his lower denture, but he indicates that it doesn't

really bother him. Kaitlin informs Mr. Ryan that she will get the dentist to check the area. Mr. Ryan becomes annoyed at her concern. He just wants to have his denture cleaned and to leave.

Questions for Consideration
1. Because Mr. Ryan has been a heavy smoker for more than 40 years, what actions are indicated to document and evaluate the lesion?
2. What are Kaitlin's obligations to the patient in communicating the possible serious nature of her findings?
3. What can be done if Mr. Ryan leaves the office without having the lesion evaluated?

COMPETENCY EXERCISES

1. Explain why regular dental hygiene maintenance care is important for edentulous patients, whether or not they are wearing complete dentures.

———————————————————————

———————————————————————

———————————————————————

2. Explain why caries-control methods are important to teach a patient with natural teeth remaining under an overdenture.

———————————————————————

———————————————————————

———————————————————————

3. After discussing several alternate treatment plans with the dentist, Mr. Bruehner has decided to have all of his remaining natural teeth extracted and immediate maxillary and mandibular dentures placed. He is very concerned, because his mother wore dentures and had lots of problems with them over the years. He has confided to Dr. Joseph that his mother's dentures didn't look like they belonged to her face and mouth, that she couldn't eat what she wanted to, that the dentures were not comfortable, and—worst of all—that his mother always had what he calls "dragon breath."

    Mr. Bruehner has an appointment with you today to begin preinsertion patient counseling

Factors To Teach The Patient

Mr. Bruehner (introduced in Competency Exercise question 3) received his immediate denture 2 days ago. This morning, he is scheduled with Dr. Joseph for a postinsertion appointment to check healing at the extraction sites; then he has an appointment with you for postinsertion education and counseling.

    Use the patient-specific dental-hygiene care plan you created for Mr. Bruehner and the example of a patient conversation in Appendix B as guides to prepare an outline for a conversation that you will have with Mr. Bruehner during this appointment.

This scenario is related to the following factors:

- Dentures and tissues must be examined at least once a year for care of the tissue-supported removable prosthesis; implant-supported dentures require more frequent examination. The frequency of maintenance appointments is geared to the individual, depending in part on that patient's ability to clean the dentures and to keep them free from biofilm, stain, and calculus.
- Dentures may need periodic replacement. Tissues under the dentures change.
- Avoid the use of drugstore remedies, reliners, and other home-applied materials unless the dentist has provided specific instructions.
- There are specific methods of care for dentures.
- Leave the dentures out of the mouth overnight in accord with the dentist's directions.

before he schedules the extraction appointment. You are developing a dental hygiene care plan before he arrives.

When you read the assessment data in his patient record, you learn that Mr. Bruehner has been receiving his dental treatment in this practice for a bit longer than 1 year. His general health status is relatively good; he is currently taking one medication for hypertension that contributes to xerostomia. He has a history of periodontal disease for which the original prognosis was rated as poor. He has a fairly high dental IQ because of education provided by the previous dental hygienist, but the counseling he received was focused on his periodontal status and the attempt to arrest the progress of oral disease.

Use a copy of the Patient-Specific Dental Hygiene Care Plan Template in Appendix C and the information in Table 50-1 in the textbook to develop a dental-hygiene care plan for a series of preinsertion and postinsertion appointments for Mr. Bruehner. Be sure to include at least one preinsertion appointment (more if you think he might need them), an appointment for instructions the day of his extractions, and a postinsertion appointment for instructions after he receives his dentures.

_____

_____

_____

_____

_____

_____

The Oral and Maxillofacial Surgery Patient

Learning Objectives

Upon successful completion of these exercises, you will be able to:

1. Identify and define key terms and concepts related to oral and maxillofacial surgery.
2. Identify causes, classifications, and treatment options for facial fractures.
3. Discuss dental hygiene interventions for patients before and after general surgery.
4. Plan dental hygiene care, oral health education, and dietary recommendations for patients before and after oral and maxillofacial surgery.

KNOWLEDGE EXERCISES

1. What is orthognathic surgery?

   _____

   _____

   _____

2. In your own words, define *intermaxillary fixation.*

   _____

   _____

   _____

3. Define *exodontics.*

   _____

   _____

   _____

4. List at least three reasons it is important to provide dental hygiene care for a patient before oral and maxillofacial surgery, even when all of the patient's teeth will be removed during the surgical procedure.

   _____

   _____

   _____

5. List three personal factors that can affect communication with your patient when you are providing oral hygiene instructions to him or her before oral surgery.

_____

_____

_____

6. List three types of printed instructions that you would provide as part of your presurgical patient education.

_____

_____

_____

7. Identify specific components to include in instructions you provide your patient immediately after a surgical procedure.

_____

_____

_____

8. List postsurgical procedures you may be asked to participate in during follow-up care for your patient.

_____

_____

_____

9. Identify two possible causes of a fractured jaw.

_____

_____

_____

10. List three clinical signs that can aid in recognition of a fractured jaw.

_____

_____

_____

11. Describe a comminuted fracture.

_____

_____

_____

12. Which type of fractured jaw is more likely to occur in a small child?

_____

_____

_____

13. What is an arch bar, and how does it immobilize the mandibular jaw?

_____

_____

14. Identify three advantages for using intermaxillary fixation (IMF) after surgical reduction of a fracture.

_____

_____

_____

15. List three contraindications for using an IMF.

_____

_____

_____

16. List three types of systems/materials used for immobilization after open surgical reduction of a skeletal fracture.

_____

_____

_____

17. List factors that make maxillary fractures more difficult to manage than mandibular fractures.

_____

_____

_____

18. Describe a maxillary alveolar process fracture. (*Hint:* Draw a diagram of what you are trying to describe.) List the components of treatment provided for the patient with this type of fracture.

_____

_____

_____

19. Identify two reasons a healthy liquid or soft diet is difficult to plan for a postsurgical patient.

_____

_____

20. List three vitamins that are essential in the diet of a patient who is healing after an oral/maxillofacial surgical procedure.

_____

_____

_____

21. Provide three examples of feeding methods used for patients after a surgical fixation procedure.

_____

_____

_____

22. List three foods that can supply needed nutrients as part of a soft diet prepared for a patient with only a single-jaw fixation appliance.

_____

_____

_____

23. When is personal oral care and thorough biofilm removal by the patient resumed after an oral surgical procedure?

_____

_____

_____

24. List three reasons why it is difficult for a postsurgical patient who has a fixation appliance or who is experiencing trismus to accomplish complete dental biofilm removal.

_____

_____

_____

COMPETENCY EXERCISES

1. Compare open and closed reduction procedures used for the treatment of a facial fracture.

_____

_____

_____

2. Mr. Bright is scheduled in 2 weeks for oral surgery to remove all of his remaining maxillary teeth and receive an immediate denture. His patient record contains assessment data indicating that teeth 1, 3, 6–9, 13, and 16 are missing; tooth 2 is extremely sensitive owing to a carious lesion; teeth 4 and 5 are mobile; and his gingival tissue is sensitive and bleeds profusely. There is visible calculus and a high level of biofilm on all the remaining teeth. He has not had any regular dental care or oral-hygiene instructions for many years. In **Infomap 51-1** below:

   ■ Identify at least two factors that can affect instrumentation techniques when you are providing presurgical scaling for Mr. Bright.
   ■ Explain why these factors are a problem.
   ■ Suggest procedures you might use to overcome each problem.

3. Your patient, Alicia Wentworth, is upset today when she comes to the office for her dental hygiene appointment. She tells you that her good friend, David, was recently injured in an automobile accident. She asks you to explain what a simple fracture of the mandible is and what a Le Fort II midfacial fracture is. Draw diagrams you can use to educate Alicia.

INFOMAP 51-1		
FACTORS AFFECTING INSTRUMENTATION	**REASON FOR THE PROBLEM**	**SOLUTION**

Everyday Ethics

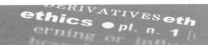

Refer to the Codes of Ethics (Appendices I, II, and III of the textbook) and Framework for Making Decisions (Table 1-2 in the textbook) as you discuss the following scenario with your classmates.

Mrs. Squires was involved in a serious automobile accident that fractured her mandible and required fixation. Fortunately, Mrs. Squires had some presurgical débridement before placement of the intermaxillary wiring. This is her first appointment with William, the dental hygienist, since the accident 10 months ago. He documents the moderate amounts of calculus and heavy dental biofilm throughout the mouth. Mrs. Squires demonstrates difficulty opening her mouth and seems apprehensive when William continually asks her to "open wide."

Questions for Consideration

1. How can William demonstrate empathy toward Mrs. Squires?
2. What steps in the decision model (Table 1-2, page 14) can help to analyze optimal oral health services to benefit this patient?
3. What is the role of the dental hygienist in coordinating preventive care with the posttreatment examinations Mrs. Squires has with the oral maxillofacial surgeon?

4. A week later, Alicia calls and leaves a message on the office voice mail. She says that David is coming home from the hospital, and she has agreed to provide meals for him every day. His fracture has been treated using an IMF appliance, and he must receive all his nutrition using a straw or a spoon-feeding technique. He is restricted to a full liquid diet. She asks you to call her back and recommend foods and preparation methods. She wants to know about how he can keep his mouth clean after he eats.

   Make notes that you can refer to when you call her back to give her the information she is asking for.

   _____

   _____

   _____

   _____

   _____

   _____

Factors To Teach The Patient

Mr. Brown is scheduled in about 2 weeks for some very serious surgery that is part of his treatment for pancreatic cancer. His physician has recommended that Mr. Brown visit his dental hygienist for a complete dental assessment before the surgery. As you go over his health history, you discover that he is very confused about why dental hygiene interventions are necessary in his case—after all, his illness has nothing to do with his mouth!

Use the information in Chapter 51 of the textbook and the example of a patient conversation in Appendix B as a guide to write a statement explaining to Mr. Brown why this dental-hygiene appointment is such an important component of his total health and well-being.
This scenario is related to the following factor:

■ Why it is necessary to have dental and dental hygiene care completed before surgery

The Patient with Cancer

Learning Objectives

Upon successful completion of these exercises, you will be able to:

1. Identify and define key terms and concepts related to the patient with cancer.
2. Identify risk factors for oral cancer.
3. Identify standard cancer treatments and the oral effects of each.
4. Plan dental hygiene care for the cancer patient before, during, and after therapy.

A Search for Prevention Word Search Puzzle

To solve the puzzle, first use the clues to determine the words; then find the words in the grid. Words in the grid can run across, down, or diagonally and can start at the right or left or top or bottom. When you have found all of the terms in the puzzle, **the unused letters in the first seven rows** will identify important risk factors related to cancer.

```
R  A  D  I  A  T  I  O  N  T  H  E  R  A  P  Y  T
O  B  A  C  C  O  ,  A  L  C  O  S  Y  U  H  O  H
L  ,  S  U  N  L  I  G  C  H  T  G  T  T  ,  E  E
N  V  I  R  O  N  N  A  M  A  O  E  A  O  N  T  M
A  L  C  A  R  C  R  E  G  L  I  N  N  L  O  G  A
E  N  S  ,  V  C  I  I  O  R  U  S  A  O  S  E  T
S  ,  P  O  I  V  N  C  E  P  R  T  P  G  A  Y  O
J  W  M  N  K  G  N  V  N  W  L  H  L  O  R  K  L
H  N  O  H  C  O  M  G  J  K  X  A  A  U  C  T  O
T  M  C  A  R  C  I  N  O  G  E  N  S  S  O  C  G
A  R  J  F  N  N  Q  R  D  T  T  F  I  M  M  V  I
B  V  W  X  E  B  T  K  M  P  N  C  A  D  A  K  C
T  N  T  B  C  H  E  M  O  T  H  E  R  A  P  Y  B
W  M  A  L  I  G  N  A  N  T  R  M  Z  W  B  Z  N
W  M  Y  K  Z  G  M  E  T  A  S  T  A  S  I  S  N
N  T  I  N  S  I  T  U  W  T  R  C  R  V  L  D  N
M  F  I  E  L  D  O  F  R  A  D  I  A  T  I  O  N
```

Word Search Clues: Terms Related to Cancer and Cancer Treatment

■ The study of tumors
■ A chemical, physical, or biologic agent that may cause cancer
■ Any new and abnormal growth; can be benign or malignant
■ The irreversible alteration in adult cells toward embryonic cell types, characteristic of tumor cells
■ The succinct, standardized description of a tumor in regard to origin and spread
■ Type of tumor that grows slowly by expansion and does not infiltrate surrounding tissue, does not spread by metastasis, and does not usually cause death unless its location interferes with vital functions
■ Confined to the site of origin (two words)
■ The spread of cancer cells from one body tissue or organ to others through blood and lymph systems
■ Type of tumor that bears little resemblance to cells of normal tissues, grows at a rapid rate, gains access to blood and lymph channels to metastasize into other areas of the body, and usually causes death unless growth can be controlled
■ Malignant tumor of epithelial origin
■ Tumor composed of cells derived from connective tissue
■ Treatment of an illness using drugs that affect rapidly developing cells
■ Treatment of disease with ionizing radiation (two words)
■ Area of the body where the external beam of radiation is applied during radiation therapy for cancer (three words)
■ Donor for this type of bone marrow transplant is the patient
■ Analysis of blood and blood-forming tissues for normal blood values (two words)

KNOWLEDGE EXERCISES

1. Match the following terms related to the physical and oral effects of cancer treatment with the correct description.

TERM	DESCRIPTION OF EFFECT
_____ Mucositis	A. Diminishment or abate-
_____ Dysgeusia	ment of the symptoms of
_____ Neurotoxicity	a disease
_____ Alopecia	B. Recurrence of a disease
_____ Palliative	after its apparent
_____ Herpes simplex	cessation
_____ *Candida albicans*	C. Treatment that provides
_____ Trismus	relief of symptoms but is
_____ Immunosuppression	not intended to cure
_____ Relapse	D. A loss of hair
_____ Remission	E. Virus that can cause oral
	infection during or after
	radiation therapy
	F. Distortion of the sense of
	taste
	G. Limited jaw opening
	because of spasm or
	fibrosis of muscles or
	joint; may occur
	3–6 months after
	radiation treatment to the
	head and neck
	H. Fungus that commonly
	causes oral infection
	related to treatment for
	cancer
	I. Inhibition of antibody
	responses resulting from
	leucopenia related to
	chemotherapy treatments
	J. Inflammation of the oral
	mucosa
	K. Can cause a bilateral
	feeling of toothache
	related to chemotherapy
	treatments for cancer

2. What is cancer?

_____

_____

_____

3. How are cancers classified and described?

_____

_____

_____

4. What are the risk factors for developing cancer?

_____

_____

_____

5. Why is it important to plan comprehensive and coordinated dental hygiene care for your patient before, during, and after treatment for cancer?

_____

_____

_____

_____

_____

_____

6. Identify the dental hygiene interventions you will most likely provide for your patient before the medical treatment for cancer begins.

_____

_____

_____

7. Radiation therapy for cancer is most likely to have oral effects if the field of radiation is concentrated in your patient's head and neck area. Identify the long-term complications of radiation treatment on oral tissues.

_____

_____

_____

8. Identify the signs and symptoms of radiation- and chemotherapy-induced stomatitis.

_____

_____

_____

9. List recommendations you can make to help your patient reduce sensitivity and increase ability to maintain daily oral hygiene measures when mucositis is a problem during cancer treatment.

_____

_____

10. Radiation to salivary glands can cause a serious reduction in secretion of saliva. Chemotherapy treatments can also induce a transient xerostomia. Identify the ways that xerostomia can affect the oral cavity.

_____

_____

_____

11. What suggestions can you make to help your patient manage xerostomia during and after cancer treatments?

_____

_____

_____

12. Identify measures that can prevent radiation caries.

_____

_____

_____

13. What are the systemic side effects of chemotherapy cancer treatment?

_____

_____

_____

14. List the types of oral infections that are common during and after radiation therapy and/or chemotherapy treatment for cancer.

_____

_____

_____

15. _____ is a destructive blood vessel compromise and necrosis of bone that can occur after high-dose radiation treatment in the head and neck area. This condition results in a decreased ability to heal and increased susceptibility to infection.

16. What oral changes can influence/restrict nutritional intake and further compromise the health status of a patient who is undergoing cancer therapy?

_____

_____

_____

17. In your own words, briefly describe a hematopoietic cell transplantation.

_____

_____

_____

_____

_____

_____

18. What is graft-versus-host disease?

_____

_____

_____

19. What patient factors can influence your patient's ability to attend to and comply with the counseling and oral hygiene instructions that you provide before, during, and after treatment for cancer?

_____

_____

_____

COMPETENCY EXERCISES

Mrs. Marge Henley is scheduled today in Dr. Singh's book as an emergency patient. After he examines her, Dr. Singh calls you in to consult with him. Mrs. Henley is currently undergoing chemotherapy for cancer treatment and is experiencing severe oral symptoms related to the treatment. Dr. Singh has already written a prescription to treat the oral candidiasis. He asks you to counsel Mrs. Henley about daily oral care and to write a dental hygiene care plan for her continuing care during the cancer treatment.

When you carefully examine her, you discover that Mrs. Henley's oral tissues are heartbreakingly inflamed, blistered, and dry. She tells you that she has been feeling a bit guilty because her mouth has been so sore that she cannot brush and floss as often or as thoroughly as she used to do. Her sense of humor has remained intact, though, and she tells you with a twinkle in her eye that she eats vanilla pudding for breakfast, lunch, and dinner every day. She asks for any suggestions you have to help her get through this difficult time.

1. Write at least two dental hygiene diagnosis statements to include in Mrs. Henley's written care plan.

Problem	Cause (Risk Factors and Origin)
_____ _related to_	_____
_____ _related to_	_____

2. Write a goal for each of the problems identified in the dental hygiene diagnosis statements in question 1. Include a time frame for meeting each goal. How will you measure whether your patient met the goal?

Goal 1

_____

_____

_____

■ *Evaluation method*

_____

_____

_____

■ *Time frame*

_____

_____

_____

Goal 2

_____

_____

_____

■ *Evaluation method*

_____

_____

_____

■ *Time frame*

_____

_____

_____

3. Using your institution's guidelines for writing in patient records, document Mrs. Henley's visit and write a statement regarding her next visit.

Date	Comments	Signature

DISCOVERY EXERCISE

The National Oral Health Information Clearinghouse (NOHIC) is a resource center for oral health information geared to patients with special needs and the healthcare providers who serve them. Visit their Web site (*www. nohic.nidcr.nih.gov*) to discover a wonderful series of education pamphlets about oral cancer and the oral complications of cancer treatment.

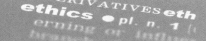

Everyday Ethics

Refer to the Codes of Ethics (Appendices I, II, and III in the textbook) and Framework for Making Decisions (Table 1-2 in the textbook) as you discuss the following scenario with your classmates.

It's the end of the day, and all of the patients, the staff, and the dentist had left the office. Ashley, the dental hygienist, was reviewing the next day's patient records at the front desk.

The telephone rang, and Ashley answered it. It was Gina, the daughter of a longtime patient, Mr. Prisby. Gina, a pediatric registered nurse, lives out of state but is visiting her 70-year-old father, who is undergoing head and neck radiation therapy and chemotherapy treatments for tongue cancer. When she arrived, she was shocked to find her father having difficulty opening his mouth completely and a white coating on the inside of his cheeks. Gina also noticed multiple sores in his mouth. Her father has been unable to eat anything but the softest of foods because of the severe discomfort and dryness. Gina is concerned that her father cannot maintain a

healthy weight during treatment. She asks Ashley what the white coating is in her father's mouth, what the sores are, and what can be done for him.

Ashley puts Gina on hold and pulls Mr. Prisby's record. She sees that he had a complete examination and all treatment performed that left him in good dental health 3 months ago, just before he started his cancer treatment. The white coating that Ashley described may be candidiasis and require medication. But she's not sure how to treat the sores Gina sees. Ashley considers whether to refer Gina back to the oncologists treating her father or phoning in the prescription in the dentist's name to save time.

Questions for Consideration
1. What advice can Ashley give to Gina, considering the stipulations of patient confidentiality?
2. Describe the ethical and legal consequences of Ashley phoning in a prescription for Mr. Prisby.
3. What decisions and/or actions are appropriate for Ashley to pursue within the scope of her duties at this time?

Factors To Teach The Patient

George Murphy, a 45-year-old construction worker, has recently been diagnosed with parotid gland cancer that has spread into his left neck. He will be having surgery to remove the left parotid gland with a left neck dissection followed by radiation therapy. He is scheduled today for a pretreatment dental examination. Mr. Murphy has not seen a dentist in more than 10 years and has dental caries lesions, moderately advanced periodontal disease, and very poor oral hygiene. You are asked to prepare a dental hygiene care plan to address Mr. Murphy's oral care needs during and after the radiation treatment.

Mr. Murphy tells you that he hates dentists because they always hurt him and that is why he never comes to see one. The only reason he is here today is because he was told that he could not proceed with his cancer treatment unless he gets his mouth into better shape.

Use the information in the "Personal Factors" section of Chapter 52 of the textbook and the example of a patient conversation in Appendix B as guides to prepare an outline for a conversation you will use to counsel Mr. Murphy regarding his oral condition.

This scenario is related to the following factors:

- Why the dental hygienist needs to conduct an oral soft-tissue screening and complete oral examination at regular, frequent intervals
- How and when to use dental biofilm control methods, gel-tray application, use of saliva substitute, and all other details of personal care to reduce oral side effects caused by the disease and/or cancer treatment
- Ideas for remembering to follow the instructions to keep the mouth healthier and more comfortable during cancer treatment
- The reasons why a routine schedule of preventive periodontal scaling, fluoride application, and oral hygiene assessment done by a dental hygienist contributes to the success of cancer treatment

QUESTIONS PATIENTS ASK

"How can I possibly keep my mouth clean when it is so sore and/or dry that it hurts to use the toothbrush? And why is that so important anyway?" "When is the best time to have my teeth worked on while I am undergoing treatment for my cancer?" "How soon after my radiation treatment can I get my new dentures and/or partial dentures?"

What sources of information can you identify that will help you answer your patient's questions? How will you use the evidence-based decision-making methods you learned from reading the EBDM Primer in Appendix A to help answer these questions for each specific patient?

CHAPTER 53

Care of Patients with Disabilities

Chapter Outline

Learning Objectives

Upon successful completion of these exercises, you will be able to:

1. Identify and define key terms and concepts relating to individuals with disabilities.
2. Identify oral conditions caused by or resulting from disabling conditions.
3. Describe procedures and factors that contribute to safe and successful dental-hygiene treatment for individuals with disabilities.
4. Describe factors that enhance the prevention of oral disease for individuals with disabilities and their caregivers.

Key Terms Crossword Puzzle

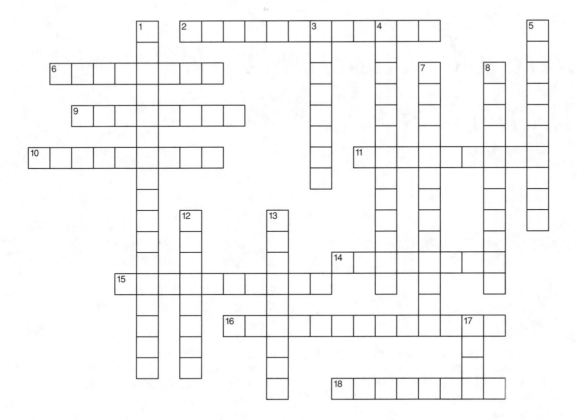

Across

2 An aid that can be used to help transfer an individual from a wheelchair to the dental chair and back again (two words).

6 Refers to the disadvantage that can limit fulfillment of a normal role for a person with an impairment.

9 A dental treatment room that is not wheelchair accessible is an example of this kind of barrier that can hinder access to oral care.

10 Person who performs or helps to perform daily life activities for the individual who is disabled; an important source of information and help during dental care.

11 The need for longer appointment time—and the dental professional's need to be reimbursed for providing that time—can constitute this type of barrier that limits oral-care options for an individual with a disability.

14 Not feeling adequately trained to provide safe treatment is an example of this characteristic of a dental professional that creates a barrier to providing oral care for disabled individuals.

15 Integration rather than segregation.

16 Refers to a disability of indefinite duration with an onset before the age of 18.

18 Stabilizes a patient in the dental chair by enclosing from neck to ankles with nylon mesh; three sizes from infant to larger child.

Down

1 Refers to providing community-based support that allows individuals with disabilities to live at home rather than custodial institutions.

3 The individual responsible for making decisions if a person is declared incapacitated in a legal process; requires written proof for decision making.

4 Standard that requires removal of architectural, transportation, and communication barriers in public places.

5 Refers to the restriction resulting from an impairment.

7 Making everyday life as close as possible to patterns in mainstream society.

8 Accessible to all without discrimination; obstacles to passage or communication have been removed (without the hyphen).

12 A term that refers to several techniques for moving a person from a wheelchair to a dental chair and back.

13 Education program about some specific topic, such as oral care for individuals with disabilities, that is provided for parents, teachers, volunteers, nurses, or other health professionals (without the hyphen).

17 The Americans with Disabilities Act, NOT the American Dental Association!

KNOWLEDGE EXERCISES

1. In your own words, briefly describe each of the two main components of the World Health Organization International Classifications of Functioning, Disability, and Health.

   ◼ *Part I: Functioning and Disability*

   _____

   _____

   _____

   _____

   _____

   _____

   ◼ *Part II: Contextual Factors*

   _____

   _____

   _____

   _____

   _____

   _____

2. List three objectives for providing quality dental and dental-hygiene care for individuals with disabilities.

   _____

   _____

   _____

3. For you to plan dental hygiene care that takes all of the needs of your patient with a disability into consideration, it is essential to gather as much information as possible before the first appointment. Identify three individuals (or groups) who can provide the needed information.

   _____

   _____

   _____

4. To avoid confusion, it is best to ask direct questions concerning the type and severity of your patient's disability. Identify four categories of information to obtain from the patient or caregiver.

   _____

   _____

   _____

5. List four factors to consider when scheduling appointments for an individual with a disability.

   _____

   _____

   _____

6. In your own words, define a barrier-free dental treatment facility.

   _____

   _____

   _____

7. What size parking space must be allowed for disabled individuals?

   _____

   _____

   _____

8. How wide must outdoor walkways and indoor passageways be to accommodate a wheelchair?

   _____

   _____

   _____

9. An appropriately constructed wheelchair ramp entrance has a handrail and a gentle slope that rises _____ for every _____ in length.

10. Lightweight doors with lever handles must open at least _____ wide for a wheelchair to pass through.

11. For providing oral-hygiene instruction for a patient who is in a wheelchair, it is ideal to have a table or sink built at a height of _____ that permits clearance underneath for knees and wheelchair arms.

12. A dental chair that is accessible for wheelchair transfers can be lowered to at least _____ from the floor.

13. Describe a way to position your wheelchair-bound patient for dental hygiene treatment if a portable headrest is not available to attach to the wheelchair.

   _____

   _____

14. List three basic types of wheelchair transfers.

_____

_____

_____

15. What is the first thing you should do before starting a wheelchair transfer?

_____

_____

_____

16. Who can give you advice as to how best to help during a wheelchair transfer?

_____

_____

_____

17. List three factors that take special consideration during a wheelchair transfer.

_____

_____

_____

18. Describe the position of the wheelchair with respect to the position of the dental chair when transferring your patient from the wheelchair to the dental chair.

■ _Mobile transfer_

_____

_____

_____

■ _Immobile transfer_

_____

_____

_____

■ _Sliding-board transfer_

_____

_____

_____

19. It makes sense, when transferring your patient back to the wheelchair after treatment, to position the seat of the dental chair slightly _____ than the seat of the wheelchair.

20. If you are helping your patient with a mobile transfer from a wheelchair to the dental chair, where are your patient's arms and hands?

_____

_____

_____

21. Describe the position of the first aide's hands/arms when two people are helping with an immobile patient transfer.

_____

_____

_____

22. What is the responsibility of the second aide during an immobile patient transfer?

_____

_____

_____

23. What is your role in assisting a patient with a walker, crutches, or a cane to seat themselves in the dental chair?

_____

_____

_____

24. List factors that contribute to safety and comfortable positioning or stabilization of your patient with a disability while in the dental chair.

_____

_____

25. What precautions are important to consider before the use of body stabilization during dental hygiene treatment?

_____

_____

_____

26. Identify two techniques for safely stabilizing a patient's head during dental hygiene treatment.

_____

_____

_____

27. List mechanisms that can be used to maintain the patient's mouth in an open position while you are providing dental hygiene treatment or during daily oral care provided by caregivers.

_____

_____

_____

28. List precautions to observe if you are using a mouth prop.

_____

_____

_____

29. In your own words, describe additional precautions you can take to ensure safety, comfort, or minimization of extreme movements during dental hygiene treatment for your patient with a significant disability.

_____

_____

_____

30. In many cases, the education component of your dental hygiene care plan for a patient with a disability will not be different from the education component of a care plan for a nondisabled patient. Identify two oral diseases found in people with disabilities that are _not_ different from those of nondisabled individuals.

_____

_____

_____

31. Identify additional oral findings that can be caused by, or be a result of, your patient's disability.

_____

_____

_____

32. List oral manifestations related to drug therapies commonly used to treat patients with disabilities.

_____

_____

_____

33. When should you recommend that the use of a dentifrice should be limited or eliminated from the oral care regimen of a patient with a disability?

_____

_____

_____

34. What recommendations can you make so that a patient who cannot use a dentifrice receives the benefits of fluoride?

_____

_____

_____

35. Identify factors to take into consideration when planning dietary recommendations for your patient with a disability.

_____

_____

_____

36. To plan oral hygiene instructions for your patient with a disability, it is important for you to understand the ability of your patient to perform daily living skills such as toothbrushing. What other terms/concepts correspond to the three functioning levels described in Chapter 53 in the textbook for patients with disabilities?

▨ _High-functioning level_

_____

_____

▨ _Moderate-functioning level_

_____

_____

▨ _Low-functioning level_

_____

_____

_____

37. What is your role in providing oral hygiene instructions for an individual who is identified as having a moderate- or low-functioning level?

_____

_____

38. In your own words, describe the position that a caregiver can use to be most effective when providing daily oral care for a person with disabilities.

_____

_____

_____

39. Self-care aids can make a difference in the ability of a patient or caregiver to maximize effectiveness of oral care. List the general prerequisites of a good oral self-care aid.

_____

_____

_____

40. Identify three general modifications that can be made to a toothbrush handle to enhance the ability of a patient with a disability to provide oral self-care.

_____

_____

_____

41. What factors will you take into consideration when recommending the use of a power-assisted toothbrush for a patient with a disability?

_____

_____

_____

42. Briefly describe modifications that can be made to help a patient with a disability care for a removable dental prosthesis.

_____

_____

_____

43. Identify three factors that, if addressed during planning, can enhance/contribute to the success of a caregivers' education/in-service program you provide in a long-term care facility.

_____

_____

_____

44. Identify ways to evaluate the success of an in-service program.

_____

_____

_____

45. Identify topics to include in an in-service presentation that teaches caregivers how to examine oral tissues.

_____

_____

_____

Everyday Ethics

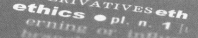

Refer to the Codes of Ethics (Appendices I, II, and III in the textbook) and Framework for Making Decisions (Table 1-2 in the textbook) as you discuss the following scenario with your classmates.

When Mrs. Becker has her dental appointment, Lauren, the dental hygienist, must rush to finish the previous patient so she can have time to go to the storage closet in the basement and get the transfer board to slide Mrs. Becker over to the dental chair from her wheelchair. Mrs. Becker has numerous medical and dental problems that she tends to complain about. She has been very difficult to motivate to perform daily biofilm control. Her current dental status indicates that she should be placed on more frequent 2- to 3-month maintenance appointments. Lauren feels overstressed to prepare for and treat Mrs. Becker in the time she is allowed for appointments. Lauren is considering ignoring the plan for more frequent maintenance visits and scheduling Mrs. Becker in 6 months to avoid another unpleasant experience for both of them.

Questions for Consideration
1. What issues could Lauren discuss with her employer to defend her request for a longer appointment time?
2. What efforts could Lauren make to improve biofilm control with Mrs. Becker?
3. What might Mrs. Becker feel about her dental experiences, including with Lauren?

47. Identify four additional oral care/disease prevention techniques to teach during staff in-service training.

_____

_____

_____

COMPETENCY EXERCISES

1. In your own words, explain the relationship between the terms *impairment, disability,* and *handicap.*

_____

_____

_____

_____

_____

_____

2. Steve McKnight is your patient with cerebral palsy. He is charming and witty. He works for a company that develops voice technology for computers. He has significant physical impairments associated with his condition and moves about with difficulty, using crutches and special leg braces to walk. He is fiercely independent, preferring to manage as many tasks as possible on his own.

    Steve moves his hands with difficulty and cannot grasp small objects very well. He feeds himself using specially adapted utensils. When you talk to him about his daily oral care, he mentions that he used a power-driven toothbrush for a while but that it was heavy, and when it started to vibrate, he could barely hold it up to his mouth. He sighs and says that he really wishes he could find a regular toothbrush that he could hold on to without dropping it in the sink all the time.

Factors To Teach The Patient

Use the information in Chapter 53 about diet instruction and the example of a patient conversation in Appendix B as a guide to write a conversation educating the mother of a child with a disability about the general concepts of maintaining a tooth-healthy diet.
This scenario is related to the following factor:

■ Practice a healthy lifestyle, including a healthy diet

Find appropriate materials and make a device to adapt a toothbrush and floss handle that would help Steve continue to be independent in his daily oral care. Share your design with your classmates. Does your design meet the general prerequisites for a self-care aid as described in the textbook?

_____

_____

_____

3. Your next patient tells you that her daughter, Sara (age 14), has a fractured right elbow and will spend the next several months handicapped by a cast that holds her arm stiff in a slightly bent position. She can maneuver her wrist about but cannot bend her arm. Describe how your patient can modify a toothbrush that will allow Sara to independently accomplish biofilm removal until her arm heals.

_____

_____

_____

The Patient who is Homebound

Chapter Outline

Learning Objectives

Upon successful completion of these exercises, you will be able to:

1. Identify and define key terms and concepts related to the homebound, bedridden, or terminally ill patient.

2. Prepare materials necessary for visiting a homebound patient.

3. Plan adaptations to dental hygiene care plans and oral-hygiene instructions for the homebound patient.

KNOWLEDGE EXERCISES

1. What characteristics help define a person who may not be able to access dental hygiene care in a traditional private practice office setting?

   _____

   _____

   _____

2. What are the barriers that prevent a homebound individual from receiving oral health services?

   _____

   _____

   _____

3. List three objectives of providing dental hygiene care in a home or nursing home setting.

   _____

   _____

   _____

4. Identify three unique objects or implements, not usually associated with providing care in a dental office, to include when planning to provide care for a homebound patient.

   _____

   _____

   _____

5. List three factors that can influence scheduling an appointment time to provide dental hygiene care for a homebound or nursing home patient.

_____

_____

_____

6. List five unhealthy mental characteristics associated with inactivity and the monotonous existence of a homebound patient.

_____

_____

_____

7. When is a firm pillow important for patient positioning during dental hygiene care?

_____

_____

_____

8. Describe a patient who is comatose.

_____

_____

_____

9. In your own words, define the concept of hospice care for the terminally ill.

_____

_____

_____

10. Define _palliative care._

_____

_____

_____

11. What common oral infection is often found in a patient with a terminal illness?

_____

_____

_____

COMPETENCY EXERCISES

1. You are one of the dental hygienists on a dental care team that visits the Nightingale Long Term Care Center each month to provide oral care for residents. Your first patient of the day is Bruce Wilkerson, a handsome 29-year-old who has been in a coma since a diving accident 8 years ago. After looking at the information in Bruce's medical record, you enter his room and greet him. As you prepare your armamentarium, position him for oral care, and place towels under his chin, you keep up a cheerful one-sided conversation. Explain why it is important to talk with this patient even though he will definitely not respond to your remarks.

_____

_____

_____

2. Miss Louise Piranian is a 96-year-old resident in the Nightingale Long Term Care Center. She is amazingly feisty and young-acting for her age, and she delights the nursing staff with her antics. Her favorite trick is to slip her upper denture out and grin widely with no front teeth! She also wears a lower partial denture, but she won't take that one out because it is too hard to get back in.

   Miss Louise loves to entertain guests at her daily tea party and can talk and talk and talk about all sorts of interesting topics while keeping everyone's teacup full. Lately she is getting a bit forgetful, though, so the Nightingale Center nursing staff is putting together a plan to make sure all her daily personal care needs are met.

   Write your recommendations for a daily oral health plan for Miss Louise that takes into account daily oral care regimens, nutrition, and care of her denture.

_____

_____

_____

3. Mrs. Malcolm has been a patient in your clinic for about 15 years. She has always had fairly good oral hygiene, and a healthy mouth has been important to her. You haven't seen her in quite a while, though, because Mrs. Malcolm has spent a lot of time in the hospital over the last year. You recently heard that she has been receiving hospice care in her home.

   Dr. Gable, the dentist you practice with, has agreed to provide some basic comfort care at home for Mrs. Malcolm, and she suggests that you accompany her. When you arrive, you find that Mrs. Malcolm, although very weak, is awake and able to speak with you. She reports having a very dry mouth, and you notice that her lips are coated with a dry-looking,

Everyday Ethics

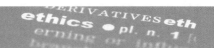

Refer to the Codes of Ethics (Appendices I, II, and III in the textbook) and Framework for Making Decisions (Table 1-2 in the textbook) as you discuss the following scenario with your classmates.

Elena is 55 years old and is dying of esophageal cancer. She has been involved in an outpatient hospice program and receives all medical services in her home. Elena's daughter contacts the dental office of Dr. Gray and asks if someone can please come to the house and check her mother's teeth.

Sandy, the dental hygienist in the practice, offers to go and provide whatever "comfort care" she can for Elena.

Questions for Consideration

1. What legal and ethical concerns need to be addressed before going to Elena's home as care will be limited?
2. Reviewing the principle of justice, if Elena's homebound status prevents her from accessing dental care, what options can the dental team offer to her at this time?
3. Describe several "virtues" that can be exhibited by the dental team to benefit this patient.

---

crusty material. She mentions that her lower partial denture does not fit very well any more and often slips around whenever she tries to eat. It is rubbing on her left cheek. She says her mouth feels and tastes bad and that her gums were bleeding when her daughter tried to help her brush her teeth a couple of days ago.

    Write at least three dental hygiene diagnosis statements for Mrs. Malcolm's care plan.

Problem	**Cause (Risk Factors and Origin)**
_____ *related to*	_____
_____ *related to*	_____
_____ *related to*	_____

4. Write a goal and evaluation method for one of the diagnosis statements you identified in question 3. Include a time frame for meeting that goal.

  ◼ *Goal*

    _____

    _____

    _____

  ◼ *Evaluation method*

    _____

    _____

    _____

  ◼ *Time frame*

    _____

    _____

    _____

5. Describe ways that you can arrange your working situation for providing dental hygiene care to Mrs. Malcolm in her home bedroom.

  _____

  _____

  _____

Factors To Teach The Patient

Today you are giving hands-on training in providing daily oral care for a group of nurse's aides at the Nightingale Long Term Care Center. You have set up a suction toothbrush at the bedside of Bruce Wilkerson (introduced in Competency Exercises question 1). Besides showing and telling the nurse's aides how to brush someone else's teeth and care for the suction toothbrush afterward, you also want to explain the reasons for providing daily oral cleansing for all of the residents/patients in the center.

    Use the example of a patient conversation in Appendix B as a guide to write an outline of information you need to present to the group of nurse's aides.

    Use the conversation you create to role play this situation with several fellow students. If you are a nurse's aide in the role play, be sure to ask questions. If you are the dental hygienist, try to anticipate questions and answer them in your explanation.

This scenario is related to the following factors:

- The contribution of good oral health to general health
- How a clean mouth can contribute to wellness and quality-of-life factors
- How to care for the patient's natural teeth: toothbrushing, flossing, rinsing, and other personal needs
- How to use a suction toothbrush, power brush, or other device to provide oral care for the patient

6. Mrs. Malcolm's daughter, Amy, mentions that she bought some lemon and glycerin swabs at the drugstore to help with the dry mouth her mother has been experiencing. What information can you provide Amy that will help her relieve her mother's dry mouth?

_____

_____

_____

DISCOVERY EXERCISES

1. Use the information in Table 54-1 in the textbook as well as additional information from dental supply catalogs and web sites to put together a plan and a budget for everything you would need for a portable dental hygiene practice.

QUESTIONS PATIENTS ASK

"There are so many agencies now that offer health and personal-care services to homebound individuals—why don't they have someone who can come to my house/nursing home so that I could get my teeth cleaned?" "Is there a dentist around here who will make house calls?" "Why doesn't the staff in my mother's nursing home help her brush her teeth every day?"

What sources of information can you identify that will help you answer these questions? What components of your state's dental/dental hygiene practice act limit—or support—the ability of homebound individuals to access professional oral health services?

The Patient with a Physical Impairment

Chapter Outline

Learning Objectives

Upon successful completion of these exercises, you will be able to:

1. Identify and define key terms and concepts related to physical impairment.
2. Describe the characteristics, complications, occurrence, and medical treatment of a variety of physical impairments.
3. Identify oral factors and findings related to physical impairments.
4. Modify a dental hygiene care plan based on assessment of needs that are specific to a patient's physical impairment.

KNOWLEDGE EXERCISES

1. Define the following terms and concepts related to movement.

   ■ *Akinesia*

   _____

   _____

   _____

   ■ *Ankylosis*

   _____

   _____

   _____

   ■ *Ataxia*

   _____

   _____

   _____

■ Athetosis

_____

_____

_____

■ Bradykinesia

_____

_____

_____

■ Diplegia

_____

_____

_____

■ Dysphagia

_____

_____

_____

■ Flaccidity

_____

_____

_____

■ Hemiplegia

_____

_____

_____

■ Kyphosis

_____

_____

_____

■ Lordosis

_____

_____

_____

■ Muscle atrophy

_____

_____

_____

■ Myopathy

_____

_____

_____

■ Orthosis

_____

_____

_____

■ Palsy

_____

_____

_____

■ Paralysis

_____

_____

_____

■ Paraplegia

_____

_____

_____

■ Paresis

_____

_____

_____

■ Parkinsonism

_____

_____

_____

■ Polyarthritis

_____

_____

_____

■ Quadriplegia

_____

_____

_____

■ Rigidity

_____

_____

_____

■ Sclerosis

_____

_____

_____

■ *Scoliosis*

_____

_____

_____

■ *Spasticity*

_____

_____

_____

■ *Tetraplegia*

_____

_____

_____

■ *Tremor*

_____

_____

_____

■ *Triplegia*

_____

_____

_____

2. Describe the sensorimotor effects of the following lesions.

    ■ *Complete spinal cord injury lesion*

    _____

    _____

    _____

    ■ *Incomplete spinal cord injury lesion*

    _____

    _____

    _____

3. Identify the appropriate descriptive term and the number of vertebrae associated with each of the following letters.

    ■ *C*

    _____

    _____

    _____

    ■ *T*

    _____

    _____

    _____

■ *L*

_____

_____

_____

4. A patient's level of disability depends on the level of the spinal cord injury. Paralysis occurs in the limbs and muscle groups innervated by nerve fibers extending at and below the injured vertebrae. The most severely disabled individuals are those with a spinal cord injury above _____.

5. Paralysis of limbs, the need for wheelchair use, and potential complications can require that you be prepared to modify standard patient care techniques, especially when your patient's spinal cord injury is located at T6 or above. Identify modifications you might make during dental hygiene treatment to accommodate your patient's comfort and safety.

    _____

    _____

    _____

    _____

    _____

6. What causes a decubitus ulcer, and how can you help prevent this condition during dental hygiene treatment of a patient with paralysis?

    _____

    _____

    _____

7. Describe hyperreflexia. What is your response to this situation?

    _____

    _____

    _____

8. Mouth-held appliances can aid your patient with a spinal cord injury in performing a variety of basic procedures that contribute to independence. List the criteria for an adequate oral orthosis.

    _____

    _____

    _____

9. In your own words, define *CVA*.

   _____

   _____

   _____

10. What is a TIA?

    _____

    _____

    _____

11. What causes a stroke to happen?

    _____

    _____

    _____

12. What patient-assessment technique, commonly used by dental hygienists, can provide information that may indicate your patient's increased risk for CVA?

    _____

    _____

    _____

13. What conditions increase an individual's risk for CVA?

    _____

    _____

    _____

14. Describe signs and symptoms commonly observed in a patient with a history of CVA.

    _____

    _____

    _____

15. What is aphasia?

    _____

    _____

    _____

16. If your patient has a history of CVA damage to the **right** side of the brain, that patient would exhibit _____ hemiplegia and have difficulty with _____.

17. If your patient has a history of CVA damage to the **left** side of the brain, that patient would exhibit _____ hemiplegia and have difficulty with _____.

18. Osteoarthritis is a chronic degenerative joint disease that is common in individuals who are _____.

19. Describe the location and progression of osteoarthritis symptoms.

    _____

    _____

    _____

20. Describe osteoarthritis symptoms that can occur in the temporomandibular joint.

    _____

    _____

    _____

21. What is rheumatoid arthritis?

    _____

    _____

    _____

22. In your own words, describe the symptoms of rheumatoid arthritis.

    _____

    _____

    _____

23. What is juvenile rheumatoid arthritis?

    _____

    _____

    _____

24. How does rheumatoid arthritis affect the temporomandibular joint?

    _____

    _____

    _____

25. What modifications to standard treatment techniques can you use to increase the comfort of your patient who has arthritic involvement of the

temporomandibular joint while you are providing dental hygiene treatment?

_____

_____

_____

26. What is the relationship between rheumatoid arthritis and periodontal disease?

_____

_____

_____

27. Drugs used for treatment of arthritis include pain medications such as NSAIDs. What additional drugs are used to control rheumatoid arthritis?

_____

_____

_____

28. If your patient has severe arthritis, what additional important question will you be sure to incorporate when you are updating his or her health history?

_____

_____

_____

29. What are the functions of the kidney?

_____

_____

_____

30. What oral findings are associated with impaired kidney function?

_____

_____

31. List the drugs, some commonly used or recommended during dental care, that use the kidney as a major pathway of elimination.

_____

_____

_____

32. Describe the medical treatments used when kidney function is very low.

_____

_____

_____

33. Which of the treatments described in question 32 has a potential effect on oral tissues?

_____

_____

_____

34. When is antibiotic premedication needed before dental treatment for your patient who has kidney dysfunction?

_____

_____

_____

35. Complete Infomaps 55-1 and 55-2 with just enough basic information to help you identify and differentiate among the listed developmental and acquired

INFOMAP 55-1	DEVELOPMENTAL CONDITIONS (Onset before age 18)			
CONDITION	**CAUSE/ OCCURRENCE**	**BASIC CHARACTERISTICS**	**MEDICAL TREATMENT**	**ORAL FINDINGS/DENTAL HYGIENE CONSIDERATIONS**
Cerebral palsy				
Muscular dystrophy, Duchenne				
Muscular dystrophy, facioscapulohumeral				
Myelomeningocele				

INFOMAP 55-2	ACQUIRED IMPAIRMENT (Onset after age 18)			
CONDITION	CAUSE, OCCURRENCE, PATHOLOGY	BASIC CHARACTERISTICS	MEDICAL TREATMENT	ORAL FINDINGS/DENTAL HYGIENE CONSIDERATIONS
Bell's palsy				
Multiple sclerosis				
Myasthenia gravis				
Parkinson disease				
Scleroderma, progressive systemic sclerosis				

disabling conditions. The following questions will require a bit more detail about each of the conditions included in the Infomaps.

36. What percent of patients with cerebral palsy also have brain damage that causes mental retardation?

37. What additional disabling conditions can sometimes accompany a diagnosis of cerebral palsy?

38. What oral characteristics are associated with cerebral palsy?

39. What symptoms of muscular dystrophy can directly affect your patient's oral health status?

40. Describe the categories that are used to identify types of multiple sclerosis.

41. What oral factor places a patient with multiple sclerosis at risk for relapse or an increase of symptoms?

42. Myasthenia gravis and scleroderma are both disabling conditions that have special significance for dental professionals. Why?

43. Care is taken when raising the dental chair after treatment of your patient with Parkinson disease who is being treated with dopamine replenishment, because of the possibility of _____.

COMPETENCY EXERCISES

1. For each spinal level, label **Figure 55-1** with suggested modifications in oral-hygiene instructions or mechanical aids that would help a patient with a spinal-cord injury at that level attain and maintain oral health. (*Hint:* Review Chapter 53, "Care of Patients with Disabilities," in the textbook.)

2. Identify the classification of cerebral palsy associated with each of the following descriptions of movement or motor activity.

   ■ *Jane Goodin comes to your treatment room in a wheelchair with an attendant. She is unable to stand, her head droops to her chest, and her hands are folded limply in her lap, but her eyes look up at you, and she tries to smile as she greets you. You must listen very carefully to understand what Jane is saying, because of her speech impairment. Her chin is wet, and you notice that she wears a towel around her neck.*

   _____

   _____

   _____

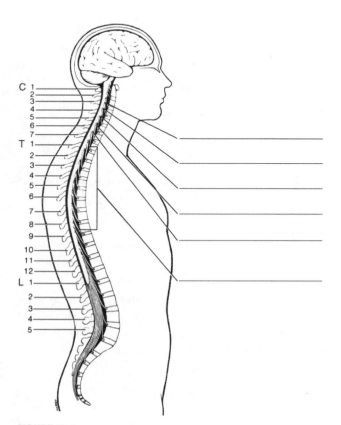

FIGURE 55-1

   ■ *While you are helping transfer Anitha Jones from her wheelchair to the dental chair, you note that she cannot control the constant disorganized movements of her arms, legs, and head. When you mistakenly startle her by reaching quickly to turn on the dental light, this uncontrolled movement becomes intensified, and her hand flings out and bumps into the instrument tray, scattering instruments all over the floor. Anitha's face muscles are in constant motion; she drools and breathes through her mouth. When you talk with her about her daily oral hygiene habits, it takes her a long time to say anything to you because of her speech defect. Besides the cerebral palsy classification, note which area of the brain is involved in this disability.*

   _____

   _____

   _____

   ■ *Steve has the ability to walk and follow you from the reception area to the treatment room, but his movements are awkward and stiff. He jokingly says that he seldom gets this much exercise, and as he walks he runs his fingers slowly along the nearby wall to balance himself. When you move the dental chair, his limbs have a strong inclination for sudden spasms, which means that you must keep your instrument tray in a different position from the one you are used to. Besides the cerebral palsy classification, note which area of the brain is involved in this disability.*

   _____

   _____

   _____

3. Sean O'Brien, age 73, is assisted to your treatment room by his wife, Moira. You watch them coming toward you down the hallway, with Mrs. O'Brien supporting Mr. O'Brien on his right side. He smiles at you as you adjust the dental chair, and you note that the muscles on the right side of his face are significantly paralyzed. When you and Mrs. O'Brien update his medical history, you are not surprised to learn that Mr. O'Brien is recovering from a cerebrovascular accident that happened about 8 months ago. He is taking a long list of medications, including an anticoagulant, an antihypertensive, a thrombolytic medication, and a vasodilator. What verbal communication skills will help you successfully provide oral hygiene instructions to Mr. O'Brien after his wife returns to the reception area?

   _____

   _____

   _____

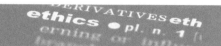

Everyday Ethics

Refer to the Codes of Ethics (Appendices I, II, and III in the textbook) and Framework for Making Decisions (Table 1-2 in the textbook) as you discuss the following scenario with your classmates.

John had an accident when diving into surf at the beach 2 years ago at age 18. He is now quadriplegic. At his biannual dental maintenance visit, Amy, the dental hygienist, was assisting in the wheelchair transfer into the dental chair. During the transfer, John's t-shirt was inadvertently lifted slightly, and Amy noticed obvious decubitus ulcers. Amy continues to safely transfer him into the dental chair and then stops to consider what to do next. Dramatic images from a lecture in dental-hygiene school flash through her mind. She will never forget those photographs of patients suffering from neglect.

Questions for Consideration

1. If John is unaware of the sores, and they are not being treated, what actions does Amy take, and what issues need to be addressed before the appointment can occur? Serious infections need to be resolved before elective treatment.
2. John came to the appointment with his mother, who is his primary caregiver. What options should Amy consider if the mother denies the existence of the problem?
3. Is the possibility that John is a victim of neglect an ethical issue or ethical dilemma? What responsibility does Amy have to inform the patient or others?

4. Mr. O'Brien has been receiving physical and occupational therapy to help him learn how use his left hand to do what he used to do with his now partially paralyzed right hand and arm. He is very proud of his growing independence and slowly tells you about how he can now comb his own hair and brush his own teeth. While you are performing an oral examination, you note that his biofilm control is very poor and that there is a bolus of leftover food pocketed in his right cheek. The paralyzed muscles on that side of his face have affected his ability to self-clean and even to detect the food that is pouching there after he eats.

   ■ *How can you counsel Mr. O'Brien about his oral health needs and encourage him to let his wife help him clean his mouth, especially on the paralyzed side, while still respecting his desire to independently care for his own personal needs?*

   _____

   _____

   _____

   ■ *Role play this situation with a student colleague.*

5. Anitha Jones (introduced in question 2) is here today for her regular 3-month periodontal maintenance visit. Anitha has enjoyed regular professional dental care throughout her life. Daily oral biofilm removal has been carefully provided by her long-time personal caregiver. Her periodontal status is currently healthy and stable.

   Today, Anitha introduces you to her new personal caregiver, Laura. Laura admits to having very

 Factors To Teach The Patient

Once a month, your employer, Dr. Tom Buckner, and his entire dental team provide care in a little dental clinic inside a nearby assisted-living residence. Your next patient, Terry Biensfield, 25 years old, sustained a level C5 spinal-cord injury in a motorcycle accident several years ago. He has worked hard in his physical-therapy sessions to maximize his level of function in activities of daily living by using adaptive aids. You have taught him how to brush his own teeth using a modified, long-handled toothbrush attached to one hand, but he still needs some caregiver support and reminders that he must complete his daily oral care routine.

Last month, Dr. Buckner and the physical therapist devised a mouthstick appliance that allows Terry to use a computer. Terry has been practicing with the computer every day, when he participates in an online discussion for people with spinal-cord injuries. He now has lots of new ideas for ways he can use his mouthstick to be more independent and creative in his daily life.

Use the example of a patient conversation in Appendix B as a guide to write a statement explaining to Terry how important it is for him to maintain his present level of oral health so that his teeth can continue to support the use of a mouthstick.

This scenario is related to following factors:

■ That daily, thorough biofilm removal is particularly necessary to reduce the occurrence of oral disease
■ That regular maintenance appointments are important to promote oral health
■ Why maintaining periodontal health has added value for teeth used as abutments for a mouth-held implement
■ How to clean and maintain the mouth-held implement
■ The need to maintain teeth in order to tolerate a mouth-held aid

little dental knowledge, but she very much wants to learn how to keep Anitha's mouth as healthy as her previous caregiver has done. Anitha asks you to include Laura when you discuss the dental-hygiene care plan you prepare.

Use the Patient Assessment Summary data for Anitha Jones (Appendix D) and a copy of the Individualized Dental-Hygiene Care Plan template (Appendix C) to complete a dental-hygiene care plan for Anitha that includes appropriate education for Laura.

The Patient with a Sensory Disability

Learning Objectives

Upon successful completion of these exercises, you will be able to:

1. Identify and define key terms and concepts related to sensory impairment.
2. Describe the causes of sensory impairments.

3. Identify factors that affect interpersonal communication and patient education.
4. Determine adaptations that enhance dental hygiene care for a patient with a sensory impairment.

KNOWLEDGE EXERCISES

1. A reference to a patient with a disability always begins with a statement about the person before defining the disability. How does the Americans with Disabilities Act (ADA) define an individual with a disability?

   _____

   _____

   _____

2. In what way does the ADA define the responsibility of the dental practitioner in meeting the needs of a patient with a hearing or vision impairment?

   _____

   _____

   _____

3. In your own words, define *visual impairment*.

   _____

   _____

   _____

4. Define *total blindness*.

   _____

   _____

   _____

5. Explain the term *legally blind*.

   _____

   _____

   _____

6. For each descriptive term for the two types of visual impairment often corrected by prescription eyeglasses, provide the medical term and characteristics associated with it.

   ■ *Farsighted*

   _____

   _____

   _____

   ■ *Nearsighted*

   _____

   _____

   _____

7. An astigmatism, also often corrected with prescription glasses, is caused by what?

   _____

   _____

   _____

8. An _____ measures visual acuity and prescribes lenses for the correction of visual defects; an _____ is the technician who prepares the adaptive lenses prescribed by the specialist.

9. An _____ is a physician specializing in treatment of defects, injuries, and diseases of the eye.

10. _____ during pregnancy is the cause of at least half of the blindness in children.

11. _____ is an inflammation of the retina.

12. What is retinopathy?

    _____

    _____

    _____

13. Identify and describe the condition that causes blindness in infants who must be treated at birth with very high concentrations of oxygen.

    _____

    _____

    _____

14. In your own words, define *glaucoma*.

    _____

    _____

    _____

15. What action during dental hygiene treatment can cause pain for your patient with glaucoma?

    _____

    _____

    _____

16. Which of the following terms refers to a visual impairment that can be caused by a vitamin deficiency?

    ■ *Braille*
    ■ *Color blindness*
    ■ *Diplopia*
    ■ *Nyctalopia*

17. Through observation, how can you identify a potential visual impairment in an older patient who does not admit to failing sight?

    _____

    _____

    _____

18. Why do you always speak to patients who have a significant visual impairment each time before you enter or leave the room and each time before you touch them during dental hygiene treatment?

    _____

    _____

    _____

19. A person can hear when the _____ vibrates and sound waves are transmitted to nerve endings by the ossicles of middle ear, to cochlea in the inner ear, and then to the brain.

20. What is tinnitus?

    ■ *A vibrating tuning fork*
    ■ *A physician specialist in ear diseases*
    ■ *A constant ringing/buzzing sound*
    ■ *A telecommunication device*

21. What is vertigo?

    _____

    _____

    _____

22. What is the abbreviation for decibel?

    _____

    _____

23. Your patient is considered deaf when the hearing impairment is at what level?

_____

_____

_____

24. What descriptive phrase is used for a patient who has a hearing impairment but uses an aid to facilitate communication?

_____

_____

_____

25. List factors that may contribute to hearing loss.

_____

_____

_____

26. What is an audiologist?

_____

_____

_____

27. How does the audiologist determine an hearing loss hearing ability?

_____

_____

_____

28. An otologist would most likely be the healthcare worker involved with treating otitis media. What is otitis media?

_____

_____

_____

29. Identify the four types of hearing loss, and briefly identify the damaged body structure(s) associated with each type.

_____

_____

_____

_____

_____

30. How does a hearing aid function?

_____

_____

_____

31. Why should you remind your patient who uses a hearing aid to either turn it off or take it out during dental hygiene treatment?

_____

_____

_____

32. Describe a cochlear implant.

_____

_____

_____

33. In your own words, what is American Sign Language (ASL)?

_____

_____

_____

34. What is speech reading?

_____

_____

_____

35. If your patient is speech reading, what can you do to enhance his or her understanding during oral hygiene instructions?

_____

_____

_____

_____

_____

36. The best way to teach skills such as biofilm removal to your patient with a hearing loss is by _____ rather than by explanation.

COMPETENCY EXERCISES

1. You have completed Mr. Corkman's dental hygiene treatment for today, and you direct him down to

Jenny, the appointment manager, so he can schedule his next visit while you clean and disinfect the treatment room for your next patient. When he gets to the end of the hallway, you hear him say, "Delighted to meet you, Benny!" You observe him at the front desk for a bit, then walk up to him and remind him that he turned his hearing aid off when you were using the ultrasonic scaler during his treatment. What did you observe that indicated Mr. Corkman had forgotten to turn it on again?

_____

_____

_____

2. Ask one of your student colleagues to role play the part of Anastasia Binghamton, 16 years old, your patient who is profoundly deaf. Her preferred method of communicating is using a combination of ASL and finger spelling. Use the pictures in Figures 56-3 and 56-4 in the textbook to help you practice asking her the following questions.

■ *Are there any changes in your health history?*
■ *Is there any pain in the area where tooth 32 was extracted last month?*
■ *Can you please open wider so that I can polish the back teeth?*
■ *I will show you how to position your toothbrush in order to get all the bacteria off the gums.*
■ *The dentist will be right in to examine your mouth.*
■ *Please make your next appointment in 6 months.*

3. Patty Ricalde, 25 years old, is one of your favorite patients. She usually arrives for her appointment clinging to the arm of her younger sister; both of

them out of breath, laughing uproariously, and looking as though they had just returned from some astonishing adventure. Sometimes they have, as you found out last year, when they came in with photographs of a desert hiking adventure in southern Utah! Sometimes, when you listen to the two of them, you forget that Patty is designated as legally blind. She also wears a hearing device that allows her to communicate with anyone who will take the time to talk slowly and clearly.

You will be developing a new dental hygiene care plan for Patty, and you want to designate her ADL level to indicate her ability to manage daily oral care (*Hint*: Refer to Table 21-3 in the textbook.)

Discuss the ADL level you will assign to Patty.

_____

_____

_____

4. What ASA classification will you assign to Patty? (*Hint*: Refer to Table 21-1 in the textbook.)

_____

_____

_____

5. Patty arrives without her sister, but with a huge golden retriever guide dog she calls Harrison. You are a bit flustered, and you hold out your hand to greet Patty without first letting her know you have come into the room with her. She bumps into you as she turns to return your greeting. You aren't quite sure what to do next, as Patty's sister has always helped guide Patty to your treatment room and

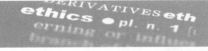

Everyday Ethics

Mr. Dolson was scheduled for 11:00 AM with Regan, the newest dental hygienist in the practice. He arrived about 15 minutes late, so Regan was ready and waiting to begin the maintenance appointment. She quickly escorted Mr. Dolson to the chair and began the oral examination without much talking. Mr. Dolson sensed that Regan was in a hurry but was uncertain of what to say. He wore a hearing aid but didn't always turn it on. He had been known to "blurt out" his thoughts rather loudly at times not realizing the volume

or tone of his voice. "Tell me if I'm doing a good job with my brushing," began Mr. Dolson. Rather startled, Regan said "You're really not brushing well at all!" Mr. Dolson grew very quiet.

Questions for Consideration
1. Professionally and ethically, how would you describe the provider-patient relationship in this scenario?
2. Was Regan's response to Mr. Dolson justified? Why or why not? Explain your rationale.
3. How should virtue ethics apply to a patient with special needs such as a hearing impairment or other loss of sensory functions?

helped her get settled in the chair, and today you will obviously have to help her yourself. You cover your distress by complimenting her on the beauty of her dog and bending down to hug him.

You gently take Harrison by the collar and lead him down the hall to the door of your treatment room. Patty follows you and her dog into the room. You raise the chair up a bit higher, so the seat is just above the level of Patty's knees, and you turn her around and gently ease her back until she is sitting against the edge of the dental chair. You tell her you will place the dog out in the hall where there is significantly more room. She seems uneasy about that, but you reassure her that no one will be going by to step on him there, as your treatment room is the last one down the hall.

As you return to the room, Patty pushes herself up and back into the chair, turns, and slides her feet up on the footrest. You wince as her head just misses the dental light, but she doesn't hit it and you breathe a sigh of relief. You notice the time, so you quickly update her health history (no significant findings), lower the chair and tell Patty to grab hold of the armrests before you tilt her back. You complete your oral assessment and begin scaling.

Later, after polishing her teeth, you squirt lots of water so she can rinse her mouth. She raises herself from the chair, swallows twice, and then apologizes and asks for a cup to rinse. After you help her rinse with a cup, you are feeling that this appointment has been very stressful for you, and you would love to have a quiet minute to recover your calm. As Patty gets out of the dental chair, you walk out into the hallway to bring Harrison back in to her.

Factors To Teach The Patient

When you have completed care for Patty Ricalde (introduced in the Competency Exercises) for the day, she tells you laughingly that her vet said she needs to clean Harrison's teeth regularly to keep him healthy. You reply that, of course, regular oral hygiene is as important for him as it is for Patty. You agree to teach her how. Because your next patient is due, you don't have time today, but you agree to meet her during your lunch hour tomorrow. She already has a toothbrush and some special chicken-flavor toothpaste. You decide that to be thorough, you had better plan this doggy oral hygiene instruction carefully before you meet with Patty tomorrow.

Keeping in mind that Patty is blind and wears a hearing aid, use the example of a patient conversation in Appendix B as a guide to prepare a conversation to teach Patty about maintaining her guide dog's oral health.
This scenario is related to the following factor:

■ The importance of oral care for the guide dog

What could you have done differently to manage Patty's care to reduce both her stress and your own during this appointment?

_____

_____

_____

_____

_____

_____

Family Abuse and Neglect

Learning Objectives

Upon successful completion of these exercises, you will be able to:

1. Identify and define key terms and concepts related to family abuse and neglect.
2. Describe various categories of family maltreatment.
3. Recognize signs and behavioral indicators of abuse.
4. Identify the dental hygienist's role in recognizing and reporting abuse and neglect.

KNOWLEDGE EXERCISES

1. Define *forensic dentistry*.

_____
_____
_____

2. What is PANDA?

_____
_____
_____

The factors involved in the recognition and management of suspected maltreatment of children, the elderly, people with disabilities, and women are similar. When answering the following questions, be sure to take all of these potential at-risk groups into consideration, unless the question specifies a particular group or groups.

3. List four major types of maltreatment that can occur in families.

_____
_____
_____

4. Identify two types of maltreatment of elders that do not usually occur in cases involving children.

_____
_____
_____

5. In your own words, define *dental neglect*.

_____

_____

_____

6. When children state that there is no one at their house to help them brush their teeth, what additional appearance and behavioral indicators might lead you to suspect that your patient is neglected?

_____

_____

_____

_____

7. Identify the signs of lice infestation.

_____

_____

_____

8. Identify personal appearance factors that might lead you to suspect that an individual is being physically abused.

_____

_____

_____

9. In your own words, describe the raccoon sign.

_____

_____

_____

10. What is an area of baldness that is caused by pulling out hair by the roots?

_____

_____

_____

11. What is the medical term used to identify a bruise?

_____

_____

_____

12. Describe what you might notice about site of an accidental injury versus the common sites you might notice if the injuries are inflicted or deliberate.

_____

_____

_____

13. Identify intraoral signs of physical abuse.

_____

_____

_____

14. Identify general signs of physical abuse and neglect in a child patient.

_____

_____

_____

15. In what way do these general signs compare with what you might notice if an elderly patient is being mistreated?

_____

_____

_____

16. Extremely aggressive behavior by a child when you try to examine his or her mouth can be a behavioral indicator for _____ as well as for physical abuse.

17. Identify intraoral signs of sexual abuse.

_____

_____

_____

18. List nonabuse-related conditions that can mimic the physical signs of abuse.

_____

_____

_____

19. One important role for the dental hygienist in cases of suspected abuse is to document the observable facts in the patient's record. What information is necessary to have available when you are reporting abuse to state authorities?

_____

_____

_____

Everyday Ethics

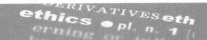

Refer to the Codes of Ethics (Appendices I, II, and III of the textbook) and Framework for Making Decisions (Table 1-2 in the textbook) as you discuss the following scenario with your classmates.

Sarah, a young, usually vivacious patient in Dr. Stuart's practice for about 2 years, presents for a maintenance appointment with Amy, the dental hygienist. Since her previous appointment, Sarah had had a big wedding. Amy was expecting to hear about it and maybe even see pictures.

When Sarah came into the treatment room, she seemed very quiet and avoided eye contact with Amy. Upon completion of Sarah's oral assessment, the following was noted: class II mobility on no. 6, no. 7, and no. 8; disto-incisal edge fractures on no. 7 and no. 8; and a 4-mm scar on the vermilion border of the upper lip. Sarah explained that she

slipped and fell on a wet kitchen floor. She could not remember how she got the scar, which was not present 6 months ago. Amy is not sure that Sarah is telling the truth. She suspects Sarah may be in an abusive relationship with her new husband. There is not enough time to have a long discussion with Sarah or with Dr. Stuart, who is in the middle of a crown-preparation procedure.

Questions for Consideration

1. Legally, what is Amy's role as a health care professional to obtain more details from the patient? Explain what documentation should be included in the patient's record.
2. Would discussion of the oral assessment with Dr. Stuart be a breach of confidentiality? Why or why not?
3. How would Amy incorporate her suspicions about Sarah into the personal oral care recommendations without violating the patient's rights?

COMPETENCY EXERCISES

1. In Knowledge Exercise question 6, you identified parent factors that can contribute to dental neglect. What is your role as a dental hygienist in addressing each of the factors you identified?

   _____

   _____

   _____

2. Read the information in the Everyday Ethics case study for this workbook chapter. Using your institution's guidelines for writing in patient records, document your findings regarding Sarah.

Date	Comments	Signature

3. Outline the thought process you will use when making a decision to report suspected child abuse to state authorities. Discuss your outline with a small group of your student colleagues. Use the results of this discussion to write a protocol for reporting expected abuse.

   _____

   _____

Factors To Teach The Patient

Johnny is 8 years old. This is his first dental hygiene visit with you, and his dental history indicates that he has not seen a dentist since a dental examination was required by the HeadStart program when he was 3 years old. His parents scheduled this dental appointment as a result of a directive from state authorities after a report by his teacher.

Johnny is very shy, but after he gets to know you a bit during his appointment, he seems interested in what you are doing and asks all kinds of questions. You note during your intraoral examination that his teeth are completely covered with dental biofilm. Johnny states he doesn't really have a very good toothbrush. He obviously is not performing daily self-care, and you suspect that his parents are not helping or encouraging him in any way. Fortunately, there are no carious lesions, but his gingival tissue is red and bleeds easily when you touch it.

Use the example of a patient conversation in Appendix C as a guide, and use language appropriate for a child to explain why Johnny needs to brush his teeth every day. *This scenario is related to the following factors:*

- The value of oral hygiene with age-appropriate materials
- What the bacterial biofilm is on teeth, using a disclosing agent
- How to use the new toothbrush the child just received
- Why it is especially important to brush the teeth and tongue just before going to sleep

_____

_____

_____

_____

DISCOVERY EXERCISES

1. Investigate the laws and the processes for reporting child, elder, or spouse abuse in your state.

2. Investigate the agencies in your area where abused elders or battered spouses can obtain help or emergency assistance.

3. Investigate programs in your area, such as the PANDA program, to learn more about recognizing and reporting family abuse and neglect.

The Patient with a Seizure Disorder

Chapter Outline

Learning Objectives

Upon successful completion of these exercises, you will be able to:

1. Identify and define key terms and concepts related to seizure disorders.
2. Identify cause, classifications, clinical manifestations, and emergency management of seizures.

3. Discuss oral considerations related to management of seizures.
4. Plan dental hygiene care for a patient with a history of seizure disorder.

Chapter 58 Crossword Puzzle

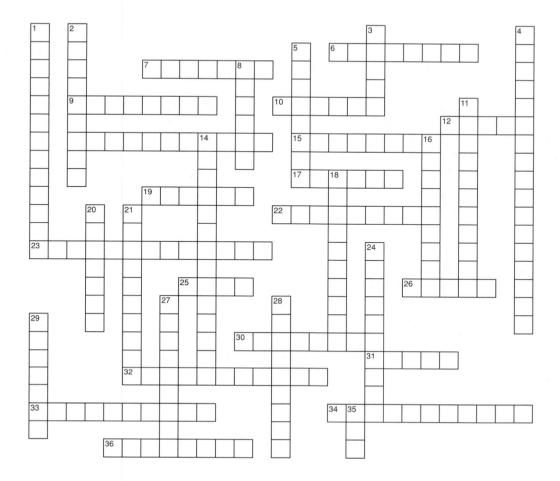

Across

6 Refers to a symptom that indicates the onset of a disease or condition.

7 Refers to a seizure that involves only part of the brain.

9 Describes a group of functional disorders of the brain characterized by recurrent seizures.

10 Type of seizure in which there is alternate contraction and relaxation of muscles.

12 Nerve that is stimulated by a pacemaker-like device implanted to reduce seizures.

13 Refers to a seizure condition that arises as a secondary symptom of a variety of neurologic and nonneurologic medical conditions.

15 The sudden recurrence or intensification of sharp spasms or convulsions.

17 Refers to irregular muscle action.

19 Refers to expression or appearance of the face.

22 Refers to the phase following a seizure when rest, reassurance, and palliative care for any oral trauma are administered.

23 Describes the degree of awareness or responsiveness.

25 A peculiar prodromal sensation experienced by some people immediately preceding a seizure.

26 Active, acute phase of an epileptic seizure.

30 Former term for absence seizure.

31 Sudden, involuntary contraction.

32 A disorder for which the cause is hidden.

33 Refers to a seizure disorder that does not resolve following treatment with a basic, single drug therapy.

34 Refers to a seizure that affects the entire brain at the same time.

36 Former term for a type of tonic–clonic epileptic seizure (two words).

Down

1 Remedy for seizures.

2 Impaired digestive function.

3 Refers to a state of continuous, unremitting muscular contractions.

4 A life-threatening emergency related to seizure disorders (two words).

5 Double vision.

8 Describes a muscle that is without normal tone or tension.

11 Abnormal burning, prickling, or tingling sensation.

14 Drug that inhibits convulsions.

16 Refers to shocklike contractions of muscles or groups of muscles.

18 Uncontrolled motor activity, such as repeated swallowing.

20 A type of seizure in which the person experiences a brief impairment of consciousness; manifests in a blank stare, fixed posture, and sometimes rhythmic face movements before a return to awareness with no recollection of the seizure.

21 Refers to a seizure condition with a primary (genetic or neurologic abnormality) etiology.

24 A term that means violent spasm.

27 Class of anticonvulsant drugs highly correlated with gingival hyperplasia.

28 Term associated with symptoms such as pallor, flushing, sweating, pupillary dilation, cardiac arrhythmia, or incontinence.

29 Unprovoked, unpredictable, and involuntary symptoms of a motor, sensory, cognitive, or emotional nature.

35 Electroencephalography; used to diagnose brain function.

KNOWLEDGE EXERCISES

1. A seizure is the result of what?

_____

_____

_____

2. Although most seizure disorders tend to be stable, some individuals experience a random pattern of seizures that disrupts their lives. List some activities that may be compromised for an individual who experiences recurrent seizures.

_____

_____

_____

3. It is important for you to ask your patient with a seizure disorder some questions about the conditions under which a seizure is more likely to occur. Identify factors that can trigger a seizure in a susceptible patient during dental hygiene treatment.

_____

_____

_____

4. If your patient has a history of seizure activity, when should you contact/consult with your patient's physician?

_____

_____

_____

5. In what three ways are epileptic syndromes classified?

_____

_____

6. List the subcategories for the partial and generalized epileptic seizures.

   ■ *Partial seizures*

_____

_____

   ■ *Generalized seizures*

_____

_____

_____

7. A partial seizure involves only part of the brain. In your own words, briefly describe the clinical manifestations of a partial seizure.

_____

_____

_____

8. A generalized seizure affects both sides of the brain at the same time. In your own words, briefly describe the clinical manifestations of an absence seizure.

_____

_____

_____

9. Describe a tonic–clonic seizure.

_____

_____

_____

10. List other medical conditions you need to consider if your patient is manifesting some clinical signs of a seizure, particularly if the patient's medical history does not indicate a seizure disorder. (*Hint:* Think "differential diagnosis.")

_____

_____

_____

11. If your patient does have a seizure during dental hygiene treatment, what emergency measures will you take to protect your patient from injury?

_____

_____

_____

12. What oral injuries are associated with generalized seizures?

_____

_____

_____

13. What action should you take in the event that your patient's tonic–clonic seizure continues for longer than 5 minutes?

_____

_____

_____

14. Describe status epilepticus.

_____

_____

_____

15. Identify surgical interventions that are used to treat patients with seizure disorders.

_____

_____

_____

16. Which treatment for seizure disorders will require you to modify the use of some dental devices during dental hygiene treatment?

_____

_____

_____

17. Your patient with a seizure disorder is likely to be taking an antiepileptic medication. Of the medications listed in Table 58-1 in the textbook, phenytoin (Dilantin) is the most likely to induce gingival hyperplasia in your patient. In your own words, describe the mechanism, incidence, appearance, and effects of phenytoin-induced gingival hyperplasia.

_____

_____

_____

_____

_____

_____

18. What medications, in addition to phenytoin, are associated with gingival overgrowth?

_____

_____

_____

19. Identify dental hygiene treatment and education interventions that can prevent or inhibit the growth of gingival tissues in your patient who is taking phenytoin or another medication that causes gingival enlargement.

_____

_____

20. What surgical options are available for treating phenytoin-induced gingival hyperplasia?

_____

_____

_____

COMPETENCY EXERCISES

1. You can tell that your new patient has a very business-like approach to his health care. Mr. Arakawa is a 45-year-old chief executive officer in a major corporation in town. As you lead him back to your treatment room, he stops briefly at the front desk to make sure of the procedure for submitting today's charges to his dental insurance. He mentions that he is on a tight schedule and wants to be sure about what time his appointment will end.

   He fills out the health history form you hand him with short, efficient strokes of his pen and hands it back to you. The only positive answers on the form are for seizure activity and medication, but he does not indicate what drug he is taking. You know that to completely understand Mr. Arakawa's condition, you must ask him more questions. Create a list of questions you will ask Mr. Arakawa as you clarify his health history information.

   _____

   _____

   _____

2. When you begin to ask Mr. Arakawa the questions you formulated, he briskly states that his history of seizures is not relevant to his dental treatment. He states that his previous dental provider never asked such questions, and, besides, he has not had a seizure for a long time. He tells you about the medication he is taking but is clearly not happy about answering the other questions you are asking.

   You know that he needs to understand why it is important for you to learn about his history of seizures. What information will you include in your discussion with Mr. Arakawa as you convince him to comply with your request for information about his seizures?

   _____

   _____

   _____

3. Your education/counseling approach is successful, and you find out that Mr. Arakawa has been experiencing seizures for almost 30 years. The severity of the tonic–clonic type seizures he experiences has

Everyday Ethics

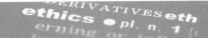

Refer to the Codes of Ethics (Appendices I, II, and III in the textbook) and Framework for Making Decisions (Table 1-2 in the textbook) as you discuss the following scenario with your classmates.

Lillian, the dental hygienist, just finished treating her last patient of the day. Diana, the patient, is a very pleasant woman with excellent oral health and a history of a car accident with concussion more than a month ago. She has no other medical findings. While passing the window, Lillian notices that Diana has collapsed in the parking lot and is convulsing. She calls for assistance from the dentist and assistant, and they rush out. By the time they reach Diana, she is getting to her feet and says she just tripped and fell.

Individuals with seizures may have their driver's license revoked because of the potential for serious automobile accidents that may occur during a seizure. Diana is about to get into her car to drive home.

Questions for Consideration

1. What actions of beneficence should Lillian and the dentist take toward Diana?
2. Given the patient's medical history, what condition could Diana be experiencing? How should this information be documented? Should it remain confidential or be shared with the patient's family, authorities, license bureau, and others?
3. Describe the rights of the patient and the professional duties of the dental hygienist having witnessed the incident. Explain your answer using the principles of autonomy and paternalism.

---

decreased since his teenage years, and in fact, the seizures are now fairly well under control.

The medication he is currently taking is an ethosuximide (Zarontin), but his previous prescription was a phenytoin (Dilantin), which he took for almost 20 years. About 10 years ago, he had gingival surgery to control gingival overgrowth he experienced from taking the phenytoin and fears that his gums are growing again.

Mr. Arakawa experienced some fairly serious dental trauma when he lost consciousness and fell during a seizure, and his maxillary anterior teeth have been replaced with a porcelain bridge. He has often bitten his lips and tongue when he is convulsing. One time when he was young, he experienced a seizure during routine dental treatment, and that is why he was at first reluctant and embarrassed to share much information about his seizures with you. He describes the aura that he experiences before a seizure, which appears as flashes of light just outside the direct view of his left eye. He also mentions that sometimes changing patterns of light have caused a seizure to happen and asks you to be careful when positioning the dental light during his treatment. His last seizure was about 2 years ago.

Using your institution's guidelines for writing in patient records, document what you have learned about Mr. Arakawa's medical condition.

Date	Comments	Signature
_____	_____	_____
_____	_____	_____
_____	_____	_____

4. You know that many medications prescribed to control seizures have numerous side effects, other than gingival hyperplasia, that are a concern for dental professionals. Refer to the list of potential side effects in the "Treatment" section of Chapter 58 in the textbook, and indicate which side effects have

Factors To Teach The Patient

Use the information provided in Chapter 58 in the textbook and the example of a patient conversation in Appendix B as a guide to prepare a conversation that you could use to provide patient education for Mr. Arakawa (introduced in Competency Exercises question 1). As you prepare the conversation, remember that you have already observed Mr. Arakawa's businesslike approach to health care. Make sure your education approach suits his personality.

Use the conversation you create to role play this situation with a fellow student. If you are the patient in the role play, be sure to ask questions. If you are the dental hygienist, try to anticipate questions and answer them in your explanation.

This scenario is related to the following factors:

■ Relationship of systemic health to oral health
■ Importance of careful daily care of mouth
■ Antiepileptic medication side effects, including gingival enlargement and how to minimize its growth
■ Seek immediate care if any oral change or injury is suspected

implications for patient education or treatment modifications during Mr. Arakawa's dental hygiene appointments.

_____

_____

_____

_____

_____

_____

5. When you examine Mr. Arakawa's mouth, you observe areas of advanced gingival hyperplasia. Use the decision tree in Figure 58-3 in the textbook to indicate what the next step would be in deciding appropriate treatment for this condition.

_____

_____

_____

_____

_____

_____

59 | CHAPTER

The Patient with a Mental Disability

Learning Objectives

Upon successful completion of these exercises, you will be able to:

1. Identify and define key terms and concepts related to the patient with a mental disability.
2. Identify the dimensions, intellectual functioning levels, risk factors, and etiologies associated with mental retardation.

3. Describe the specific characteristics of a person with Down syndrome and autistic spectrum disorders.
4. Plan modifications necessary for dental hygiene care and effective oral hygiene instruction for persons with mental disabilities.

Key Words and Concepts Crossword Puzzle

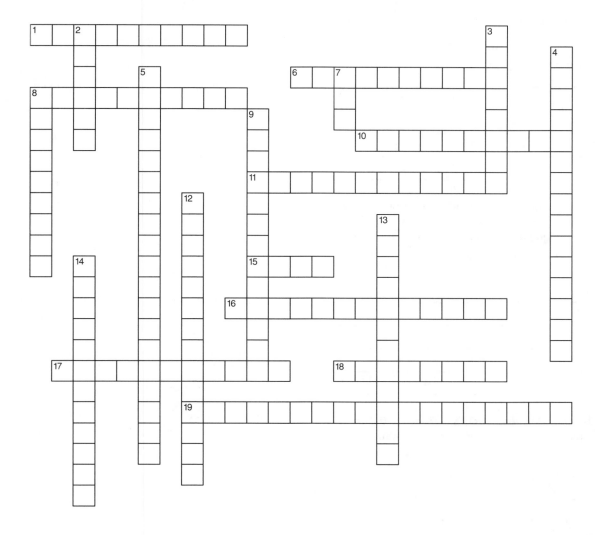

Across

1 Repeated regurgitation of food.
6 A behavior-management approach for dental professionals to use specifically for patients with autistic spectrum disorders.
8 A vertical fold of skin on either side of the nose; a normal characteristic of persons of some races that is associated with Down syndrome.
10 Involuntary utterance of vulgar or obscene words.
11 One of the autism spectrum disorders that occurs only in girls; characterized by repetitive hand movements (two words).
15 Persistent craving/eating of nonnutritive substances or unnatural articles of food.
16 Common characteristics or typical symptoms of a particular disease or syndrome.
17 Abnormality in morphologic development.
18 Category of mental retardation in which the individual would most likely need to have daily oral hygiene measures provided by a caregiver.
19 One of the autistic spectrum disorders that is characterized by no significant delays in language, cognitive ability, or developmental age-appropriate skills (two words).

Down

2 Inability or refusal to speak.
3 Category of mental retardation in which the individual could most likely attend to personal oral care with some reminders from a caregiver.
4 The reflection or transmission of ultrasonic waves in body tissues; can be used to examine a fetus to determine birth defects.
5 Expresses the results of tests that are used to determine an individual's level of intellectual functioning (two words).
7 An involuntary, recurrent, nonrhythmic motor movement or vocal sound.
8 The involuntary repetition of a word or sentence just spoken by another person.
9 Small size head in relation to the rest of the body.
12 Having a short, wide head.
13 Very large tongue.
14 Trisomy 21 syndrome (two words).

KNOWLEDGE EXERCISES

1. Identify the mental disorders that are usually first diagnosed before or during adolescence.

   _____

   _____

   _____

   _____

   _____

   _____

2. In your own words, write a description of mental retardation that includes a description of the five interrelated dimensions that contribute to testing an individual's functioning ability.

   _____

   _____

   _____

   _____

   _____

3. In your own words, briefly summarize the characteristics that describe each level of intellectual functioning.

   ◾ *Mild retardation*

   _____

   _____

   _____

   ◾ *Moderate retardation*

   _____

   _____

   _____

   ◾ *Severe retardation*

   _____

   _____

   _____

   ◾ *Profound retardation*

   _____

   _____

   _____

4. Identify the four types of risk factors for mental retardation.

   _____

   _____

   _____

5. What types of maternal behavior during pregnancy may result in an infant who has a mental disorder?

   _____

   _____

   _____

6. What can happen during the infant's birth that can lead to mental retardation?

   _____

   _____

   _____

7. When an infant is born normal, what two early childhood situations can lead to mental retardation?

   _____

   _____

   _____

8. Identify three characteristic anomalies you might note when performing your extraoral examination for your patient with mental retardation.

   _____

   _____

   _____

9. List five intraoral findings common in individuals with mental retardation.

   _____

   _____

   _____

10. List five characteristics that can help you identify an individual with Down syndrome.

    _____

    _____

    _____

11. What level of functioning do individuals with Down syndrome usually reach?

    _____

    _____

12. Most individuals with Down syndrome have pleasant personalities. Identify three personal characteristics that make these individuals likable and easy to be around.

_____

_____

_____

13. Why do patients with Down syndrome often present for dental treatment with very cracked and dried lips?

_____

_____

_____

14. What oral feature appears larger than it actually is in a patient with Down syndrome?

_____

_____

_____

15. Identify two physical/medical health problems commonly found in individuals with Down syndrome that require special consideration or modifications during dental hygiene treatment.

_____

_____

_____

16. Autistic spectrum disorders occur four times more frequently in _____ than in _____.

17. Briefly describe the characteristics that distinguish each of the five variations of pervasive development disorder.

_____

_____

_____

_____

_____

_____

_____

18. Describe two types of treatment used to manage symptoms and increase the ability of the patient with autism to live a normal life.

_____

_____

_____

19. Identify the five steps from the D-TERMINED program that you can use to help your patient with an autistic spectrum disorder learn how to cooperate with your dental hygiene interventions and self-care recommendations.

_____

_____

_____

COMPETENCY EXERCISES

1. Briefly summarize the strategies you can use to aid in providing clinical dental hygiene care for a patient with an autistic spectrum disorder.

_____

_____

_____

_____

_____

2. Next week you will be starting a new part-time position as the dental hygienist for 50 resident patients in a small private nursing center. You will go once a week to work with Dr. Sally Roderick, the dentist who has been providing dental care at the residence for 25 years. The individuals living in the residence are classified as having severe or profound mental retardation. You are excited about the opportunity to work with Dr. Roderick and to learn about this population, which you have only read about in your textbook.

   As you prepare for this new challenge, you create a list of planning measures you can take and modifications you can make to your usual treatment procedures so you can increase your effectiveness when providing dental hygiene care for these patients..

_____

_____

_____

_____

_____

3. On the first day at the nursing center, you find that Dr. Roderick has done very well providing her

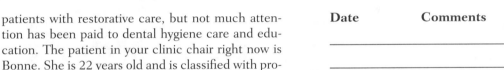

Everyday Ethics

Refer to the Codes of Ethics (Appendices I, II, and III in the textbook) and Framework for Making Decisions (Table 1-2 in the textbook) as you discuss the following scenario with your classmates.

At the Caring Community Dental Health Clinic, the first and third Mondays of each month are reserved for special-needs patients referred by health professionals in the local area. Adults and children with Down syndrome, autistic spectrum disorder, and other mental retardation are scheduled frequently for dental hygiene appointments. With only one full-time and one part-time dental hygienist, more hygiene appointment time has been needed. Dental hygiene students from a nearby dental hygiene program have been invited to rotate through the clinic as a community practicum experience.

Questions for Consideration
1. Two days before a scheduled assignment, Ellie, a student, confides to her classmate, Julie, that she cannot participate in this field experience because she is too afraid of people with mental disabilities. What are the ethical issues in this situation?
2. When arriving at the assignment, the students are greeted and oriented by the part-time hygienist, Ms. Gray. She advises the students, "Just get 'em in and get 'em out. They don't understand anything anyway, and it's a waste of your time to try to talk to them for patient instruction." What are the ethical principles applicable to this situation?
3. How might the students handle these ethical issues using the decision model in Table 1-2 (page 14) to determine an acceptable course of action?

---

patients with restorative care, but not much attention has been paid to dental hygiene care and education. The patient in your clinic chair right now is Bonne. She is 22 years old and is classified with profound mental retardation.

One of the nurse's aides, who is Bonne's regular caregiver, helps you place Bonne in the papoose board and sits by the side of the dental chair to help when she can. You have some difficulty examining Bonne's mouth, but you can readily see that she has extensive biofilm buildup and significant amounts of calculus in all areas of her mouth.

You know that it will take more than one appointment to assess Bonne's dental hygiene needs thoroughly and to make a full plan for care. However, Dr. Roderick asks you to write up a formal dental hygiene care plan for what you will accomplish in the next three or four appointments so that it can be recorded in Bonne's medical record. You know that you must plan enough time for the complete assessment that you need to accomplish before you can fully understand Bonne's oral condition. You must also plan for daily biofilm control.

Use the Dental Hygiene Care Plan Template in Appendix B to develop a formal, written care plan for clinical procedures and educational interventions you will provide during the four appointments you will schedule in the next few weeks for Bonne and her caregiver.

4. Today when you saw Bonne in the clinic, you reviewed her medical history, provided a limited intra-oral assessment examination, and developed a written care plan. Use your institution's guidelines for writing in patient records to document these procedures.

Date	Comments	Signature

Factors To Teach The Patient

Use information in Chapter 59 in the textbook and the example of a patient conversation in Appendix B as guides to develop a conversation you will use to provide oral hygiene instructions for a patient who is classified with moderate mental retardation. Include the patient's caregiver as you discuss strategies for daily oral care.

Use the conversation you create to role play this situation with a fellow student. If you are the patient or the caregiver in the role play, be sure to ask questions. If you are the dental hygienist, try to anticipate questions and answer them in your explanation. Modify your conversation based on what you learned.

This scenario is related to the following factors:
For the patient:

- How to perform oral self-care procedures
- Why assistance from others is an important supplement to the patient's own efforts
- How to use and show cooperation skills

For the caregiver:

- Why a total preventive program is important
- How to incorporate behavior modification into oral care procedures
- The importance of repeating "show-tell-do" instructions often

CHAPTER 60

The Patient with a Psychiatric Disorder

Chapter Outline

Learning Objectives

Upon successful completion of these exercises, you will be able to:

1. Identify and define key terms and concepts related to psychiatric disorders.
2. Describe the symptoms, treatment, and oral implications of a variety of psychiatric and mood disorders.

3. Plan dental hygiene care and oral health education for a patient with a psychiatric disorder.

KNOWLEDGE EXERCISES

1. Why is it more appropriate to refer to your patient as "an individual with bulimia" rather than as "a bulimic"?

   _____

   _____

   _____

2. In what way are agitation, bradykinesia, akinesia, and catatonia related? How are they different?

   _____

   _____

   _____

   _____

   _____

   _____

3. What is a psychotropic medication?

   _____

   _____

4. In your own words, define *schizophrenia*.

   _____

   _____

   _____

5. List three phases of schizophrenia.

   _____

   _____

   _____

6. Identify five behavioral characteristics that can pre-cede or follow the active phase of schizophrenia (see Box 60-2 in the textbook).

   _____

   _____

   _____

   _____

   _____

   _____

7. List five types of profoundly unusual behavior that are considered symptoms of the active phase of schizophrenia.

   _____

   _____

   _____

8. Identify the concept or term defined by each of the following statements.

   ▪ *A false sensory perception in the absence of an actual external stimulus*

   _____

   _____

   _____

   ▪ *A mental impression derived from misinterpretation of an actual sensory stimulus; a false perception*

   _____

   _____

   _____

   ▪ *A false belief firmly held though contradicted by social reality*

   _____

   _____

   _____

▪ *A psychiatric disorder characterized by delusions of persecution, illusions of grandeur, or a combination of both*

   _____

   _____

   _____

9. Unfortunately, many people diagnosed with schizo-phrenia also qualify for a diagnosis of _____. This condition can aggravate psychiatric symptoms and complicate treatment.

10. Schizophrenia is associated with an excess of dopamine at specific synapses in the brain. List the brand names of three antipsychotic medications that block dopamine receptors.

    _____

    _____

    _____

11. In your own words, define *dysarthria*.

    _____

    _____

    _____

12. What is tardive dyskinesia?

    _____

    _____

    _____

13. During a scaling and root planing procedure, how can you facilitate safety and comfort of your patient with tardive dyskinesia?

    _____

    _____

    _____

14. Major depressive disorder and bipolar disorder are the primary _____ disorders discussed in the textbook chapter.

15. List reasons why the elderly are more susceptible to major depressive episodes.

    _____

    _____

16. List five characteristics that, if demonstrated by your patient, can help you identify a major depressive episode.

_____

_____

_____

17. Identify five types of medications that are prescribed to stabilize the mood for individuals with depression.

_____

_____

_____

18. What oral condition is a frequent side effect of medications used to treat depression?

_____

_____

_____

19. What preventive measures can you recommend for your patient to help combat the effects of the medications used to treat depression?

_____

_____

_____

20. Why might you offer tinted protective eyewear for a patient who is taking medications to treat depression?

_____

_____

_____

21. If your patient's depression is not well controlled by medication, what personal/emotional factors can influence the way in which you need to approach oral hygiene instructions?

_____

_____

_____

22. List two specific behaviors you should avoid in your approach to oral health education for a patient with depression.

_____

_____

23. Identify three situations in which electroconvulsive therapy is used to treat an individual with depression.

_____

_____

_____

24. Define _euphoria_.

_____

_____

_____

25. In what way is bipolar disorder different from major depressive disorder?

_____

_____

_____

26. How is bipolar depression treated?

_____

_____

_____

27. What drug used to treat bipolar disorder can impart a metallic taste in your patient's mouth?

_____

_____

_____

28. Provide five characteristics common to the manic phase of bipolar disorder.

_____

_____

_____

29. Define _postpartum depression_.

_____

_____

_____

30. Compare postpartum blues and postpartum psychosis.

_____

_____

_____

31. List the four types of anxiety disorders described in the textbook.

_____

_____

_____

32. Briefly describe each of the three types of treatment provided for a patient with anxiety disorder.

_____

_____

_____

_____

_____

_____

33. What oral problems are associated with anxiety disorders?

_____

_____

_____

34. List three risk factors for the occurrence of a dental psychiatric emergency during a dental hygiene appointment.

_____

_____

_____

35. In your own words, describe measures you can take to prevent or prepare for a psychiatric emergency.

_____

_____

_____

_____

_____

36. If your patient has a panic attack while you are providing dental hygiene care, what should you do?

_____

_____

_____

37. Identify and briefly describe the three types of serious eating disorders.

_____

_____

_____

_____

_____

_____

_____

38. Discuss the effects of perimylolysis as it relates to bulimia.

_____

_____

_____

COMPETENCY EXERCISES

1. Study the list of potential effects of antipsychotic medications in Table 60-1 in the textbook. Identify at least three modifications you would make beyond your usual clinical routines to ensure the comfort and safety of your patient, who is taking an antipsychotic medication.

_____

_____

_____

_____

_____

2. When you check his health history before calling Jack into your treatment room at the VA hospital, you note that he has been diagnosed with schizophrenia. You greet him cheerfully and talk to him brightly all the way down the hall to your room about how beautifully the sun is shining today. You ask him, with a smile, if there have been any changes in his medications since he was last seen in the dental clinic.

   You suspect that he is displaying the negative symptoms of the active phase of his disorder. Describe the type of responses that Jack displays in this situation. Make sure you don't just list the symptoms mentioned in Box 60-2 in the textbook, but rather describe what you might observe about Jack's demeanor or behavior based on the symptoms.

_____

_____

_____

_____

_____

_____

_____

_____

_____

3. Shaun Kennedy, a newspaper reporter, has been your patient for several years. You always enjoy the stories he tells about working for the newspaper. His oral hygiene has never been particularly good, and you have been really working with him each time he comes in to make sure he understands how his risk for oral disease increases when he doesn't thoroughly remove the dental biofilm from his teeth every day. You know that he is receiving treatment for bipolar disorder but, so far, you have not noticed that he ever displays any symptoms of either the manic phase or the depressive phase of his disease.

   Today Shaun is talking a mile a minute about a new novel he has started writing. As he gets more excited about telling you the plot of the novel, he actually pushes your hands aside, leaps up from the chair, and walks back and forth in your small treatment space! You would really like to convince him to get back in the dental chair so you can complete your oral hygiene instructions in a timely manner. What can happen if you pressure him to comply? Given Shaun's behavior today, how can you sensitively and realistically approach this situation?

_____

_____

4. Compare and contrast the four types of anxiety disorders. (_Hint:_ Create an Infomap with identifying symptoms, severity, and predisposing factors for each type.)

_____

_____

_____

_____

_____

_____

5. Isabella Stamos, 13 years old, is a beautiful girl with long curly blond hair, huge green eyes, and an already successful modeling career. You still have not started your intraoral examination, but after talking with her and observing her for several minutes, you suspect that she has an eating disorder. What clinical clues or signs can you look for to help confirm your impressions? What questions will you ask Isabella to help you determine if your suspicions are correct?

_____

_____

_____

Everyday Ethics

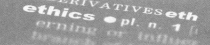

Refer to the Codes of Ethics (Appendices I, II, and III in the textbook) and Framework for Making Decisions (Table 1-2 in the textbook) as you discuss the following scenario with your classmates.

Samuel, age 28, suffers from panic disorder and generally requests short appointments because he becomes very anxious while receiving dental care. Even with a moderate amount of generalized deposits, Ginny, the dental hygienist, usually schedules two visits to complete the treatment.

   During his visit today, Samuel appears in an almost dream-like state. He was asked by the receptionist at the check-in about any new medications, but he stated that only a sleep aid was added to his pills, which he takes at night. Ginny suspects the patient may have taken his

medication incorrectly and is concerned that Samuel is driving home after the appointment.

Questions for Consideration
1. Without breaching confidentiality, what ethical or other responsibility does Ginny have in verifying the type and amount of medication Samuel took, and how does that influence the current day's dental hygiene appointment procedures?
2. If Ginny feels he might harm himself or others, how would Samuel be deemed competent to drive a car after leaving the dental office?
3. What would be the appropriate documentation for this patient given his change of behavior compared with previous appointments? How would decisions for treatment be adjusted?

Factors To Teach The Patient

You have talked with Isabella (introduced in Competency Exercise question 5) about some ways she can receive help with her eating disorder, but as a dental hygienist, you know that the most important thing you can do is educate her about the risks to her oral health.

Use the example of a patient conversation in Appendix B as a guide, taking into account the personal factors that often accompany this disorder, educate Isabella about the negative oral findings common in a patient with bulimia. Discuss strategies for protecting her teeth and gums until she gets her eating behaviors under control.
This scenario is related to the following factors:

■ The causes and effects of enamel erosion; the high acidity of the vomitus from the stomach
■ How to rinse after vomiting but not brush immediately; demineralization begins promptly after the acid from the stomach reaches the teeth, and brushing can cause abrasion of the demineralizing enamel
■ The need for multiple fluoride applications through use of home dentifrice, rinse, and brush-on gel, as well as professional application of varnish or gel-tray at regular dental hygiene appointments

6. After you have questioned Isabella and completed an intraoral examination, it becomes clear that she is battling with bulimia nervosa. What ethical factors will you take into consideration when you discuss your assessment findings and Isabella's oral health needs with her mother at the end of the appointment?

_____

_____

_____

_____

The Patient with a Substance-Related Disorder

Learning Objectives

Upon successful completion of these exercises, you will be able to:

1. Identify and define key terms and concepts related to alcohol and drug use.
2. Identify physical and behavioral factors associated with alcohol and drug use.

3. Describe health-related effects of alcohol and drug use, abuse, and withdrawal.
4. Plan dental hygiene care for the patient with a substance-related disorder.

KNOWLEDGE EXERCISES

1. Define the following terms and concepts in your own words to help you differentiate them and understand what they mean.

   ▪ *Abuse*

   _____

   _____

   _____

   ▪ *Dependence*

   _____

   _____

   _____

   ▪ *Addiction*

   _____

   _____

   _____

■ *Tolerance*

_____

_____

_____

■ *Alcoholism*

_____

_____

_____

■ *Polysubstance dependence*

_____

_____

_____

2. What are the differences between chemical, physical, and psychologic dependence?

_____

_____

_____

3. Identify the levels in the spectrum of alcohol use.

_____

_____

_____

4. Identify the signs of alcoholism.

_____

_____

_____

5. What is *acne rosacea?*

_____

_____

_____

6. What factors contribute to the etiology of alcoholism?

_____

_____

_____

7. How is the concentration of alcohol in the blood measured?

_____

_____

_____

8. What behavioral characteristics, if you observe them in an otherwise healthy patient, might indicate that your patient is intoxicated?

_____

_____

_____

9. Define *nystagmus.*

_____

_____

_____

10. The liver is the organ most severely affected by chronic alcohol abuse. Briefly describe the adverse effects of excessive or prolonged alcohol use on each of the following body systems.

■ *Immune system*

_____

_____

■ *Digestive system*

_____

_____

_____

■ *Cardiovascular system*

_____

_____

■ *Nervous system*

_____

_____

■ *Reproductive system*

_____

_____

_____

11. In what ways does excessive alcohol consumption affect nutritional intake?

_____

_____

12. Describe the two types of complications that can occur if an individual abruptly withdraws from alcohol use.

    ◼ *Alcohol hallucinosis*

    _____

    _____

    _____

    ◼ *Alcohol withdrawal delirium (DTs)*

    _____

    _____

    _____

13. Identify factors that can increase the severity of the symptoms that a person with alcoholism may experience if he or she abruptly ceases drinking.

    _____

    _____

    _____

14. What is the overall objective of treatment provided to support an individual who is recovering from alcoholism?

    _____

    _____

    _____

15. List the four components of an alcohol treatment program.

    _____

    _____

    _____

16. Your patient who is participating in an alcohol recovery program may be taking an alcohol-sensitizing agent such as Antabuse because these drugs act as a deterrent to consuming alcohol. If alcohol is taken, this drug interferes with the conversion of _____ to _____ in the liver and makes the patient very ill.

17. Identify the drug that is prescribed for the recovering alcoholic to help inhibit or decrease the desire to consume alcohol.

    _____

    _____

    _____

18. Use of alcohol during pregnancy can seriously threaten the health of the baby because

    _____

    _____.

19. The mother's general health status, _____, _____, and _____ are additional factors linked with alcohol intake that may influence the baby's health.

20. Describe the facial features that are observed in an infant with FAS.

    ◼ *Eyes*

    _____

    _____

    _____

    ◼ *Ears*

    _____

    _____

    _____

    ◼ *Nose*

    _____

    _____

    _____

    ◼ *Lips*

    _____

    _____

    _____

21. Identify behavioral, cognitive, and psychomotor factors associated with FAS.

    _____

    _____

    _____

22. What is FAE?

    _____

    _____

    _____

23. What is ARBD?

    _____

    _____

    _____

24. List the categories of drugs that are most commonly abused.

_____

_____

_____

25. Identify oral manifestations associated with the use of each of the following drugs.

   ■ _Methamphetamine_

   _____

   _____

   ■ _Other amphetamine-based drugs_

   _____

   _____

   ■ _Cocaine_

   _____

   _____

   ■ _Cannabis_

   _____

   _____

   _____

26. Which body systems can be adversely affected by excessive use of drugs?

   _____

   _____

   _____

27. Identify medications commonly used to assist in lessening withdrawal symptoms during treatment for drug abuse.

   _____

   _____

   _____

COMPETENCY EXERCISES

1. Explain observations you can make—while greeting a patient in the waiting room and as he or she is being seated in your treatment room—that can help you to identify a patient who has a substance-related disorder.

   _____

   _____

   _____

   _____

   _____

   _____

2. Explain why it is especially important to inspect intraoral tissues each time you assess a patient who has a past or current history of excessive alcohol consumption or other drug use.

   _____

   _____

   _____

3. Your next patient is Justin Townsley, age 21. He has just returned home from his first year away at college. His mother has made a dental hygiene appointment for him because he has not had his teeth examined in at least 3 years. She also wants him to have his wisdom teeth extracted before he is no longer covered under her dental insurance plan. When you go to greet Justin in the reception area, you overhear the end of a cell phone conversation in which he is planning to meet his buddies later on this evening to go out partying. "And, we'll stay out all night so we can have even more fun _this_ time than we did _last_ time," he says just before he hangs up the telephone to greet you. He stumbles just a bit as he rises from the chair but recovers quickly to follow you to the treatment room. As he walks past you into the chair, you distinctly catch the odor of alcohol on his breath.

   Justin's health history is unremarkable except for having an arm broken in an automobile accident last year. He states that he does not take any regular medications. When you take his pulse and blood pressure today, both are slightly elevated.

   Your intraoral findings include generalized poor oral hygiene, significant calculus deposits, coated tongue, dry oral mucosa, red and swollen gingiva, generalized 4- to 6-mm probing depths, and generalized bleeding on probing. Justin states that "the left side of my jaw has been aching a lot lately, probably from grinding my teeth." A front tooth and the cusp of an upper premolar are both slightly chipped, findings that were not previously noted. As you are working to complete your oral assessment, Justin keeps up a constant conversation about how much fun he has had this year while he was away at college. He sheepishly admits that his daily oral care has suffered, saying, "I stay up all night sometimes—to

Everyday Ethics

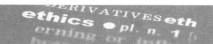

Refer to the Codes of Ethics (Appendices I, II, and III in the textbook) and Framework for Making Decisions (Table 1-2 in the textbook) as you discuss the following scenario with your classmates.

Adam Morse arrives at Dr. Greene's dental office late on a Friday afternoon as an emergency patient. He states that he has a very painful tooth and asks to be checked. The receptionist asks him to complete the necessary forms and a medical history.

Leslie, the hygienist, reviews the medical history and learns that Adam is allergic to several drugs. He seems nervous and restless in the chair and comments that Percocet usually works well when he is in pain. After taking a radiograph of tooth no. 14, Leslie consults with Dr. Greene.

She returns to tell Adam the dentist will be in shortly. Adam states that he really can't wait. He is on business in town and just needs a prescription for the pain to get him through the weekend. He will have his own dentist take care of the restoration on Monday morning.

Dr. Greene refuses to prescribe Percocet, but offers the patient a nonsteroidal anti-inflammatory drug.

Questions for Consideration

1. Has the patient disclosed enough information to Leslie and/or Dr. Greene to refuse further treatment based on accepted standards of care? Why or why not?
2. What documentation is needed for Adam's record for the appointment?
3. Discuss the indicators that this patient may be a substance abuser.

---

study for all those midterm and final exams, you know. Sometimes I just forget to brush."

You decide that you need ask Justin about his drinking and the possible use of stimulant drugs. Identify the assessment findings that lead you to this decision.

_____

_____

_____

4. What other signs and symptoms will you look for as you continue your assessment?

_____

_____

_____

5. What additional follow-up questions will you ask Justin to help you determine his patterns of alcohol and/or drug use?

_____

_____

_____

6. Your careful and sensitive questioning leads you to believe that Justin's level of alcohol consumption and possible use of street drugs is probably having some detrimental impact on his health status. You are concerned enough that you discuss the matter with him,

Factors To Teach The Patient

Discussing your concerns about potential substance abuse with a patient like Justin Townsley (introduced in Competency Exercises question 3) requires building trust. You will be more successful in educating Justin and changing his health behaviors if you approach him without disapproval or judgment, but instead give him important information that motivates him to make changes in his own behaviors.

Use information in Chapter 61 of the textbook and the example of a patient conversation in Appendix B as guides to develop a conversation you will use to discuss the negative effects that alcohol and other drugs can have on Justin's health status.

Use the conversation you create to role play this situation with a friend or fellow student. If you are the patient in the role play, be sure to ask questions. If you are the dental hygienist, try to anticipate questions and answer them in your explanation. Modify your conversation based on what you learned.

This scenario is related to the following factors:

- Drug abuse is a great risk to overall health.
- The risk of oral cancer is increased by the use of alcohol.
- Routine oral screening is needed at least twice a year to check for signs of early cancer.
- Drinking alcohol and using other drugs (prescription or over-the-counter) can lead to medical emergencies. Always check each drug and its action before using it in combination with alcohol or in combination with another drug.

and you give him a brochure about the oral effects of alcohol. You plan to bring your concerns for his health up again at his subsequent appointments. When you write a dental hygiene care plan for Justin, you will plan two additional visits for scaling and root planing his entire mouth. What education/counseling and oral hygiene instructions/home-care interventions will you plan to help Justin maximize healing and tissue response during and after oral débridement? (*Hint:* When you write dental hygiene diagnosis statements for Justin, it will help you decide on your planned interventions.)

_____

_____

_____

7. Using your institution's guidelines for writing in patient records, document progress notes for your first appointment with Justin.

Date	Comments	Signature

CHAPTER 62

The Patient with a Respiratory Disease

Chapter Outline

Learning Objectives

Upon successful completion of these exercises, you will be able to:

1. Identify and define key terms and concepts related to respiratory diseases.
2. Differentiate between upper and lower respiratory tract diseases.

3. Describe a variety of respiratory diseases.
4. Plan dental hygiene care and oral hygiene instructions for patients with compromised respiratory function.

KNOWLEDGE EXERCISES

1. What should you do if you recognize that your patient is experiencing symptoms of respiratory distress during dental hygiene treatment?

   _____

   _____

   _____

2. A patient in respiratory distress may experience hypoxia. What patient signs and symptoms characterize hypoxia?

   _____

   _____

   _____

3. _____ is defined as a breathing rate of greater than 20 breaths per minute. A patient

who is breathing very rapidly can experience
_____, which may lead to dizziness and
possible syncope.

4. What body structures are considered to be in the
   upper respiratory system?

   _____

   _____

   _____

5. What body structures compose the lower respiratory
   system?

   _____

   _____

   _____

6. What are the pleura?

   _____

   _____

   _____

7. Identify two functions of the mucus secreted from
   goblet cells in respiratory mucosa.

   _____

   _____

   _____

8. What happens when an inflammatory disease
   causes an overproduction of mucus?

   _____

   _____

   _____

9. _____ is the profuse mucous membrane dis-
   charge that often accompanies upper respiratory
   infections.

10. Identify three upper respiratory diseases that are
    more likely to be viral rather than bacterial infec-
    tions.

    _____

    _____

    _____

11. What medication is used primarily to treat bacterial
    respiratory infections but is not prescribed for infec-
    tions caused by a virus or fungus?

_____

_____

_____

12. How are upper respiratory infections transmitted?

    _____

    _____

    _____

13. How can you best prevent transmission of pathogens
    while you are providing dental hygiene treatment?

    _____

    _____

    _____

14. What type of upper respiratory infection can cause
    tooth pain?

    _____

    _____

    _____

15. Identify two oral side effects of medications com-
    monly used to treat upper respiratory infections.

    _____

    _____

    _____

16. What oral lesions can accompany the infectious
    stage of an upper respiratory infection?

    _____

    _____

    _____

17. Is pneumonia considered an upper or a lower respi-
    ratory tract disease?

    _____

    _____

    _____

18. Identify three types of organisms that can cause
    pneumonia.

    _____

    _____

    _____

19. What medical treatment is provided for each type of pneumonia identified in question 18?

_____

_____

_____

20. What pathogen causes a type of pneumonia most often associated with immune-impaired individuals?

_____

_____

_____

21. What signs and symptoms are associated with tuberculosis?

_____

_____

_____

22. How is clinically active tuberculosis diagnosed?

_____

_____

_____

23. What diagnostic test is used to determine a latent tuberculosis infection?

_____

_____

_____

24. What medication regimen is used to treat the clinically active stage of tuberculosis?

_____

_____

_____

25. Define *dyspnea*.

_____

_____

_____

26. Identify and explain the two traditional classifications of asthma.

_____

_____

_____

27. List and briefly explain the four NAEPP classifications of asthma.

_____

_____

_____

_____

_____

28. What are the signs and symptoms of an asthma attack?

_____

_____

_____

29. What types of drugs are used in the treatment of asthma?

_____

_____

_____

30. List the drugs an individual with asthma should avoid.

_____

_____

_____

31. What ingredient in local anesthetic solutions can cause an asthma attack?

_____

_____

_____

32. What oral condition may occur in patients being treated for asthma?

_____

_____

_____

33. What is the primary cause of COPD?

_____

_____

34. Patients with COPD who are chronic smokers have an increased risk for which oral conditions?

_____

_____

_____

35. The term *blue bloater* is related to _____.

_____

_____

_____

36. Describe the cough of an individual with chronic bronchitis.

_____

_____

_____

37. What are the symptoms of emphysema?

_____

_____

_____

38. Cystic fibrosis is a complex genetic condition that limits the life span and involves the lungs, _____, and _____.

39. Complete **Infomap 62-1** below to compare three types of hypersensitivity reactions.

40. What oral changes are likely to occur as cystic fibrosis progresses?

_____

_____

_____

COMPETENCY EXERCISES

1. Charles Marcin, a handsome blond gentleman who is 67 years old, has been a patient in this dental practice for many years; but this is the first time you have met him. His health history confirms your first impression of Mr. Marcin as a patient with COPD, and you remember the term *pink puffer* from your textbook. You observe Mr. Marcin carefully as he walks the short distance from the reception room to your treatment room. He rests with his head bent and his hands on the back of the dental chair to catch his breath before he sits down.

   Describe what you observe as you watch Mr. Marcin's breathing pattern, and explain how it is different from the breathing pattern of an individual with other respiratory diseases.

   _____

   _____

   _____

   _____

   _____

   _____

2. When he can talk again, Mr. Marcin reminds you to call him Charlie. He says he has recently had a bit of a cold but is feeling somewhat better now. He tells you that his cough has pretty much gone away, and he isn't blowing his nose every 5 minutes any more. He reports that this is already his second cold this year, and once he was treated for a sinus infection. He mentions his teeth are stained because he has been drinking so much hot tea lately, and he is excited about being in your office today so that he can have an especially bright smile for his daughter's wedding this coming weekend. You think back to everything you learned about respiratory diseases as you plan Mr.

INFOMAP 62-1		
CONDITION	**PATHOGENESIS**	**SIGNS/SYMPTOMS**
Allergic Rhinitis (Hay Fever)		
Atopic Asthma		
Anaphylaxis		

Everyday Ethics

Refer to the Codes of Ethics (Appendices I, II, and III in the textbook) and Framework for Making Decisions (Table 1-2 in the textbook) as you discuss the following scenario with your classmates.

On a beautiful spring day, Lana Thomas arrived for her 3-month preventive maintenance visit. Vicki, the dental hygienist, noticed a labored breathing pattern as they walked down the hall to the dental hygiene treatment room. She rechecked the patient history before beginning the intraoral assessment but found the information unremarkable.

Lana offered that she was taking an OTC product for seasonal allergies but it didn't seem to be helping with her nasal and chest congestion. The patient also requested that she not be placed so far back in the dental chair because it was difficult for her to breathe. Vicki began to reconsider her plan to use the ultrasonic scaler given the patient's current condition.

Questions to Consider
1. What baseline information is needed about the patient before proceeding?
2. Under what circumstances would a medical consultation be needed?
3. How can certain dental hygiene "core values" apply in the clinical adaptations that are needed during Lana's treatment? (Refer to Table II-1, page 20.)

Marcin's appointment for today. What safety and comfort factors will you need to assess and consider as you provide care during Mr. Marcin's dental hygiene appointment today?

_____

_____

_____

_____

_____

3. Mr. Mitch Angelo is currently taking several medications to treat his asthma. When you are examining his mouth, you notice enamel erosion on the lingual areas of the anterior teeth. Explain what is happening that may be contributing to this oral condition.

_____

_____

_____

4. When you have completed the first quadrant of scaling and root planing, you mention to Mr. Angelo that the gingival tissue in that area might be a bit sensitive later on today. He asks you what he should do if he feels pain. Which analgesics does a patient with asthma need to avoid?

_____

_____

_____

5. When you update his medical history, Mr. Ben Samuelson, a 45-year-old businessman, tells you that he has been taking a new medication called isoniazid. When you question him further, he states that he does not know why he is taking it. What follow-up questions will you ask Mr. Samuelson?

_____

_____

_____

Factors To Teach The Patient

Because of Mr. Marcin's chronic emphysema (patient introduced in Competency Exercises case study), you are concerned about his recurring upper respiratory infections. Use the information in Chapter 62 in the textbook and the example of a patient conversation in Appendix B as guides to write a statement explaining ways that Mr. Marcin can reduce his risk for reinfection or his risk for more serious respiratory diseases.
This scenario is related to the following factors:

- The need for frequent handwashing to help prevent transmission of respiratory disease
- The need for thorough daily cleaning of toothbrushes to help prevent spread of infections
- How using a new toothbrush and cleaning dentures/orthodontic appliances after bacterial infections can decrease the possibility of reinfection
- Why elderly patients and those with chronic cardiovascular disease, diabetes, and other immunosuppressed conditions should receive a pneumonia vaccine and annual influenza immunizations

6. What additional steps will you take before beginning your assessment of Mr. Samuelson's oral condition?

_____

_____

_____

7. Explain the role of oral bacteria as a potential pathogenic agent in pneumonia, particularly if the patient is debilitated or chronically ill.

_____

_____

_____

CHAPTER 63

The Patient with a Cardiovascular Disease

Chapter Outline

Learning Objectives

Upon successful completion of these exercises, you will be able to:

1. Identify and define key terms and concepts related to cardiovascular disease.
2. Describe the cause, symptoms, prevention, and treatment of major cardiovascular diseases.

3. Identify clinical considerations and oral health factors related to cardiovascular conditions.
4. Plan dental hygiene care for a patient with cardiovascular disease.

Heartfelt Dental Hygiene Care Crossword Puzzle

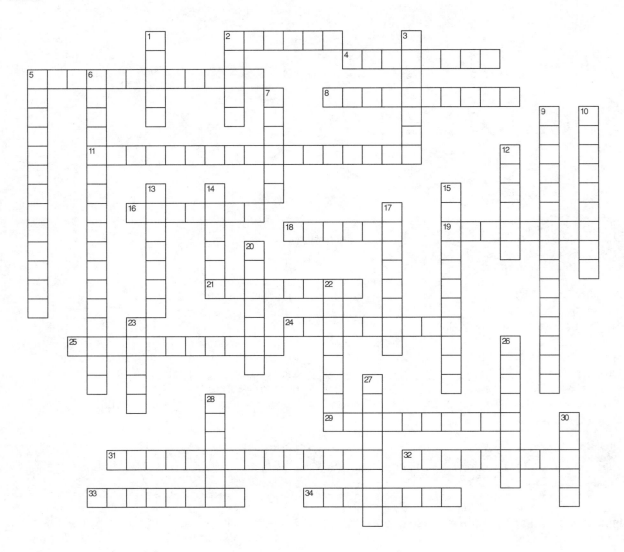

Across

2 Dividing wall between left and right ventricles in the heart.
4 Refers to narrowing or constriction (of an artery).
5 Refers to the lipid plaque that deposits on the lining of an artery.
8 The middle layer of the heart wall.
11 Congenital cyanotic malformation of the heart that includes four specific disease conditions (three words).
16 Labored or difficult breathing that may be a symptom of cardiovascular disease.
18 Irregularity of heartbeat caused by turbulent flow of blood flowing through a valve that has failed to close.
19 Bluish coloration caused by reduced hemoglobin in the blood.
21 Deficiency of oxygen and increase of carbon dioxide in the blood.
24 Natural or artificial mechanism that maintains a reliable heart rhythm.
25 Slowing of pulse to less than 60 beats per minute.
29 Variation (of the heart) from its normal rhythm.

31 The record that is produced when a beam of ultrasonic waves is directed to record the position and motion of structures in the heart.
32 Refers to the blockage or closing (of a blood vessel).
33 Caused by an object (blood clot, air bubble, or clump of bacteria) that suddenly blocks an artery.
34 Refers to a localized dilation of the wall of a blood vessel.

Down

1 Refers to the channel inside a blood vessel.
2 A term meaning passageway (as in patent ductus arteriosus).
3 Localized area of ischemic necrosis in the heart.
5 A substance that interferes with coagulation of the blood.
6 The record that is produced by recording electric currents generated by the heart; EKG.
7 The nonoxygenated blood that returns from body tissues to the heart and is pumped from the heart to the lungs.
9 Narrowing of the lining of a blood vessel by fatty deposits containing cholesterol.

10 Characterized by hardening, thickening, and loss of elasticity.
12 A disease that causes acute, spasmodic pain attack.
13 Diminished availability of oxygen to blood tissues.
14 Related to absence of oxygen in tissues; symptoms include deep respirations, cyanosis, increased pulse rate, and reduced coordination.
15 Abnormally rapid heart rate; usually more than 100 beats per minute.
17 Oxygenated blood that flows from the heart to nourish body tissues.
20 An anticoagulant.
22 Deficiency of blood to supply oxygen (to the heart); result of constriction or obstruction of a blood vessel.
23 Abnormal accumulation of fluid in body tissues.
26 Refers to the downward displacement of the mitral valve between the left atrium and the left ventricle of the heart.
27 Refers to a blood clot attached to the interior of a blood vessel.
28 A term that refers to the surgical procedure that redirects blood flow around a narrowed heart artery.
30 Temporary cessation of breathing.

KNOWLEDGE EXERCISES

1. Identify two ways to classify heart diseases.

    _____

    _____

    _____

2. Identify the various tissues in the heart that can be affected by cardiovascular disease.

    _____

    _____

    _____

3. Refer to Figure 63-1 in the textbook to help you visualize the veins, arteries, and chambers of a healthy heart. Describe the sequence of the normal flow of blood.

    _____

    _____

    _____

4. Congenital heart disease is the result of anatomic anomalies that occur during the first _____ weeks of fetal development. The exact cause is often unknown but is either _____, _____, or a combination of the two.

5. Refer to Figures 63-2 and 63-3 from the textbook to help you describe how the normal path of blood flow is compromised in each of the two types of congenital heart disease.

    ■ *Ventricular septal defect*

    _____

    _____

    _____

    ■ *Patent ductus arteriosus*

    _____

    _____

    _____

6. What is the etiology of rheumatic heart disease?

    _____

    _____

    _____

7. Describe the flow of blood through the heart when there is a mitral valve prolapse.

    _____

    _____

    _____

8. In your own words, describe the progression and diagnosis of infective endocarditis.

    _____

    _____

    _____

9. List steps you can take to prevent infection during oral assessment and dental-hygiene treatment if you suspect your patient is at risk for infective endocarditis.

    _____

    _____

    _____

10. Identify conditions that put your patient at risk for infective endocarditis.

    _____

    _____

    _____

11. Recording a patient's blood pressure is an essential step in patient assessment before dental hygiene care. Blood pressure is recorded as a fraction: systolic/diastolic pressure in millimeters of mercury. In your own words, define systolic and diastolic blood pressure.

    ■ *Systolic*

    _____

    _____

    ■ *Diastolic*

    _____

    _____

12. Patient screening and early detection of hypertension are important components of dental hygiene care because, in early stages, this condition is often unrecognized owing to lack of clinical symptoms. Identify the symptoms and sequelae of long-standing hypertension.

    ■ *Symptoms*

    _____

    _____

■ *Sequelae*

_____

_____

_____

13. List the systolic and diastolic values that determine normal adult blood pressure, prehypertension, and stage 1 and stage 2 hypertension.

_____

_____

_____

14. What is malignant hypertension?

_____

_____

_____

15. What blood pressure level triggers concern for your child patient?

_____

_____

_____

16. List anatomical or physical factors that influence an individual's blood pressure.

_____

_____

_____

17. Treatment of primary hypertension includes patient education and counseling regarding reduction of risk factors. Identify the modifiable patient risk factors associated with essential hypertension.

_____

_____

_____

18. List the causes of secondary hypertension.

_____

_____

_____

19. Your patient, who is taking an antihypertensive medication, is susceptible to what condition after dental hygiene treatment?

_____

_____

_____

20. Ischemic heart disease arises from _____ to the heart muscle.

21. What is the principal cause of ischemic heart disease?

_____

_____

_____

22. What are the modifiable (lifestyle) risk factors for ischemic heart disease?

_____

_____

_____

23. If your patient's medical history indicates ischemic heart disease, angina pectoris is one manifestation you should be prepared for during dental hygiene treatment. What are the signs and symptoms of angina pectoris?

_____

_____

_____

24. What is the difference between stable and unstable angina?

_____

_____

_____

25. If your patient's medical history indicates medication for angina pectoris, where should the container with nitroglycerin be kept during a dental hygiene appointment?

_____

_____

_____

26. The vasodilator (nitroglycerin) tablet is placed under the patient's tongue. What can you do to help the tablet dissolve more quickly?

_____

_____

_____

27. If your patient experiences an angina attack during dental hygiene treatment, what will you do? The steps are listed below. Number the list in the correct order (1 = first step; 9 = last step).

    ▨ _____ *Administer vasodilator (nitroglycerin)*

    ▨ _____ *Administer oxygen*

    ▨ _____ *Readminister vasodilator (if indicated)*

    ▨ _____ *Call for staff/colleague assistance*

    ▨ _____ *Call for medical assistance*

    ▨ _____ *Position patient in upright position*

    ▨ _____ *Check patient response*

    ▨ _____ *Check purchase date/potency of nitroglycerin*

    ▨ _____ *Terminate dental hygiene treatment*

28. When do you record vital signs after an angina attack that has been resolved by administering the patient's nitroglycerin?

    _____

    _____

    _____

29. Myocardial infarction is the most extreme manifestation of ischemic heart disease. What is the cause of myocardial infarction?

    _____

    _____

    _____

30. What is the most common artery associated with myocardial infarction?

    _____

    _____

    _____

31. The symptoms of myocardial infarction are similar to the symptoms of angina pectoris. What circumstances indicate that you should summon immediate medical assistance for a patient experiencing these symptoms and be ready to administer CPR?

    _____

    _____

    _____

    _____

32. If your patient, who is experiencing symptoms of angina, suddenly becomes unconscious, what should you do?

    _____

    _____

    _____

33. After a myocardial infarction, your patient's elective dental and dental hygiene treatment may be postponed for 6 months or _____.

34. What is congestive heart failure?

    _____

    _____

    _____

35. Identify the underlying causes and precipitating factors associated with congestive heart failure.

    _____

    _____

    _____

36. If your patient's medical history indicates chronic congestive heart failure, what symptoms can you observe that will indicate whether the right or the left side of the heart is affected?

    ▨ *Left side of heart*

    _____

    _____

    _____

    ▨ *Right side of heart*

    _____

    _____

    _____

37. Most sudden deaths in individuals with cardiovascular disease are attributed to _____.

38. What is the purpose of an artificial pacemaker?

    _____

    _____

    _____

39. Describe the two general types of artificial pacemakers.

    _____

    _____

    _____

40. What types of dental equipment are most likely to interfere with the functioning of your patient's pacemaker?

_____

_____

_____

41. List the symptoms experienced by the patient during a pacemaker malfunction.

_____

_____

_____

42. If your patient indicates that he or she has a pacemaker, what additional information will you document during the health history review?

_____

_____

_____

43. What surgical interventions can be used to treat ischemic heart disease?

_____

_____

_____

44. Identify the clinical procedures that will protect your patient who is receiving anticoagulant therapy for a cardiovascular condition.

_____

_____

COMPETENCY EXERCISES

1. Review your school's dental clinic policy and guidelines for screening and treating patients with hypertension, and answer the following questions.

   ■ _At what intervals are patient's blood pressure readings recorded in the patient record? At what level are patients referred for a physician consult?_

   _____

   _____

   _____

   ■ _At what level is administration of local anesthetic compromised?_

   _____

   _____

   _____

   ■ _At what blood pressure classification or level will you suspend planned dental-hygiene treatment and reschedule your patient after medical intervention?_

   _____

   _____

Everyday Ethics

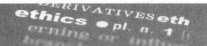

Refer to the Codes of Ethics (Appendices I, II, and III in the textbook) and Framework for Making Decisions (Table 1-2 in the textbook) as you discuss the following scenario with your classmates.

Leonard is a 68-year-old, obese black male with a history of hypertension and hypercholesterolemia. He reminds Kerstin, the dental hygienist, that he has an extreme dislike of dental appointments as he grasps very tightly to the arm rests of the dental chair.

   Upon medical history review, Leo admits that he usually remembers to take his blood pressure medications but that he doesn't feel well after the cholesterol-lowering medication, so he does not take it regularly. Kerstin takes his right arm blood pressure of 165/95. Leo then starts rubbing his left arm, and Kerstin asks him how he is feeling. Leo says he is having heartburn from a spicy dinner last night and his arm is sore, probably from doing some yard work a couple of days ago.

Questions for Consideration
1. What are Kerstin's responsibilities to inform Leonard of the serious nature of his problems?
2. Professionally, what are the choices of actions needed relative to the dental-hygiene appointment?
3. Which ethical principles apply to Kerstin's concerns for her patient?

2. What is the goal of providing dental hygiene treatment before and after cardiac surgery?

_____

_____

_____

3. When you update her health history at her 3-month dental hygiene visit, Mrs. LaShawn Peal tells you that her physician has recently prescribed anticoagulant therapy to treat a cardiac condition. She states that she doesn't really understand what the medication is for, exactly, and that the prothrombin time test you ask her about was not recommended by her physician. She minimizes the issue and tells you that if her doctor isn't worried about this kind of thing, then neither is she. She protests vehemently when you mention that you need to contact her physician for a consultation before you begin her dental hygiene maintenance treatment. Explain why you will require a physician consult before you begin dental hygiene treatment for Mrs. Peal.

_____

_____

_____

4. When you contact Mrs. Peal's physician, he tells you that he will order the test. Mrs. Peal can stop by any time to have it done. You return to the treatment room to explain the situation to her. Write a statement explaining to Mrs. Peal why her dental hygiene appointment must be rescheduled, when she should schedule the prothrombin time test, and how you will determine whether you can provide dental hygiene care following the test.

_____

_____

_____

 Factors To Teach The Patient

When you read the patient record before seating Mr. Pedro Valdez (age 58) for his dental hygiene maintenance appointment, you note that he has a very complex history of cardiovascular disease, including myocardial infarction 6 years ago. When you call his name in the reception area, he looks up at you while coughing into a tissue. He comments that you are not the dental hygienist he usually sees for his appointment. He rises wearily from the chair, complains briefly he has been waiting quite a long time, and walks with you to your treatment room.

As you stroll slowly beside him, you notice he is pale, and the back of his neck is sweating. When he reaches the dental chair, he collapses into it breathing heavily. While you take his blood pressure, you note that his skin feels quite cold, his fingernail beds look bluish, and his wrists and ankles appear quite swollen. You record a blood pressure of 135/95 mm Hg on his right arm and a resting pulse of 83 beats per minute. When you begin to lower the dental chair for your intraoral examination, he becomes agitated, leans forward in the chair, and tells you that he has to sit up straight to be comfortable.

Use the information in Chapter 63 in the textbook and the example of a patient conversation in Appendix B as guides to prepare an outline for a conversation that you might use to discuss the ways you will help Mr. Valdez to be comfortable and safe during his dental hygiene treatment.

5. Using your institution's guidelines for writing in patient records, document why Mrs. Peal was dismissed today and her dental hygiene appointment rescheduled.

Date	Comments	Signature

The Patient with a Blood Disorder

Chapter Outline

Learning Objectives

Upon successful completion of these exercises, you will be able to:

1. Identify and define key terms and concepts related to hematologic conditions.
2. Recognize blood components and normal reference values.

3. Describe the causes, symptoms, and oral effects of red and white blood cell disorders, bleeding disorders, and clotting deficiencies.
4. Plan dental hygiene education and treatment for patients with a blood disorder.

Terminology Crossword Puzzle

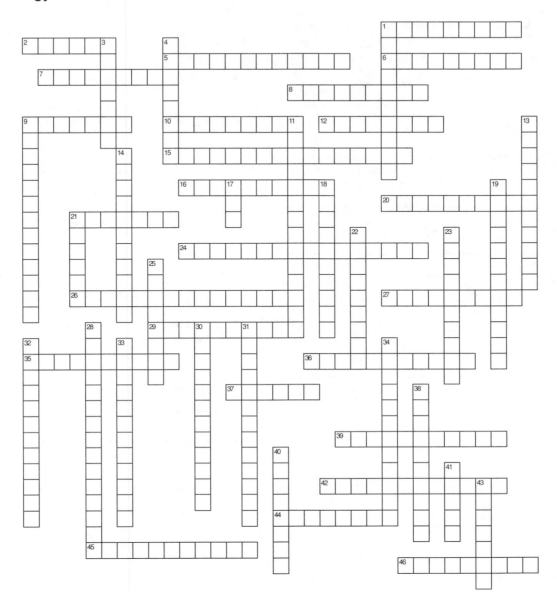

Across

1 Rupture of erythrocytes with release of hemoglobin into plasma.
2 Some general signs and symptoms of this condition are paleness, weakness, headache, vertigo, and brittle nails.
5 Increase in total number of leukocytes.
6 Abnormally small erythrocyte.
7 Loss of structural differentiation with revision to a more primitive type of cell.
8 Inflammation of the tongue.
9 Diminished availability of oxygen to body tissues.
10 White blood cell.
12 Large agranulocyte with indented nucleus that is actively phagocytic.
15 A lowered number of platelets caused by decreased production in the bone marrow.
16 Granulocyte that increases markedly during allergic conditions.
20 Most numerous of all white blood cells; first line of defense of the body.
21 Hemorrhage into tissues.

24 Occurs if 100% oxygen is not administered at the conclusion of a nitrous-oxide sedation procedure (two words).
26 Rare serious disease involving distruction of bone marrow; malignant neutropenia.
27 Abnormally large blood cell.
29 Nonelevated blue or purplish spot on skin or mucous membrane.
35 Reduction in leukocytes in blood to less than 500 per mL.
36 Pain in the tongue.
37 Darker color blood containing only 20-70% oxygen.
39 Diminished number of neutrophils.
42 Type of purpura; circulating platelets are decreased.
44 Pinpoint-size hemorrhage.
45 Red blood cell.
46 Young cell found circulating in the blood in certain diseases.

Down

1 Measure of red blood cells in whole blood; normal range is 37-54%.
3 Defective development or congenital absence of an organ or tissue.

4 Small element without a nucleus, about one fourth the size of a red blood cell, that has a role both in clotting and clot dissolution after healing.
9 Formation/development of blood cells, usually in the bone marrow.
11 Formation of red blood cells.
13 Factor in blood plasma that is essential to normal blood clotting.
14 A group of congenital disorders of the blood-clotting mechanism; related directly to the level of clotting factor in the circulating blood.
17 Type of bleeding time test; normal range less than 5 minutes.
18 Small, round agranulocyte with a large nucleus that nearly fills the cell; can multiply as immunologic need arises.
19 Engulfing of microorganisms by phagocytes.
21 Blood fluid composed of 90% water and 10% proteins, inorganic salts, gases, and other substances.
22 Nose bleed.
23 A condition in which cell production cannot keep pace with turnover rate, resulting in a decreased total number of white blood cells.

25 The most extreme abnormal cause of leukocytosis.
28 Test used for blood evaluation; normal range 11-15 seconds (two words).
30 Blood in a joint cavity.
31 Bright red blood; 97% saturated with oxygen.
32 Test used for blood evaluation; normal range 4-8 minutes (two words).
33 Condition that can be caused by a variety of factors; characterized by an increase in the number of circulating white blood cells.
34 Condition characterized by an increase in number and concentration of red blood cells; hemoglobin and hematocrit values are raised.
38 Transmits molecular oxygen to body cells; normal range is 12–18 g/100 mL.
40 Functions to increase vascular permeability during inflammation.
41 Destruction of decomposition of a cell wall.
43 Temporary treatment that can limit the spread of a hematoma.

KNOWLEDGE EXERCISES

1. Early signs of systemic conditions are often recognized first by a dental hygienist. Identify five oral signs associated with blood disorders.

   _____

   _____

   _____

2. List seven formed elements that make up blood.

   _____

   _____

   _____

   _____

   _____

   _____

3. What is the composition of plasma?

   _____

   _____

   _____

4. Identify the functions of three of the plasma proteins.

   _____

   _____

   _____

5. Why are red blood cells termed *corpuscles*?

   _____

   _____

   _____

6. What is the purpose of red blood cells?

   _____

   _____

   _____

7. Identify two main types of disorders in which red blood cells are destroyed.

   _____

   _____

   _____

8. Identify two causes of diminished production of red blood cells.

   _____

   _____

9. What genetic disorders are characterized by absent or decreased production of normal hemoglobin?

   _____

   _____

   _____

10. What is a normal hemoglobin value?

   _____

   _____

   _____

11. When the diagnosis is anemia, what has happened to the hemoglobin value?

   _____

   _____

   _____

12. Identify five basic causes of anemia.

   _____

   _____

   _____

13. Iron-deficiency anemia is more often seen in younger people than in older people; and more often in _____ than in _____.

14. What can cause iron-deficiency anemia?

   _____

   _____

   _____

15. What is an oral effect of liquid ferrous iron therapy sometimes prescribed for children with anemia?

   _____

   _____

   _____

16. Which megaloblastic anemia is caused by a vitamin B_{12} deficiency?

_____

_____

_____

17. Which foods can you suggest to your patients as good sources of vitamin B$_{12}$?

_____

_____

_____

18. Dietary factors are important in the treatment of folate-deficiency anemia, but this type of megaloblastic anemia may be more frequently related to _____ than to inadequate intake.

19. What severe condition affecting newborns is also a result of folic-acid deficiency?

_____

_____

_____

20. Sickle cell disease is a form of _____ anemia.

21. Individuals from which two ethnic populations are most at risk for sickle cell disease?

_____

_____

_____

22. In your own words, briefly describe the clinical course of the chronic and acute phases of sickle cell disease.

■ *Chronic*

_____

_____

_____

■ *Acute*

_____

_____

_____

23. Briefly describe preventive and disease-state treatments for sickle cell disease.

■ *Preventive*

_____

_____

_____

■ *Disease state*

_____

_____

_____

24. List bone changes associated with sickle cell disease that can be identified by the dental hygienist.

_____

_____

_____

25. A red blood cell count higher than normal levels is characteristic of _____.

26. What causes the relative form of the condition described in question 25?

_____

_____

_____

27. What causes the primary form of the condition described in question 25?

_____

_____

_____

28. Identify three factors that can contribute to the secondary form of the condition described in question 25.

_____

_____

_____

29. Which of the three types of the condition described in question 25 can result in purplish red tongue, mucous membrane, and gingiva?

_____

_____

_____

30. Identify two main types of white blood cells.

_____

_____

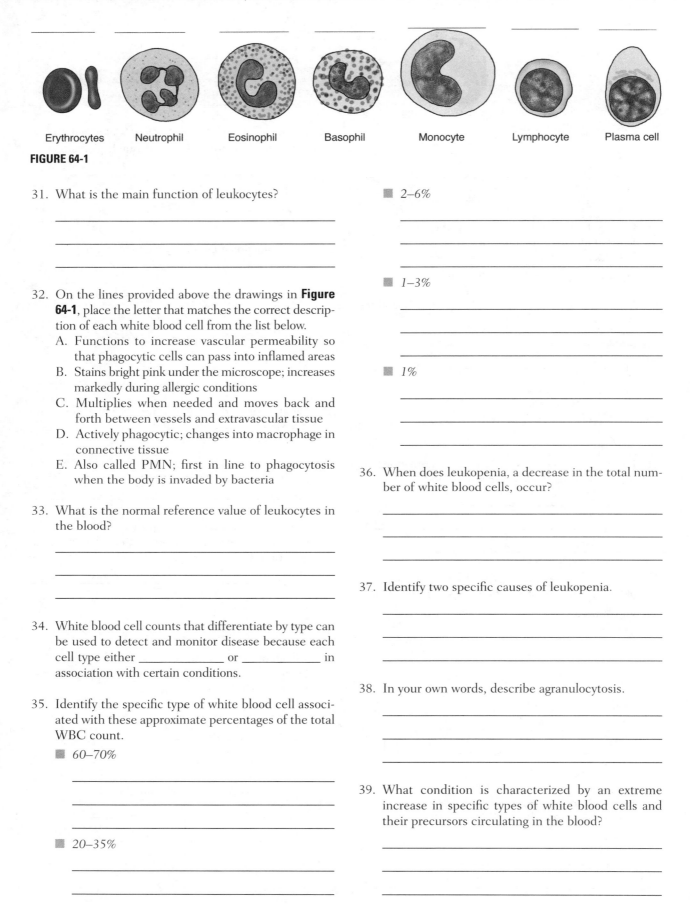

Erythrocytes   Neutrophil   Eosinophil   Basophil   Monocyte   Lymphocyte   Plasma cell

FIGURE 64-1

31. What is the main function of leukocytes?

_____

_____

_____

32. On the lines provided above the drawings in **Figure 64-1**, place the letter that matches the correct description of each white blood cell from the list below.
   A. Functions to increase vascular permeability so that phagocytic cells can pass into inflamed areas
   B. Stains bright pink under the microscope; increases markedly during allergic conditions
   C. Multiplies when needed and moves back and forth between vessels and extravascular tissue
   D. Actively phagocytic; changes into macrophage in connective tissue
   E. Also called PMN; first in line to phagocytosis when the body is invaded by bacteria

33. What is the normal reference value of leukocytes in the blood?

_____

_____

_____

34. White blood cell counts that differentiate by type can be used to detect and monitor disease because each cell type either _____ or _____ in association with certain conditions.

35. Identify the specific type of white blood cell associated with these approximate percentages of the total WBC count.

▪ *60–70%*

_____

_____

_____

▪ *20–35%*

_____

_____

_____

▪ *2–6%*

_____

_____

_____

▪ *1–3%*

_____

_____

_____

▪ *1%*

_____

_____

_____

36. When does leukopenia, a decrease in the total number of white blood cells, occur?

_____

_____

_____

37. Identify two specific causes of leukopenia.

_____

_____

_____

38. In your own words, describe agranulocytosis.

_____

_____

_____

39. What condition is characterized by an extreme increase in specific types of white blood cells and their precursors circulating in the blood?

_____

_____

40. Identify three general types of bleeding disorders.

    _____

    _____

    _____

41. Acquired coagulation disorders are related either to liver disease or to a deficiency in _____.

42. The normal level of blood clotting factor in the circulating blood is _____%.

43. Spontaneous bleeding can occur, at least occasionally, in a patient with < _____% concentration of a clotting factor in his or her blood.

44. Identify the clotting factor associated with each of the following coagulation disorders.

    ▨ *Hemophilia A*

    _____

    _____

    _____

    ▨ *Hemophilia B*

    _____

    _____

    _____

    ▨ *von Willebrand disease*

    _____

    _____

    _____

    ▨ *Christmas disease*

    _____

    _____

    _____

    ▨ *Classic hemophilia*

    _____

    _____

    _____

45. Which is more common: hemophilia A or hemophilia B?

    _____

    _____

    _____

46. What is the most common hereditary platelet dysfunction?

    _____

    _____

    _____

47. Which hemophilia occurs in both men and women?

    _____

    _____

    _____

48. In your own words, describe the effects of hemophilia.

    _____

    _____

    _____

COMPETENCY EXERCISES

1. Unless they are carefully educated, some patients with hemophilia will be afraid to brush and floss their teeth. How will you educate them?

   _____

   _____

   _____

2. When you update his health history, Jeremiah Bell tells you that that his gums, which have always been healthy, have been bleeding profusely when he flosses. Once he woke up in the morning with blood in his mouth and on his pillow. What questions will you ask him?

   _____

   _____

   _____

3. Mr. Bell replies that he has seen his physician to be tested for a blood disorder and hands you a sheet of paper reporting the results of four tests. Which four blood evaluation tests would you expect to see included in the report Mr. Bell has handed you?

   _____

   _____

   _____

Everyday Ethics

Refer to the Codes of Ethics (Appendices I, II, and III in the textbook) and Framework for Making Decisions (Table 1-2 in the textbook) as you discuss the following scenario with your classmates.

Just as Dena, the dental hygienist, begins to probe for recording the gingival examination for her patient, Mr. Bennett, the receptionist interrupts to give Dena a medical clearance form that has been faxed from the patient's physician. As Dena reviews the information, she understands that the patient has a blood disorder but is unclear as to its extent from the laboratory values in the report. She briefly questions Mr. Bennett about any medical tests, and he indicates that he was in the hospital 4 days last month.

As Dena continues the probing, she notices considerable bleeding with oozing around the gingival margins.

Questions for Consideration

1. What action, if any, does Dena need to take to ensure she is performing beneficently on behalf of this patient?
2. It appears that Mr. Bennett has not given sufficient information about his medical condition before this maintenance appointment. What obligation does a patient have to update the medical history at each appointment? And what obligation does the professional person have to help the patient understand this obligation?
3. While Dena quietly acknowledges to herself that she used to know the information about bleeding conditions, she is currently uncertain of the meaning of the laboratory values in this patient's report. Ethically, how can this realization be assessed? What is the immediate need? What can be done to prevent such a situation from occurring again in the future?

4. If the report handed to you by Mr. Bell indicates a diagnosis of leukemia, what results would you expect to see for the blood tests?

_____

_____

_____

5. You and the attending dentist decide together to postpone clinical dental hygiene treatment for Mr. Bell until you can arrange a telephone consultation with his physician. You provide oral hygiene instruction for Mr. Bell with an emphasis on what he can do on a daily basis to minimize oral effects of his blood disorder. Using your institution's guidelines for writing in patient records, document this appointment.

Date	Comments	Signature

6. Mrs. Jarell is 93 years old. She is fairly frail and has some trouble walking, but her son brings her in for her periodontal maintenance appointment every 3 months. You notice that she has lost weight. She looks even more frail than usual and sounds tired and confused. She has more trouble walking than normal and mentions that it is because her feet are cold. She trembles as you help her sit in the dental chair.

You and she have worked hard together for several years to set and attain goals that help her keep her mouth healthy. Her past health history is unremarkable for a woman her age; she has no serious medical conditions and lists no medications. But today her son tells you that she is receiving regular Vitamin B_{12} injections.

Factors To Teach The Patient

When Mr. Bell (introduced in Competency Exercises question 2) returns in a few weeks for his follow-up appointment, he tells you that he has just started treatment for leukemia. He has been advised that it is very difficult to control all of the symptoms of his condition. He is very concerned about his oral health.

Use the information in Chapter 64 in the textbook the example of a patient conversation in Appendix B to outline your education plan for Mr. Bell.

Use the outline you created to role play this situation with a fellow student. If you are the patient in the role play, be sure to ask questions. If you are the dental hygienist, try to anticipate questions and answer them in your explanation.

This scenario is related to the following factors:

■ Meticulous hygiene techniques to practice daily: toothbrushing, flossing, and other interdental cleaning devices

■ How to self-evaluate the oral cavity for deviations from normal; any changes should be reported to the dentist and dental hygienist

Write at least three dental hygiene diagnosis statements concerning potential oral factors related to Mrs. Jarell's blood disorder or concerning factors that indicate treatment modifications you will need to provide to increase her safety and comfort.

Problem	Cause (Risk Factors and Origin)
_____ *related to* _____	
_____ *related to* _____	
_____ *related to* _____	

7. Write a goal for one of the problems identified in the dental hygiene diagnosis statements in question 6. Include a time frame for meeting the goal. How will you measure whether the goal was met?

▨ *Goal*

_____

_____

_____

▨ *Evaluation method*

_____

_____

_____

▨ *Time frame*

_____

_____

_____

65 CHAPTER

The Patient with Diabetes Mellitus

Chapter Outline

Learning Objectives

Upon successful completion of these exercises, you will be able to:

1. Identify and define key terms and concepts related to diabetes.
2. Explain the function and effects of insulin.
3. Identify risk factors for diabetes.
4. Describe etiologic classifications, signs and symptoms, diagnostic procedures, complications, and common medical treatment for diabetes.
5. React appropriately in a diabetic emergency.
6. Explain the relationship between diabetes and oral health.
7. Plan dental hygiene care and oral hygiene instructions for patients with diabetes.

KNOWLEDGE EXERCISES

1. What type of diabetes is related to genetics, obesity, and hormones during pregnancy?

   _____

   _____

   _____

2. Identify five health-related factors besides pregnancy that can result in diabetes.

   _____

   _____

   _____

INFOMAP 65-1	DESCRIPTIONS OF TYPE 1 AND TYPE 2 DIABETES	
TYPE 1 CHARACTERISTICS	**TYPE 2 CHARACTERISTICS**	

3. What genetic syndromes are sometimes associated with diabetes?

   _____

   _____

   _____

4. Descriptions of type 1 and type 2 diabetes are listed below. Complete **Infomap 65-1** by writing each description in the appropriate column.

   - ▪ *The most prevalent type of diabetes*
   - ▪ *Symptoms result from defective cell receptors that prevent glucose transfer into the cell*
   - ▪ *Symptoms result from lack of insulin circulating in the blood*
   - ▪ *Pancreas does not produce insulin*
   - ▪ *Blood glucose levels lead first to increased production and later to decreased production of insulin*
   - ▪ *Patient tends to be underweight*
   - ▪ *Patient tends to be overweight*
   - ▪ *Usually arises in childhood*
   - ▪ *Typical onset after age 30*
   - ▪ *Often identified by screening after risk factors are identified*
   - ▪ *Usually identified by acute symptoms*
   - ▪ *Formerly named IDDM*

   - ▪ *Formerly named ketosis-resistant diabetes*
   - ▪ *Formerly named brittle diabetes*
   - ▪ *Insulin deficiency*
   - ▪ *Insulin resistance*
   - ▪ *Depends on exogenous insulin*
   - ▪ *Requires use of oral hypoglycemic agents*
   - ▪ *Frequent occurrence in families*
   - ▪ *Less frequently hereditary*
   - ▪ *Rapid onset of symptoms enhances diagnosis*
   - ▪ *Slow onset; frequently goes undiagnosed*
   - ▪ *Acute complications possible*
   - ▪ *Acute complications rare*
   - ▪ *Prevention/delay with lifestyle changes*
   - ▪ *Prevention methods unclear*
   - ▪ *More often diagnosed in ethnic populations*
   - ▪ *Most common in whites*

5. Diabetes is characterized by hyperglycemia. In your own words, define the *normal glucose blood level* and *hyperglycemia* using milligrams per deciliter and millimole per liter measurements.

   _____

   _____

   _____

6. Define the following symptoms of hyperglycemia.
   ■ *Polyuria*

   _____

   _____

   _____

   ■ *Polydipsia*

   _____

   _____

   _____

   ■ *Polyphagia*

   _____

   _____

   _____

7. In your own words, describe the oral glucose tolerance test used to screen patients who have signs or
   symptoms of diabetes.

   _____

   _____

   _____

8. Describe the two tests considered *best* for monitoring blood glucose levels during treatment of
   diabetes.

   _____

   _____

   _____

9. If your patient tells you that the result of his fasting
   plasma glucose test this morning was _____,
   you know that his diabetes is well controlled, and it
   is safe to provide dental hygiene treatment today.

10. If your patient tells you that her postprandial glu-
    cose level this morning was >200 mg/dL, you know
    that her diabetes is _____.

11. What is the role of insulin in the human body?

    _____

    _____

    _____

12. Where is insulin produced in the human body?

    _____

    _____

    _____

13. What is exogenous insulin?

    _____

    _____

    _____

14. How is exogenous insulin administered?

    _____

    _____

    _____

15. What factors determine the dose of insulin adminis-
    tered for each patient?

    _____

    _____

    _____

16. Identify the duration of peak action for each of the
    four classes of insulin.

    _____

    _____

    _____

17. If too much insulin is circulating in the blood because
    of inadequate nutritional intake, _____,
    sometimes referred to as _____, can occur.

18. If too little insulin is administered to control hyper-
    glycemia, _____ or _____ can
    occur.

19. Oral hypoglycemic agents act differently from
    insulin to control blood glucose levels. What is the
    mechanism of action of biguanides and thiazolidine-
    diones?

    _____

    _____

    _____

20. If your patient is taking sulfonylureas or megli-
    tinides to control type 2 diabetes, what side effect is
    important for you to watch for during dental hygiene
    treatment?

    _____

    _____

    _____

21. Your patient with uncontrolled diabetes is at risk for
    many long-term health complications. List the body

systems or organs (other than the mouth) that can be affected.

_____

_____

_____

22. Diabetes can be controlled, but to date, there is no known cure. List five factors important for maintaining the overall good health and well-being of an individual with diabetes or at risk for diabetes.

_____

_____

_____

23. It is important to monitor your patient with diabetes for signs of depression. Why is this emotional condition a significant concern?

_____

_____

_____

24. In one sentence, describe the relationship between poorly controlled diabetes and periodontal disease.

_____

_____

_____

25. Uncontrolled glucose levels place your patient at risk for _____, an opportunistic oral infection.

26. What is the role of the dental hygienist in planning care for patients who are at risk for diabetes or who are exhibiting signs and symptoms of diabetes?

_____

_____

_____

27. Why is stress prevention an important component of a dental hygiene care plan for a patient with diabetes?

_____

_____

_____

28. Identify three ways the dental hygienist can reduce stress while providing care for the patient with diabetes.

_____

_____

_____

_____

29. Why should you be very careful to avoid undue tissue trauma when providing dental hygiene care for your patient with diabetes?

_____

_____

_____

_____

Everyday Ethics

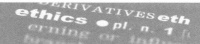

Refer to the Codes of Ethics (Appendices I, II, and III in the textbook) and Framework for Making Decisions (Table 1-2 in the textbook) as you discuss the following scenario with your classmates.

Ed Smith a 45-year-old restaurant owner, presents for an appointment with Susan, the dental hygienist. She has treated this patient before, but he has not had an appointment for more than 2 years. The review of his medical history determines he is overweight, reports dry mouth, has excessive thirst, and has not seen his physician in several years. An intraoral exam reveals candidiasis on his hard palate. Susan suggests that he see

his physician, but he refuses to even talk about it. He insists that he just wants clean teeth for his daughter's upcoming wedding.

Questions for Consideration
1. What options should be considered before treating this patient, and how should the patient be informed of the protocol?
2. Given the medical and dental assessment of this patient, would Susan be violating the patient's rights if she denies Ed's access to dental hygiene care?
3. Describe how each of the core values apply to this scenario.

COMPETENCY EXERCISES

1. In your own words, explain what can happen at the cellular level when glucose needed to supply energy cannot be accessed owing to either decreased supply or action of insulin.

   _____

   _____

   _____

   _____

   _____

   _____

2. While you are waiting for Mrs. Adamson, your first patient of the day, you look over her health history and note that she has type 1 diabetes. She arrives 15 minutes late for the appointment. She is extremely anxious and states she is late because of the traffic. Her morning, it seems, has not gone well, and everything is off schedule. As you bring her back to your treatment room, you notice that she is pale and trembling. She is perspiring profusely and seems agitated as she sits in the chair.

   What questions will you ask Mrs. Adamson when you update her medical history?

   _____

   _____

   _____

3. Mrs. Adamson responds irritably to your questions and gives vague answers. "You know my health history," she says. "I have been having my teeth cleaned here for years." When you take her vital signs, you note that her pulse is 85 beats per minute. You are really conscious of your appointment time slipping away, so you tilt the dental chair back to do an intra-oral examination and begin dental hygiene treatment. After 10 minutes, Mrs. Adamson stops you and says "Please sit me upright. I need a drink of water right now."

   What is most likely to be happening? What will your response be?

   _____

   _____

   _____

Factors To Teach The Patient

Use the information from Chapter 65 in the textbook and the example of a patient conversation in Appendix B as guides to prepare a conversation that you might use to educate Mr. Smith (introduced in Everyday Ethics) about his high risk for diabetes, how diabetes can affect his oral health, and what he can do to prevent further health complications.

Use the conversation you create to role play this situation with a fellow student. If you are the patient in the role play, be sure to ask questions. If you are the dental hygienist, try to anticipate questions and answer them in your explanation.

This scenario is related to the following factors:

- Recognizing early warning signs of diabetes and seeking medical treatment
- Reviewing practice of meticulous oral hygiene to prevent dental and periodontal disease

4. Afterward, Mrs. Adamson insists that she has to get up out of the dental chair to go to the ladies room. As she stands, she gets dizzy and slumps back into the chair. You support her so she doesn't fall and note that her breath smells sweet and is coming in rapid gasps. What will you do?

   _____

   _____

   _____

5. Using your institution's guidelines for writing in patient records, document what happened during Mrs. Adamson's appointment.

Date	Comments	Signature

Emergency Care

Learning Objectives

Upon successful completion of these exercises, you will be able to:

1. Identify and define key terms, abbreviations, and concepts related to emergency care.
2. List factors and procedures essential for preventing and preparing for a medical emergency in a dental setting.
3. Describe basic life support, rescue breathing, and external chest compression.
4. Describe oxygen administration and AED defibrillation, and identify contraindications for use.
5. Recognize signs and symptoms of a medical emergency, and identify an appropriate response.

KNOWLEDGE EXERCISES

1. Identify the patient-assessment components that will help you know enough about your patient to help prevent an emergency during dental hygiene treatment.

_____

_____

_____

2. List five *patient* factors that contribute to increased risk for medical emergency in a dental setting. (*Hint:* These are identified in several places in Chapter 66 in the textbook; some are psychosocial and some are specific to patient health status.)

_____

_____

_____

3. Identify two dental treatment–related factors that contribute to greater risk for emergencies.

_____

_____

_____

4. Recognizing the signs of patient stress is one important way to prevent medical emergencies. Identify ways you can reduce your patient's stress during dental hygiene treatment.

_____

_____

_____

5. Where in the patient's dental record is medical information listed indicating that the patient is predisposed to medical emergencies?

_____

_____

_____

6. What additional information should you document in the patient record about your patient's risk for medical emergency?

_____

_____

_____

7. When your patient arrives for a dental hygiene appointment, what is a _main indicator_ that suggests you need to be alert and prepare for a potential emergency?

_____

_____

_____

8. What information must be clearly posted by the telephone in a dental clinic?

_____

_____

_____

9. What does EMS stand for?

_____

_____

_____

10. When a medical emergency happens in the dental setting, it is mandatory to document all pertinent information in writing during the event and in the patient's record after the event. Why?

_____

_____

_____

11. List the eight vital signs mentioned in Chapter 66 in the textbook.

_____

_____

_____

12. Indicate the normal adult range of the following characteristics.

■ _Blood pressure_

_____

_____

■ _Pulse_

_____

_____

■ _Respiration_

_____

_____

■ _Temperature_

_____

_____

13. In a medical emergency, your patient is "compensating" if the vital signs _____.

14. In your own words, describe what happens if your patient goes into shock.

_____

_____

_____

15. When a patient is in shock, he or she is placed in the Trendelenburg position. What does this mean?

_____

_____

_____

16. In your own words, describe the purpose of basic life support (BLS) in the dental setting.

_____

_____

_____

17. If an emergency situation occurs in which you will be responsible for providing basic life support, you will first quickly _____ the situation and then _____ to provide rescue breathing and/or external chest compressions.

18. Describe two ways to open your patient's airway.

_____

_____

_____

19. Describe what happens if an unconscious person's airway is not adequately opened.

_____

_____

_____

20. How do you check for your patient's breathing?

_____

_____

_____

21. If your patient becomes unconscious, but is still breathing, what should you do next?

_____

_____

_____

22. List the steps for performing rescue breathing.

_____

_____

_____

23. How frequently are the ventilations repeated during rescue breathing?

_____

_____

_____

24. How do you identify whether each breath in rescue breathing is effective?

_____

_____

_____

25. How frequently do you check for pulse during rescue breathing?

_____

_____

_____

26. Where do you check for the pulse?

_____

_____

_____

27. What determines the need for external chest compressions?

_____

_____

_____

28. What is the purpose of CPR?

_____

_____

_____

29. Describe the patient's position when you perform CPR.

_____

_____

_____

30. In your own words, describe the landmarks used to determine hand placement during CPR.

_____

_____

_____

31. Chest compressions during CPR are intended to move the sternum downward with a firm, steady vertical pressure. How far down do the compressions move the thorax before releasing to allow the chest to return to normal?

_____

_____

_____

32. How long do you continue CPR?

_____

_____

_____

33. What is the recovery position?

_____

_____

_____

34. Identify and define five key words from Box 66-1 in the textbook related to the automatic external defibrillator (AED).

_____

_____

_____

_____

_____

_____

35. In your own words, describe what the AED does.

_____

_____

_____

36. List three contraindications for using the AED.

_____

_____

_____

37. Identify three measures you can take to prevent aspiration of objects during dental treatment.

_____

_____

_____

38. What is happening if your patient suddenly looks distressed, tries to up in the dental chair, and touches his or her neck?

_____

_____

_____

39. What does FBAO stand for?

_____

_____

_____

40. Define *dyspnea*.

_____

_____

_____

41. Describe the actions of a patient with a "mild" airway obstruction.

_____

_____

_____

42. What are the signs of a "severe" airway obstruction?

_____

_____

_____

43. If your patient is in distress and coughing but appears to have good air exchange, what should you do?

_____

_____

_____

44. Your patient begins gasping and making sounds when breathing in, but the cough is not strong enough to expel the object and the patient is starting to panic. What should you do?

_____

_____

_____

45. In your own words, briefly describe an abdominal thrust.

_____

_____

_____

46. What happens to your patient's body when an abdominal thrust is applied?

_____

_____

_____

47. Under what circumstances is it appropriate to use a thrust that is positioned directly backward from the sternum rather than upward from the abdomen?

_____

_____

_____

48. In your own words, describe a finger sweep.

_____

_____

_____

49. What two special considerations must be given when using the finger sweep to remove an object from the mouth of an infant or small child?

_____

_____

_____

50. What series of steps will you follow if you are responding to a foreign body airway obstruction (FBAO) emergency and the patient becomes unconscious just as you arrive at her side?

_____

_____

_____

_____

_____

_____

51. What is the term for insufficient oxygenation of the blood?

_____

52. What is the term for diminished oxygen in body tissues?

_____

53. Direct delivery of oxygen is useful in most emergencies, but it is contraindicated in which two situations?

_____

_____

_____

54. If your patient is not breathing, _____ oxygen delivery is indicated, and a bag mask or _____ is used to deliver 90–100% oxygen.

55. If a regular face mask oxygen delivery system is used, _____ L/min and _____% oxygen is delivered to the patient.

56. If the patient is breathing and needs only low levels of oxygen, the use of a _____ device is indicated. Supplemental oxygen is started at _____ L/min.

57. If a bag mask device is used, the bag is compressed at _____-sec intervals for an adult and _____-sec intervals for a child.

58. What should you do if your patient's chest does not rise and fall after applying bag mask oxygen?

_____

_____

_____

59. What size oxygen cylinder is recommended for emergency use in a dental setting?

_____

_____

_____

COMPETENCY EXERCISES

1. Describe two ways that you and your student colleagues can prepare to respond to potential medical emergencies in the dental clinic at your school.

_____

_____

_____

2. The only real way to become competent in responding to emergencies in the dental setting is to practice, practice, practice, and then practice some more. This exercise should be ongoing and include everyone in your dental clinic.

Everyday Ethics

Refer to the Codes of Ethics (Appendices I, II, and III in the textbook) and Framework for Making Decisions (Table 1-2 in the textbook) as you discuss the following scenario with your classmates.

A 12-year-old patient, Jonathan, had just received local anesthesia in Dr. Spar's treatment room in preparation for a restorative procedure. Suddenly Jonathan started to have a rhythmic twitching of the eyelids and appeared pale. Dr. Spar's assistant, Loraine, called the usual emergency alarm, and Elisa, the dental hygienist, joined in the team protocol for medical emergencies.

In a few minutes the generalized absence (petit mal) seizure was over and the patient was conscious with no other symptoms evident. Dr. Spar went about the dental procedure as if nothing had happened. Neither Loraine nor Dr. Spar made an entry in the record at the time. Elisa glanced over the patient's record and nothing she could find in the history showed that Jonathan had a susceptibility to seizures. As Elisa went back to her own treatment room, she wondered if she should record the emergency or ask Dr. Spar about it.

Questions for Consideration
1. Which of the dental hygiene core values apply in this situation?
2. Who needs to be informed of the event, and what potential ethical responsibilities are related to the patient?
3. What considerations for future treatment appointments are needed? From an ethical point of view, in what way were the patient's best interests compromised?

First, all students, faculty, and support personnel should study Table 66-4 in the textbook. Next, refer to Figure 66-2 in the textbook, and write the list of duties assigned to each emergency team member on three small cards (or use your school's emergency protocols and procedures). Finally, write the signs and symptoms of each emergency health situation listed in Table 66-4 on a small card. If you'd like, write the list of procedures to follow for each emergency on the back side of its signs and symptoms card so that you will have a handy reference for evaluating everyone's response to that situation.

When everything is ready, randomly give three people one of the three emergency team member cards and one person one of the emergency situation cards. The person who receives the emergency situation card is the patient and should act out the signs and symptoms listed. The emergency team must respond appropriately to the situation.

It is a great idea to practice this in your clinic setting, if possible. Try to initiate a round of this game when it is not expected to add to the reality of the situation. When you and your colleagues become proficient at responding, try doing this role play when patients are in the clinic receiving treatment. If you do this, talk quietly to each patient and make sure he or she knows what is going on; you will find that the patients are delighted to see you are practicing your emergency response. Some of them might even be willing to participate as the patient who is experiencing the emergency!

DISCOVERY EXERCISES

1. Locate the emergency cart or kit in your school clinic. Use the emergency equipment list in Table 66-1 in the textbook to identify what items are included in the kit.

2. Does your school have a written plan for medical emergencies in the dental clinic? Is the procedure outlined similar to or different from the example in Figure 66-1 in the textbook? In what ways is your school's emergency report form similar to or different from Figure 66-2 in the textbook?

3. How do you activate emergency services in your community?

Factors To Teach The Patient

It is clear that Mr. Montgomery is an extremely anxious dental patient. He is scheduled with you today for presentation of the dental hygiene care plan you have developed. His health history indicates that he has type 2 diabetes, hypertension, and angina. He has a past history of alcohol abuse, and he still uses tobacco.

Mr. Montgomery is extremely overweight and has trouble catching his breath after walking from the reception area to your treatment room. His periodontal status is poor, and he will require multiple appointments for scaling and root planing. In your dental hygiene care plan, there are several dental hygiene diagnosis statements that address his risk for medical emergencies during treatment.

To minimize the risk of a medical emergency, you plan to educate Mr. Montgomery carefully about how his treatment will proceed. Use the example of a patient conversation in Appendix B as a guide to prepare a conversation that you can use when you are talking to Mr. Montgomery about ways to reduce his stress during his dental hygiene treatment. *This scenario is related to the following factor:*

■ Stress minimization to prevent emergencies

Patients with Special Needs

■ Chapters 45–66

COMPETENCY EXERCISES

1. The best way to become competent in planning and providing dental hygiene care for patients with special needs is, of course, to practice planning and providing care. The learning that comes from practicing your skills is always enhanced by taking time to record the process in some sort of written format so that you can later reflect on what you have done, how you did it, and why things did or did not work out as you had planned.

   Select one or more patients for whom you provide care in your school clinic who have one (or more) of the special needs identified in the textbook. To complete this exercise, gather the assessment data from each patient's record, a copy of the patient-specific dental hygiene care plan template in Appendix B, the information from the appropriate chapters in the textbook, and any other source of information you think might be important (such as a drug reference book).

   Use the patient-specific care plan template to develop a comprehensive written dental hygiene care plan for each patient you select.

DISCOVERY EXERCISES

1. Gather as much information as you can about a specific special-need condition that interests you. Use the Primer on Evidence-based Decision Making at the front of this workbook to help you search the professional literature and/or look for online sources of information about the condition. The information in the scientific literature will probably be the most valid and reliable about the condition you select. Online sources can be variable, and it is important to determine that the host of the Web site is a reliable source of data and provides information about the condition that is supported by scientific principles.

2. Use the information you gathered in your search to create a mock patient case. You and your student colleagues can share information and learn from each other if you each present a different type of case and discuss the cases in a sort of case-presentation seminar. Each patient case you create should contain the following information:

   ■ *Patient background and demographics*
   ■ *A general description of your patient, including name, age, race, sex, height, weight, blood pressure, pulse, and respiration*
   ■ *Other information about your patient that is important for understanding the special condition*
   ■ *A statement describing the significance of these data for planning and providing dental hygiene care*
   ■ *Medical history*
   ■ *A definition of each medical problem with an explanation of its significance to the delivery of dental care*
   ■ *A description of your patient's ASA level*
   ■ *A statement of the physical and oral manifestations of your patient's conditions*
   ■ *A note about the anticipated complications associated with patient management during dental hygiene care*
   ■ *A statement of the anticipated complications or potential emergency situations that are related to your patient's medical history*
   ■ *A description of the actions needed to prevent complications and emergencies during dental hygiene care*
   ■ *Pharmacological and therapeutic considerations (Hint: Refer to a Physician's Desk Reference or other accepted drug information reference as a guide)*
   ■ *Identification of specific medications your patient is taking currently and how they relate to the medical history*
   ■ *A list containing the commercial and generic name of each drug, class or mechanism of action, usual dosage, indications for use, and anticipated adverse side effects for dentistry*

- *An evaluation of your patient's local anesthesia considerations*
- *Dental hygiene care delivery considerations*
- *A description of the general physical and oral manifestations of your patient's condition that affect dental hygiene care*
- *A description of your patient's ADL and IADL levels*
- *A description of your patient's OSCAR considerations*
- *Identification of and rationale for modifications to standard dental hygiene treatment procedures needed to meet your patient's special needs during dental hygiene care*
- *Identification of and rationale for modifications in providing oral hygiene instructions*
- *Identification of and rationale for modifications of oral hygiene aids*
- *A description of behavioral and psychosocial considerations for planning and providing care for your patient*
- *Identification of communication issues and needed actions to ensure that your patient is fully informed before he or she consents to the planned dental hygiene treatment*

3. Use the information you gathered in your information search and/or developed for your mock patient case to develop a table clinic summarizing the dental hygiene care considerations for patients with the condition you have studied. (*Hint:* Check out the American Dental Hygienists' Association Web site [adha.org] for information and guidelines for constructing and presenting a table clinic.)

FOR YOUR PORTFOLIO

1. Include your written responses to the Everyday Ethics questions from any of the chapters in this section.

2. It is likely that while you are a student, you will develop many dental hygiene care plans for a variety of patients with a wide range of special needs. Include all of these written care plans in your portfolio. Also include the care plans you developed using the patient-assessment data summaries when completing the Competency Exercises in this workbook; be sure to indicate which care plans were developed for practice patient cases and which were developed for individuals for whom you provided dental hygiene care in your school clinic.

3. An effective way to document your growing knowledge about planning patient care is to include a written reflection that describes, in detail, how the care plans you developed later in your student career are different from the care plans you developed when you were first providing patient care.

   Cite specific examples from your earlier and later care plans that document your increased competency in planning individualized, patient-specific dental hygiene care. The examples should show how your later plans are more complete, more comprehensive, and more professional than your earlier plans.

4. Include a description of the mock patient case you developed in Section VII Competency Exercise 2.

5. If you develop and present a table clinic, include your presentation outline, along with any handouts you created to accompany the table clinic. Or include a photograph that shows you and your coauthor colleagues presenting your table clinic in a professional setting. A brief written reflection of what you learned from the experience of preparing and presenting the table clinic will add depth to your documentation.

ADEA Competencies for Entry into the Profession of Dental Hygiene

CORE COMPETENCIES (C)

C1 Apply a professional code of ethics in all endeavors.

C2 Adhere to state and federal laws, recommendations, and regulations in the provision of dental hygiene care.

C3 Provide dental hygiene care to promote patient health and wellness using critical thinking and problem solving in the provision of evidenced-based practice.

C4 Use evidence-based decision making to evaluate and incorporate emerging treatment modalities.

C5 Assume responsibility for dental hygiene actions and care based on accepted scientific theories and research as well as the accepted standard of care.

C6 Continuously perform self-assessment for life-long learning and professional growth.

C7 Promote the profession through service activities and affiliations with professional organizations.

C8 Provide quality-assurance mechanisms for health services.

C9 Communicate effectively with individuals and groups from diverse populations both verbally and in writing.

C10 Provide accurate, consistent, and complete documentation for assessment, diagnosis, planning, implementation, and evaluation of dental hygiene services.

C11 Provide care to all clients using an individualized approach that is humane, empathetic, and caring.

HEALTH PROMOTION AND DISEASE PREVENTION (HP)

HP1 Promote the values of oral and general health and wellness to the public and organizations within and outside the profession.

HP2 Respect the goals, values, beliefs, and preferences of the patient/client while promoting optimal oral and general health.

HP3 Refer patients/clients who may have a physiologic, psychological, and/or social problem for comprehensive patient/client evaluation.

HP4 Identify individual and population risk factors and develop strategies that promote health-related quality of life.

HP5 Evaluate factors that can be used to promote patient/client adherence to disease-prevention and/or health maintenance strategies.

HP6 Evaluate and use methods to ensure the health and safety of the patient/client and the dental hygienist in the delivery of dental hygiene.

American Dental Education Association (ADEA), Section on Dental Hygiene Education, Competency Development Committee: Competencies for Entry into the Profession of Dental Hygiene (As approved by the 2003 House of Delegates). *J Dent Educ* 2006(70):760.

COMMUNITY INVOLVEMENT (CM)

CM1   Assess the oral health needs of the community and the quality and availability of resources and services.

CM2   Provide screening, referral, and educational services that allow clients to access the resources of the healthcare system.

CM3   Provide community oral health services in a variety of settings.

CM4   Facilitate client access to oral health services by influencing individuals and/or organizations for the provision of oral healthcare.

CM5   Evaluate reimbursement mechanisms and their impact on the patient's/client's access to oral healthcare.

CM6   Evaluate the outcomes of community-based programs, and plan for future activities.

PATIENT/CLIENT CARE (PC)

ASSESSMENT

PC1   Systematically collect, analyze, and record data on the general, oral, and psychosocial health status of a variety of patients using methods consistent with medicolegal principles.

This competency includes:

a. Select, obtain, and interpret diagnostic information, recognizing its advantages and limitations.

b. Recognize predisposing and etiologic risk factors that require intervention to prevent disease.

c. Obtain, review, and update a complete medical, family, social, and dental history.

d. Recognize health conditions and medications that affect overall patient/client care.

e. Identify patients/clients at risk for a medical emergency, and manage the patient care in a manner that prevents an emergency.

f. Perform a comprehensive examination using clinical, radiographic, periodontal, dental charting, and other data collection procedures to assess the patient's/client's needs.

DIAGNOSIS

PC2   Use critical decision-making skills to reach conclusions about the patient's/client's dental hygiene needs based on all available assessment data.

This competency includes:

a. Determine a dental hygiene diagnosis.

b. Identify patient/client needs and significant findings that affect the delivery of dental-hygiene services.

c. Obtain consultations as indicated.

PLANNING

PC3   Collaborate with the patient/client and/or other health professionals to formulate a comprehensive dental hygiene care plan that is patient centered and based on current scientific evidence.

This competency includes:

a. Prioritize the care plan based on the health status and the actual and potential problems of the individual to facilitate optimal oral health.

b. Establish a planned sequence of care (educational, clinical, and evaluation) based on the dental hygiene diagnosis; identified oral conditions; potential problems; etiologic and risk factors; and available treatment modalities.

c. Establish a collaborative relationship with the patient/client in the planned care to include etiology, prognosis, and treatment alternatives.

d. Make referrals to other healthcare professionals.

e. Obtain the patient's/client's informed consent based on a thorough case presentation.

IMPLEMENTATION

PC4   Provide specialized treatment that includes preventive and therapeutic services designed to achieve and maintain oral health. Assist in achieving oral health goals formulated in collaboration with the patient/client.

This competency includes:

a. Perform dental hygiene interventions to eliminate and/or control local etiologic factors to prevent and control caries, periodontal diseases, and other oral conditions.

b. Control pain and anxiety during treatment through the use of accepted clinical and behavioral techniques.

c. Provide life-support measures to manage medical emergencies in the patient-care environment.

EVALUATION

PC5   Evaluate the effectiveness of the implemented clinical, preventive, and educational services and modify as needed.

This competency includes:

a. Determine the outcomes of dental hygiene interventions using indices, instruments, examination techniques, and patient/client self-report.

b. Evaluate the patient's/client's satisfaction with the oral healthcare received and the oral health status achieved.

c. Provide subsequent treatment or referrals based on evaluation findings.

d. Develop and maintain a health-maintenance program.

PROFESSIONAL GROWTH AND DEVELOPMENT (PGD)

PGD1   Identify alternative career options within healthcare industry, education, and research, and evaluate the feasibility of pursuing dental hygiene opportunities.

PGD2   Develop management and marketing strategies to be used in the delivery of oral healthcare.

PGD3   Access professional and social networks and resources to pursue professional goals.

Guidelines for Conversation during Patient-Education Instructions

Created by **Tina Daniels, RDH, BS, and Charlotte Wyche, RDH, MS**

Between 30% and 70% of dental patients do not comply with personal oral care and diet recommendations because they are not motivated by the interpersonal communication skills of the dental health educator. You can do better than that if you follow these 10 rules.

1. Always talk to your patient in an upright, eye-level, and face-to-face position.
2. Begin with a positive comment, a pleasant facial expression, and an attitude of concern.
3. Use everyday words rather than professional lingo.
4. Know or ask about your patient's level of understanding, their culturally related values regarding health and wellness, and any current oral health practices. Be able to make adjustments to accommodate your patient.
5. Work with your patient to reach the oral health goals your patients set for themselves rather than impose unrealistic goals solely because you, the health provider, are the authority.
6. Actively listen and acknowledge your patient often by nodding your head.
7. Do not interrupt or make unsolicited comments when your patient is speaking.
8. Encourage the patient to stop you and ask questions any time.
9. Provide a summary and written information for later review.
10. End your instructions with a warm smile and a positive comment to encourage and motivate your patient.

AN EXAMPLE CONVERSATION FOR TEACHING TOOTHBRUSHING

INSTRUCTIONS

Practice this conversation with a student colleague or a friend before you provide instruction to a clinical patient. If possible, it is best to work in a separate patient-education room with a sink and well-lit mirror. Assemble the armamentarium:

- *Disclosing agent and cotton-tip applicators*
- *Large mirror (a wall-mounted mirror leaves hands free to demonstrate)*
- *Toothbrush in an unopened package for patient*
- *Patient education pamphlets*
- *Typodont for demonstration (if needed)*

Step 1

Record and calculate a "plaque score" and provide your patient with an individualized summary of biofilm accumulation before you begin instructions. Use the mirror to help your patient identify areas of biofilm colored by the disclosing agent on his or her teeth.

Step 2

Seat your patient in an upright position, position yourself at eye level, and explain the *purpose* of the toothbrushing method being taught.

"Mr. Santi, I am concerned with how you are removing dental biofilm from around your teeth. Biofilm first begins to develop near the gum line (gingival margin). Bacteria in biofilm cause inflammation and bleeding gums. Proper toothbrushing helps remove the biofilm *directly* beneath the gum line. Do you have any concerns you would like to share with me or any questions for me before we begin, Mr. Santi?"

Listen attentively to what your patient has to say, nodding and asking questions as appropriate.

Step 3

Open the toothbrush package, hand the toothbrush to the patient, and adjust the unit light to illuminate the mirror.

"To help us evaluate how well you are brushing your teeth, please show me how you usually brush your teeth."

Step 4

Instruct the patient to begin brushing from the back of mouth and then to demonstrate brushing in the front of the mouth as you observe.

"I can see you have been brushing; however, your plaque index score shows that you are missing biofilm in the _____ area. Let me show you how you might brush to remove the biofilm in these areas."

Step 5

Example: Bass method. With gloves on, hold the toothbrush in your hand, and demonstrate in your patient's mouth before having the patient demonstrate in his or her mouth. (You can use the typodont and a toothbrush to demonstrate; however, demonstrating in the patient's own mouth is more effective.)

"Mr. Santi, first place the sides of the toothbrush bristles straight [*up* for maxillary, *down* for mandibular] on the tooth against the gums (gingiva), and slowly direct the tips under the edge of the gum line (sulcus) at an angle. [Demonstrate a 45° angle.] Then gently, without bending the bristles, press lightly, and vibrate [or jiggle] at least 10 *very short* strokes. Now reposition the bristles to the next two or three teeth, and repeat the same brushing strokes."

Step 6

As the patient looks in the mirror, encourage, guide, and correct technique as he or she is brushing.

"Now take the brush and try brushing in your mouth using the same brushing strokes I demon-

strated. Great job, Mr. Santi, I see you have caught on to this method very well; now try vibrating the short strokes without pulling the bristle tips away from the gingival margins before moving to the next area [or now try the same thing in another area of your mouth that might be a bit more difficult to reach]."

Step 7

With gloves on, hold the toothbrush in your hand, and demonstrate in the patient's mouth how to brush the occlusal surfaces and the tongue while the patient looks in the mirror.

"Now that you have brushed the inside [lingual] and outside [facial] of all your teeth, let me demonstrate how to brush the tops [occlusal surfaces] of your teeth. Mr. Santi, look into the mirror and watch as I place the toothbrush with the bristles pointed down into the pits and grooves of your chewing surfaces. Vibrate the brush head in a circular movement, keeping the bristles in contact with the teeth while counting to 10; move the brush to the next few teeth and begin again. The dental biofilm also forms on the tongue; bring your tongue outward and hold the toothbrush in a vertical position with the bristles pointed downward toward tongue; using light pressure pull the brush forward gently over the tip of the tongue. Now show me in your mouth the way I demonstrated brushing your tongue and chewing surfaces."

Step 8

Reinforce the sequence.

"Again, you have caught on very well. Do you have any questions, Mr. Santi?

"Let me review with you the order in which you will brush all your teeth surfaces; remember to brush twice daily, especially before you go to sleep. Start with brushing the teeth in the back of your mouth on the tongue side then go to the facial side; repeat on the opposite side of the mouth. You may start with your upper teeth or your lower teeth. You may want to start with the areas you find most difficult to brush. Continue by brushing the teeth in the front of your mouth; both the tongue side and the facial side. Finish by brushing your chewing surfaces and tongue. Remember, Mr. Santi, it is best to floss your teeth before you begin your brushing routine.

"Do you have any questions for me, Mr. Santi?"

Step 9

Summarize and provide your patient with written instructions to be taken home.

"Today, you have learned about brushing your teeth to prevent oral infection caused by biofilm bacteria. So that you can remember everything we talked about, I would like to provide you with a pamphlet that explains everything again. Let me show you what I have for you to take home."

Step 10

End the patient's education with a positive, encouraging comment.

"Mr. Santi, you are already off to a good start. I am sure with the few changes you have made today we will see an improvement in your oral health by your next appointment."

Patient-Specific Dental Hygiene Care Plan

Patient-Specific Dental Hygiene Care Plan

Patient Name: _____   Age: _____   Gender: M   F   Initial Therapy

Student (Clinician) Name: _____   Date: _____   or Maintenance

Chief Complaint:

ASSESSMENT FINDINGS		
Medical History	**Significant Findings**	**At Risk For:**
• Systemic disease • Other conditions • Medications • ASA classification • ADL/IADL level		
Dental History		
• Treatment history • Dental knowledge		
Dental Examination		
• Extraoral examination • Intraoral examination • Teeth/restorations • Periodontal examination		

Periodontal Diagnosis / Case Type and Status:

DENTAL HYGIENE DIAGNOSIS

Problem		Cause (risk factors and etiology)
Extraoral:	Related to	
Intraoral:	Related to	
Restorative:	Related to	
Periodontal:	Related to	
Systemic health:	Related to	
Physical ability:	Related to	

PLANNED INTERVENTIONS

(to **arrest or control** disease and **regenerate, restore, or maintain** health)

Clinical	Education / Counseling	Oral Hygiene Instruction/Home Care

EXPECTED OUTCOMES

Goals	Evaluation methods	Time frame
1.		
2.		
3.		
4.		

APPOINTMENT PLAN
(**sequence** of planned interventions)

Appt #	Plan for Treatment and Services	Quadrant	Plan for Education, Counseling, and Oral Hygiene Instruction
1.			
2.			
3.			
4.			

REEVALUATION FINDINGS

Re-treat   Refer   Maintain (interval _____)

Description of findings:

Patient-Specific Dental Hygiene Care Plans and Patient Assessment Summaries

EXAMPLE 1	PATIENT-SPECIFIC DENTAL HYGIENE CARE PLAN

Patient Name: *Mrs. Lorna Patel* Age: 49 Gender: M (F) (Initial Therapy) or Maintenance

Student (Clinician) Name: D.H. Student Date: Today

Chief Complaint:

Gum tissues bleed when brushing and flossing. Mouth is dry all the time.

ASSESSMENT FINDINGS

Medical History	Significant Findings	At Risk For:

Medical History

- Systemic disease
- Other conditions
- Medications
- ASA classification
- ADL/IADL level

Significant Findings

- History of high blood pressure managed by medication
- Cholesterol managed by medication
- Mitral valve prolapse
- Allergy to penicillin
- Zocor 20 mg 1× per day
- Caltrate: 1 per day
- Enapril 10 mg/hydrochlorothiazide 25 mg 1× per day
- Multiple vitamin 1 per day
- Clindamycin 2.0 g taken 1 hour before appointment
- ASA II
- ADL level 0

At Risk For:

- Heart disease and stroke
- Xerostomia
- Postural hypotension

Dental History

- Treatment history
- Dental knowledge

- 1.5 years since last recall
- Localized 4–5-mm probing depths
- Flosses daily
- Rinses with Listerine
- Uses mints and candy for dry mouth
- Uses bottled water with no fluoride content
- Mouth dry all the time

- Increased incidence of oral disease (periodontal conditions)

Dental Examination

- Extraoral examination
- Intraoral examination
- Teeth/restorations
- Periodontal examination

- Moderate dental biofilm along cervical margins and proximal surfaces
- Generalized supra- and subgingival calculus
- Light yellow stain
- Posterior gingiva red and bleeding on probing
- Generalized moderate attrition (evidence of bruxism)
- Numerous faulty MOD amalgam restorations
- Localized 4–5-mm maxillary and mandibular probing depths

- Increased incidence of dental caries and periodontal conditions
- Increased risk for TMJ problems
- Increased risk for heart disease and stroke

Periodontal Diagnosis/Case Type and Status:

Generalized biofilm-induced gingivitis with localized chronic slight periodontitis

DENTAL HYGIENE DIAGNOSIS

Problem		Cause (Risk Factors and Etiology)
Current gingivitis and periodontitis	related to	Inadequate dental biofilm removal Faulty restorations that provide trap for biofilm
Increased caries risk	related to	Xerostomia Inadequate dental biofilm removal Faulty restorations
Risk for TMJ problems	related to	Attrition (evidence of bruxism)
Management of positioning during dental hygiene procedures	related to	Medications
Increased risk for heart disease and stroke	related to	Periodontal infection History of hypertension and high cholesterol

PLANNED INTERVENTIONS
(to **arrest or control** disease and **regenerate, restore, or maintain** health)

Clinical

- Scaling and root planing
- Selective polishing
- Fluoride application

Education/Counseling

- Importance of management of xerostomia
- Increased risk of dental caries because of faulty restorations
- Increased risk of dental caries because of lack of fluoride and use of sugar-based candies
- Correlation of risk for heart disease and periodontal disease

Oral Hygiene Instruction/Home Care

- Reinforce sulcular brushing technique
- Review flossing technique
- Discuss the use of Listerine vs. nonalcoholic mouthwash (because of xerostomia)
- Frequent use of water and/or saliva substitutes
- Use of sugarless candies
- Reinforce the need for premedication
- Reinforce the need for further dental intervention to manage faulty restorations and attrition

EXPECTED OUTCOMES

Goals	Evaluation Methods	Time Frame
1. Eliminate gingivitis/control periodontitis	1. Reduction of dental biofilm, gingival redness, gingival bleeding, and periodontal probing depths	1. 4-week re-evaluation 1a. Reassessment at maintenance appointment (3 months)
2. Increase use and frequency of sugarless mints and gum	2. Patient discussion	2. 4-week re-evaluation
3. Increase fluoride exposure; use of daily fluoride rinse and fluoridated water	3. Patient discussion	3. 4-week re-evaluation
4. Reduce attrition	4. Refer for night guard fabrication	4. 4-week re-evaluation 4a. Reassessment at maintenance appointment (3 months)
5. Eliminate faulty restorations	5. Refer for restorative dental care	5. 4-week re-evaluation 5a. Reassessment at maintenance appointment (3 months)
6. Maintain patient comfort and safety during dental treatment throughout treatment	6. Patient discussion	6. At all appointments

APPOINTMENT PLAN
(**sequence** of planned interventions)

Appt. No.	Plan for Treatment and Services	Quadrant		Plan for Education, Counseling, and Oral Hygiene Instruction
1	Assessment, scaling/root planing	X		▪ Importance of managing xerostomia ▪ Systemic impact of periodontal disease ▪ Importance of biofilm removal ▪ Reinforce sulcular brushing technique
		X		
2	Complete scaling/root planing, selective polishing, fluoride treatment		X	▪ Importance of fluoride ▪ Importance of managing xerostomia ▪ Importance of biofilm removal ▪ Demonstrate flossing technique ▪ Importance of follow-up for management of attrition and faulty restorations
			X	
3	Re-evaluation assessment—in 4 weeks			

RE-EVALUATION FINDINGS

Re-treat   Refer   Maintain (interval 3 months)

Description of findings:

EXAMPLE 2	**PATIENT-SPECIFIC DENTAL HYGIENE CARE PLAN**

Patient Name: *Mrs. Diane White*   Age: 27   Gender: M (F)   Initial Therapy
or
Student (Clinician) Name: D.H. Student   Date: Today   (Maintenance)

Chief Complaint:

Gum tissues bleed when brushing and flossing.
First trimester of pregnancy with nausea.

ASSESSMENT FINDINGS

Medical History

- Systemic disease
- Other conditions
- Medications
- ASA classification
- ADL/IADL level

Significant Findings

- First trimester of first pregnancy
- Husband smokes cigarettes in house and car
- ASA II and ADL level 0

At Risk For:

- Embryo susceptible to injuries and malformations
- Infant at risk for second- hand-smoke exposure

Dental History

- Treatment history
- Dental knowledge

- One year since last recall
- Generalized 4-mm probing depths
- Infrequent flossing
- Several white spot lesions on cervical surfaces of posterior teeth
- Uses bottled water with no fluoride content
- Smell of fluoridated toothpaste makes her nauseated
- Uses frequent, high-carbohydrate snacking to control nausea

- Increased incidence of dental caries and periodontal conditions

Dental Examination

- Extraoral examination
- Intraoral examination
- Teeth/restorations
- Periodontal examination

- Moderate dental biofilm along cervical margins and proximal surfaces
- Posterior gingiva red and bleeding on probing
- No radiographic bone changes

- Increased incidence of dental caries and periodontal conditions

Periodontal Diagnosis/Case Type and Status:

Biofilm-induced gingivitis

DENTAL HYGIENE DIAGNOSIS

Problem		**Cause (Risk Factors and Etiology)**
Current gingivitis and risk for additional periodontal condition	related to	Inadequate dental biofilm removal
Increased caries risk	related to	Evidence of demineralized areas High-sucrose snack intake Inadequate fluoride intake Inadequate dental biofilm removal
Risk for enamel erosion	related to	Nausea and vomiting
Infant at risk for effects of second-hand smoke	related to	Husband's tobacco use
Management of maintenance interval and positioning during dental hygiene procedures	related to	Advancing pregnancy

PLANNED INTERVENTIONS
(to **arrest or control** disease and **regenerate, restore, or maintain** health)

Clinical	Education/Counseling	Oral Hygiene Instruction/Home Care
▨ Scaling and root planing	▨ Importance of recall care during second trimester of pregnancy	▨ Sulcular brushing technique
▨ Selective polishing	▨ Effect of hormonal changes during pregnancy on gingival health	▨ Flossing
▨ Fluoride varnish application	▨ Increased risk of dental caries because of frequent snacking	▨ Rinsing but not brushing immediately after vomiting
	▨ Increased risk of dental caries because of lack of fluoride	▨ Daily fluoride rinse
	▨ Increased risk of enamel erosion because of nausea and vomiting	
	▨ Effects of second-hand smoke on infants	

EXPECTED OUTCOMES

Goals	Evaluation Methods	Time Frame
1. Eliminate gingivitis	1. Reduction of dental biofilm, gingival redness, gingival bleeding, and periodontal probing depths	1. 4-week re-evaluation
2. Reduce frequency of carbohydrate intake	2. Weekly diet analysis	2. 4-week re-evaluation
3. Increase fluoride exposure; use of daily fluoride rinse and fluoridated water	3. Patient discussion	3. 4-week re-evaluation
4. Increase maintenance frequency	4. Maintenance appointment kept	4. 3 months
5. Maintain patient comfort and safety during dental treatment throughout advancing pregnancy	5. Patient discussion	5. Until infant is born

APPOINTMENT PLAN
(**sequence** of planned interventions)

Appt. No.	Plan for Treatment and Services	Quadrant		Plan for Education, Counseling, and Oral Hygiene Instruction
1	Assessment, scaling/root planing, selective polishing, fluoride varnish on white-spot lesions	X X	X X	▨ Reinforce previous information ▨ Importance of fluoride ▨ Importance of minimizing dietary carbohydrate intake ▨ Importance of biofilm removal ▨ Reinforce sulcular brushing technique ▨ Demonstrate flossing
2	Re-evaluation assessment—in 4 weeks			▨ Reinforce previous information ▨ Explain effects of second-hand smoke on fetus and provide written material

RE-EVALUATION FINDINGS

Re-treat   Refer   Maintain (interval 3 months): during second trimester of pregnancy

Description of findings:

EXAMPLE 3	PATIENT-SPECIFIC DENTAL HYGIENE CARE PLAN

Patient Name: *Melody Crane*   Age: 15 months   Gender: M (F)   Initial Therapy
or
Maintenance

Student (Clinician) Name: D.H. Student   Date: Today

Chief Complaint:

Gum tissues bleed when mother brushes Melody's teeth.
Melody fights with mother when she brushes her teeth.

ASSESSMENT FINDINGS

Medical History

- Systemic disease
- Other conditions
- Medications
- ASA classification
- ADL/IADL level

Significant Findings

- Frequent ear infections—three since birth
- Liquid antibiotics—contain sweeteners

At Risk For:

- Early childhood caries

Dental History

- Treatment history
- Dental knowledge

- Melody's initial dental visit
- Teeth present at 6 months
- Fluoridated water supply—but family drinks mostly bottled water
- Fluoride toothpaste used 4× per week—unspecified amount of paste
- Bottle-fed two times daily at naptime and bedtime
- At-will use of sippy cup for juice
- Five-year-old brother with restorations on all primary molars and some anteriors
- Parental lack of dental knowledge

- Early childhood caries
- Fluorosis

Dental Examination

- Extraoral examination
- Intraoral examination
- Teeth/restorations
- Periodontal examination

- Moderate dental biofilm along cervical margins of maxillary incisors
- White-spot lesions cervical of four maxillary incisors
- Red maxillary anterior gingiva

- Early childhood caries
- Gingivitis

Periodontal Diagnosis/Case Type and Status:

Gingivitis

DENTAL HYGIENE DIAGNOSIS

Problem		Cause (Risk Factors and Etiology)
Early childhood caries	related to	Inadequate dental biofilm removal High, frequent sucrose exposure Lack of daily fluoride intake
Fluorosis risk	related to	Inadequate supervision of fluoride toothpaste intake
Mild gingivitis	related to	Poor oral hygiene Parental lack of dental knowledge

PLANNED INTERVENTIONS
(to **arrest or control** disease and **regenerate, restore, or maintain** health)

Clinical

- Toothbrushing and oral wiping with gauze
- Fluoride varnish application

Education/Counseling

- Decrease frequency of sucrose in diet
- Weaning from bottle—use during bedtimes
- Lack of fluoride in bottled water—availability of fluoridated options
- Benefits/protocols for use of fluoride varnish
- Supervised toothpaste amounts
- Importance of routine maintenance appointments for this child
- Optimum oral health of parent prevents transfer of infection to child

Oral Hygiene Instruction/Home Care

- Teach mother to lift the lip; examination of oral tissues
- Teach mother proper child management during toothbrushing
- Teach mother thorough toothbrushing techniques

EXPECTED OUTCOMES

Goals	Evaluation Methods	Time Frame
1. Thorough daily oral biofilm removal	1. Mother's report of 2X daily brushing, daily examination of effectiveness	1. 4-week re-evaluation
2. Reduce frequency of sucrose intake	2. Mother's report of weaning from bottle, sippy cup use, daily juice intake	2. 4-week re-evaluation
3. Increase use of fluoridated water	3. Mother's report	3. 4-week re-evaluation
4. Decreased gingival redness/bleeding	4. Dental hygienist's oral inspection	4. 4-week re-evaluation
5. Healthy oral tissues/no increase in white spot lesions	5. Dental hygienist's oral inspection	5. 4-month maintenance appointment

APPOINTMENT PLAN
(**sequence** of planned interventions)

Appt. No.	Plan for Treatment and Services	Quadrant		Plan for Education, Counseling, and Oral Hygiene Instruction
1	Toothbrush and gauze removal of oral biofilm; application of fluoride varnish	X	X	<ul><li>Decrease frequency of sucrose in diet</li><li>Weaning from use of bottle—use during bedtimes</li><li>Lack of fluoride in bottled water—availability of fluoridated options</li><li>Benefits/protocols for use of fluoride varnish</li><li>Supervised toothpaste amounts</li><li>Teach mother to lift the lip; examination of oral tissues</li><li>Teach mother proper child management during toothbrushing</li><li>Teach mother thorough toothbrushing techniques for self and child</li></ul>
		X	X	
2	Re-evaluation Assessment—in 4 weeks Re-application of fluoride varnish	X	X	<ul><li>Assess change in feeding patterns, home care, and use of fluoride</li><li>Evaluate for referral for dental treatment</li><li>Assess condition of gingival tissues</li><li>Explain importance of routine maintenance appointments for this child</li><li>Establish maintenance interval (4 months)</li></ul>
		X	X	

RE-EVALUATION FINDINGS

Re-treat   Refer   Maintain (interval 4 months):

Description of findings:

DENTAL HYGIENE CARE PLAN—PATIENT ASSESSMENT SUMMARY 1

Patient Name: *Christopher Michaels*   Age: 10   Gender: (M) F   Initial Therapy
or
Student (Clinician) Name: D.H. Student   Date: Today   Maintenance

Chief Complaint:

Toothache and swollen area in lower left jaw.

ASSESSMENT FINDINGS

Medical History	Significant Findings	At Risk For:
▓ Systemic disease	▓ No current findings	▓ N/A
▓ Other conditions	▓ ASA II and ADL level 0	
▓ Medications		
▓ ASA classification		
▓ ADL/IADL level		

Dental History

▓ Treatment history	▓ No dental exam in 5 years	▓ Increased incidence of dental caries and
▓ Dental knowledge	▓ High sucrose intake (juice, candy)	periodontal conditions
	▓ Poor dental biofilm control	

Dental Examination

▓ Extraoral examination	▓ Enlarged submandibular lymph node	▓ Increased incidence of dental caries
▓ Intraoral examination	▓ Numerous small carious lesions/large lesion on	▓ Further pain and endodontic infection
▓ Teeth/restorations	mandibular left primary second molar	from dental caries
▓ Periodontal examination	▓ Generalized gingivitis	▓ Gingival infection

Periodontal Diagnosis/Case Type and Status:

Gingivitis

DENTAL HYGIENE CARE PLAN—PATIENT ASSESSMENT SUMMARY 2

Patient Name: *Charen Woodmacher*   Age: 15   Gender: M (F)   Initial Therapy
or
Student (Clinician) Name: D.H. Student   Date: Today   (Maintenance)

Chief Complaint:

"Tooth on lower right has been bothering me and my mother says my teeth need cleaning"

ASSESSMENT FINDINGS

Medical History

- Systemic disease
- Other conditions
- Medications
- ASA classification
- ADL/IADL level

Significant Findings

- Recent diagnosis of bulimia—currently under medical and psychological treatment
- Iron-deficiency anemia
- Contraceptive pills
- Daily iron supplement
- ASA classification: II
- ADL level: 0

At Risk For:

- Enamel erosion
- Increased susceptibility to dental caries
- Increased gingival response to oral biofilm

Dental History

- Treatment history
- Dental knowledge

- Regular dental care until 2 years ago when she started refusing to come to the dentist
- Good general knowledge, but admits to recent general neglect of oral hygiene
- Had orthodontic bands until 6 months ago, but all appliances were removed and treatment discontinued

- Increased susceptibility to dental caries
- Demineralization
- Periodontal infection

Dental Examination

- Extraoral examination
- Intraoral examination
- Teeth/restorations
- Periodontal examination

- Deep caries no. 30 with abscess visible on radiograph
- Evidence of lingual erosion on maxillary incisors
- General biofilm accumulation
- Heavy calculus in all areas
- Generalized erythema, bulbous papilla, and bleeding on probing
- Probing depths generalized 4 mm with several 6–8-mm pockets in molar areas

- Oral pain
- Dental caries
- Gingival or periodontal infection/abscess

Periodontal Diagnosis/Case Type and Status:

Localized aggressive periodontitis

DENTAL HYGIENE CARE PLAN—PATIENT ASSESSMENT SUMMARY 3

Patient Name: *Rosalee Ayers*   Age: 55   Gender: M (F)   Initial Therapy
                                                                                    or
Student (Clinician) Name: D.H. Student   Date: Today   (Maintenance)

Chief Complaint:

"It's time for my regular prophylaxis."

ASSESSMENT FINDINGS

Medical History

- Systemic disease
- Other conditions
- Medications
- ASA classification
- ADL/IADL level

Significant Findings

- Menopausal—menses ceased 1 year ago
- No medications
- General good health
- High stress
- ASA classification: I
- ADL level: 0

At Risk For:

- Xerostomia
- Exaggerated response to dental biofilm/stomatitis
- Oral-tissue changes

Dental History

- Treatment history
- Dental knowledge

- Regular care for 15 years
- High dental knowledge
- Low biofilm index
- Brushes and flosses daily

- N/A

Dental Examination

- Extraoral examination
- Intraoral examination
- Teeth/restorations
- Periodontal examination

- Slight generalized recession
- General periodontal health
- Xerostomia
- Burning sensation on tongue, palate, lips

- Root caries

Periodontal Diagnosis/Case Type and Status:

Healthy tissues

DENTAL HYGIENE CARE PLAN—PATIENT ASSESSMENT SUMMARY 4

Patient Name: *Marie Tonawonda*   Age: 89   Gender: M (F)   Initial Therapy
                                                                         or
Student (Clinician) Name: D.H. Student   Date: Today   Maintenance

Chief Complaint:

Her nephew states: "I brought her in today for her regular cleaning appointment."

ASSESSMENT FINDINGS

Medical History

- Systemic disease
- Other conditions
- Medications
- ASA classification
- ADL/IADL level

Significant Findings

- Taking calcium-channel blocker for hypertension
- Sublingual nitroglycerine tablet as needed for occasional angina
- Recent antidepressant prescription
- Osteoporosis—exhibits curvature of upper back
- Increasing mental confusion and cognitive disability
- Decreased visual acuity even when corrected with glasses
- Wears a hearing aid
- ASA classification: II
- ADL level: 2

At Risk For:

- Decreased tolerance to stress of dental appointment
- Problems with vasoconstrictor
- Xerostomia
- Increased periodontal bone loss related to osteoporotic changes

Dental History

- Treatment history
- Dental knowledge

- Recent increase in sucrose intake
- Decreasingly able to provide daily self-oral care
- Previous knowledge high—but cognitive capacity is slowly decreasing
- Daily care provided by caregivers with little dental knowledge

- Root caries
- Increased risk for developing gingivitis and periodontal infection

Dental Examination

- Extraoral examination
- Intraoral examination
- Teeth/restorations
- Periodontal examination

- Xerostomia
- Generalized recession: 3–5 mm
- Several class I and class II furcations in molar areas
- Evidence of osteoporotic bone loss on panoramic radiograph
- Very few restorations—all in good condition

- Root caries
- Increasing periodontal bone loss

Periodontal Diagnosis/Case Type and Status:

History of generalized chronic periodontitis/currently controlled

DENTAL HYGIENE CARE PLAN—PATIENT ASSESSMENT SUMMARY 5

Patient Name: *Ms. Anitha Jones*   Age: 30   Gender: M (F)   Initial Therapy
                                                                                                          or
Student (Clinician) Name: D.H. Student   Date: Today   (Maintenance)

Chief Complaint:

Patient presents for routine 3-month maintenance prophylaxis and examination.

ASSESSMENT FINDINGS

Medical History

- Systemic disease
- Other conditions
- Medications
- ASA classification
- ADL/IADL level

Significant Findings

- Diagnosis of cerebral palsy
- Spasticity, athetosis, facial movements
- Mitral valve prolapse with regurgitation
- Takes antiseizure medication
- ASA classification: III
- ADL level: 3

At Risk For:

- Attrition from bruxing
- Risk for injury during dental treatment from flailing arms and legs
- Oral trauma injury from falls
- Infective endocarditis

Dental History

- Treatment history
- Dental knowledge

- Previous history of excellent professional dental care
- Personal dental knowledge high
- New caregiver with low dental knowledge

- Increased rate of dental caries and periodontal infection because of need for help with daily oral care

Dental Examination

- Extraoral examination
- Intraoral examination
- Teeth/restorations
- Periodontal examination

- Jaw and face movements
- Bruxism
- Mouth breathing
- Increased gag reflex
- Incisal attrition and history of anterior fractures
- Restorations in good repair
- Healthy gingival tissues
- Evidence of lip- and cheek-biting trauma

- Injury during dental treatment
- Increased risk for aerosol inhalation and choking
- Increased risk of incisal and occlusal dental caries
- Dry anterior gingiva
- Gingivitis
- Oral trauma/biting lesions and infection

Periodontal Diagnosis/Case Type and Status:

Generally healthy/stable periodontal health

DENTAL HYGIENE CARE PLAN—PATIENT ASSESSMENT SUMMARY 6

Patient Name: *Harold Wilmot*   Age: 44   Gender: (M) F   (Initial Therapy)
                                                                                                              or
Student (Clinician) Name: D.H. Student   Date: Today   Maintenance

Chief Complaint:

"I need my teeth cleaned—my breath is really bad lately."

ASSESSMENT FINDINGS

Medical History   **Significant Findings**   **At Risk For:**

- Systemic disease   - Asthma
- Other conditions   - Uses steroid inhaler
- Medications   - Hypertension (148/82)
- ASA classification   - Beta blocker for hypertension
- ADL/IADL level   - Tobacco use ½ to 1 pack per day for about 25 years
                                       - Does not use alcohol or other drugs
                                       - ASA classification II
                                       - ADL level 0

Dental History

- Treatment history   - Regular preventive dental visits—at least one per year
- Dental knowledge   - Has been educated regarding tobacco use and oral health at dental
                                         visits for the last 5 years
                                       - Has tried twice to quit smoking and relapsed because of the
                                         withdrawal symptoms

Dental Examination

- Extraoral examination   - Upper denture
- Intraoral examination   - Lower partial denture (replaces 23–26, 19 and 30)
- Teeth/restorations   - Probing depths 5 mm on 31 mesial and on mesial and distal surfaces of
- Periodontal examination   all premolars
                                       - No bleeding on probing or other signs of inflammation
                                       - Moderate calculus and stain on both natural teeth and on dentures
                                       - Proximal biofilm in lower premolars
                                       - Soft tissue leukoplakia approximately 3–4 mm on alveolar ridge distal
                                         to tooth no. 18

Periodontal Diagnosis/Case Type and Status:

Chronic periodontitis

DENTAL HYGIENE CARE PLAN—PATIENT ASSESSMENT SUMMARY 7

Patient Name: *Nicholas Diamond*   Age: 57   Gender: (M) F   ⟨Initial Therapy⟩
                                                                                                or
Student (Clinician) Name: D.H. Student   Date: Today   Maintenance

Chief Complaint:

Patient presents for new patient examination.

ASSESSMENT FINDINGS

Medical History

- Systemic disease
- Other conditions
- Medications
- ASA classification
- ADL/IADL level

Significant Findings

- Type 1 diabetes—blood sugar levels are not well controlled
- No other diagnosed health issues
- No medical visits for 2 years
- Tobacco use: 1–2 packs per day for 35 years
- ASA classification III
- ADL level 0

At Risk For:

Dental History

- Treatment history
- Dental knowledge

- 25 years in previous dental practice
- No previous periodontal therapy—only received "dental cleanings" every 6 months
- Limited dental knowledge

Dental Examination

- Extraoral examination
- Intraoral examination
- Teeth/restorations
- Periodontal examination

- Generalized 6–8-mm probing depths
- Generalized recession on mandibular anterior and lingual of maxillary molars
- Generalized slight mobility
- Generalized poor biofilm control
- Generalized bleeding on probing
- Generalized erythematous tissue
- Numerous large amalgam fillings with proximal overhangs evident on bitewing radiographs

Periodontal Diagnosis/Case Type and Status:

Generalized chronic periodontitis